Advances in DNA Vaccines

Advances in DNA Vaccines

Editors

Maria G. Isaguliants
Karl Ljungberg

MDPI • Basel • Beijing • Wuhan • Barcelona • Belgrade • Manchester • Tokyo • Cluj • Tianjin

Editors
Maria G. Isaguliants
Riga Stradins University
Latvia

Karl Ljungberg
Eurocine Vaccines AB
Sweden

Editorial Office
MDPI
St. Alban-Anlage 66
4052 Basel, Switzerland

This is a reprint of articles from the Special Issue published online in the open access journal *Vaccines* (ISSN 2076-393X) (available at: https://www.mdpi.com/journal/vaccines/special_issues/advances_DNA_vaccines).

For citation purposes, cite each article independently as indicated on the article page online and as indicated below:

LastName, A.A.; LastName, B.B.; LastName, C.C. Article Title. *Journal Name* **Year**, *Volume Number*, Page Range.

ISBN 978-3-0365-0300-4 (Hbk)
ISBN 978-3-0365-0301-1 (PDF)

Contents

About the Editors

Maria G. Isaguliants Ph.D., Associated Prof. I started my research career as a bioorganic chemist, and throughout the years developed a profile of immunology and vaccinology research. My main research interests lie in: (i) The design of DNA vaccines using consensus, chimeric genes, protein domain reshuffling, site mutagenesis against chronic viral infections and cancer, and the development of immunization techniques providing predetermined specificity and polarity of the immune response; (ii) Molecular factors of viral pathogenicity and carcinogenicity, oxidative stress, and oxidative stress response and its regulation in viral infections and cancer. Since 2000, I have been working at the Department of Microbiology, Tumor and Cell Biology, Karolinska Institutet, Stockholm, developing experimental DNA vaccines against HIV and hepatitis C virus. In 2014, I started at the Riga Stradins University, and from 2016 was the coordinator of the Twinning project "DNA vaccines against cancer". The latter shifted my research interests towards the development of vaccines against cancer associated with chronic viral infections. In 2019, my group received a grant from the Latvian Research Council on the immunotherapy of hepatitis C-related liver cancer. In the frame of this project, we developed a novel cancer vaccine candidate based on telomerase reverse transcriptase. I have a research affiliation in Russia at the Gamaleya Research Center for Epidemiology and Microbiology. In Russia, my group has pioneered the field of DNA immunization (first paper published 1999). The focus of our latest studies lies in the development of a therapeutic DNA vaccine against cancer associated with infection with human papilloma viruses for HIV-infected individuals. Our results have featured in 86 publications in peer-reviewed international and national journals. I have a passion for vaccine-related research and work hard towards the coordination of efforts of vaccinologists around the world to promote multiple perspectives of vaccine technologies. To this end, from 2002 to 2013, I served as the coordinator of the Baltic partnership "Baltic Network against life-threatening viral infections", uniting 12 institutes from Sweden, Lithuania, Latvia, Poland, Finland, and Russia; and in 2017–2018, the initiation project on innovative strategies of vaccination and immunotherapy for five Baltic countries. I am an active member of the International Society for Vaccines, acting as a Board member in 2018–2019, an editor of our professional journal Vaccines (MDPI), and (co)organizer of the yearly conferences on perspective technologies of vaccination and immunotherapy 2016–2020, the latest being held on Zoom on October 27–29, 2020 (www.techvac.org).

Karl Ljungberg, Ph.D. I am a passionate advocate for vaccines as a means of improving public health and have designated my career to vaccine research and development. I have spent the past 20 years at academic and public health institutions in Sweden and the US to study and develop vaccines, adjuvants, and antivirals against diseases caused by Chikungunya virus, influenza, HIV, and SARS, as well as immunotherapeutic vaccination against cancer. The focus of these studies has been on antigen and vector design, delivery, and immunogenicity of gene-based and viral-vectored vaccines. I have worked with several vaccine candidates that are in or are on their way into clinical trials. Currently, I am Director of Preclinical Development at Eurocine Vaccines AB. Eurocine Vaccines is a vaccine company based at Karolinska Institutet campus, Stockholm, Sweden. Eurocine Vaccines acts through partnering with vaccine companies, academic groups, and non-profit organizations during the late-stage discovery phase and facilitating development, manufacturing, and proof-of-concept in humans. We have experience from vaccine development up to and including conducting clinical trials up to phase II.

vaccines

MDPI

Editorial

DNA Vaccine Development at Pre- and Post-Operation Warp Speed

Karl Ljungberg [1] **and Maria Isaguliants** [2,3,4,5,*]

[1] Eurocine Vaccines AB, Fogdevreten 2, 17165 Solna, Sweden; karl.ljungberg@eurocine-vaccines.com
[2] Department of Microbiology, Tumor and Cell Biology, Karolinska Institutet, 171 77 Stockholm, Sweden
[3] Department of Research, Riga Stradins University, LV-1007 Riga, Latvia
[4] N.F. Gamaleya Research Center for Epidemiology and Microbiology, 123098 Moscow, Russia
[5] M.P. Chumakov Federal Scientific Center for Research and Development of Immune-and-Biological Products of Russian Academy of Sciences, 108819 Moscow, Russia
* Correspondence: maria.issagouliantis@ki.se or maria.issagouliantis@rsu.lv

Received: 17 November 2020; Accepted: 17 November 2020; Published: 4 December 2020

DNA is a rapidly developing vaccine platform for combatting cancer, infectious and noninfectious diseases. Plasmid DNA used as immunogens encode proteins to be synthesized in the cells of the vaccine recipients. Introduction of DNA vaccines into the host induces antibody and cellular responses against the encoded protein. In this way, the induction of immune response mimics the events occurring during natural infection with an intracellular pathogen. There are a few distinct ways in which the vaccine antigen can be processed and presented, which shape the resulting immune response and which can be manipulated. Characteristically, the antigen synthesized within the host cell is processed by the proteasome, loaded onto, and presented on MHC Class I molecules. Processing can be re-routed to the lysosome, or the immunogen can be secreted for further presentation on MHC Class II. Vaccine efficacy is also highly dependent on DNA delivery. DNA immunogens are often administered by intramuscular or intradermal injections, but the immune response can be significantly enhanced by subsequent electroporation of the injection site, which enhances the delivery up to 1000-fold, thereby facilitating dose sparing. Other techniques may also be employed. For instance, noninvasive introduction by biolistic devices such as gene guns and biojectors, skin applications with plasters and microneedles/chips, sonication, magnetofection, and even tattooing has been shown to improve the efficacy of delivery. The debate regarding the pros and cons of different routes of delivery is intense but the answer to which route of administration is better for a DNA vaccine is too complex to give a straightforward answer. It depends on multiple factors such as the choice of antigen and vector, expressing tissues and cells, and the disease it targets. A number of studies have compared the effect of delivery methods on the level of immunogen expression, and the magnitude and specificity of the resulting immune response. According to some, the delivery route determines the immunogenic performance; according to others, it can modulate the level of response but not its specificity or polarity. All in all, research on the optimization of DNA vaccine design, delivery, and immunogenic performance has led to a marked increase in their efficacy in larger species and humans.

This Special Issue describes the continuing efforts to increase the potency of DNA vaccines by manipulating plasmid DNA, adding adjuvants or immunomodulators (also delivered in the form of plasmid DNA), and by using a wide panel of novel delivery systems. These efforts are described in seven experimental papers and four reviews.

When we launched the "Advances in DNA Vaccines" Special Issue, little did we know that the world would face a new infectious disease threat just months after the submission deadline, a threat which would change the entire game plan for vaccine development. The current SARS-CoV-2 pandemic has forced vaccinology into a new intense phase of development, transformation, and innovation. Hit by the COVID-19 epidemics, the world has come to realize the importance of efficient vaccines against viral infections. It is comforting that the contributing authors were working hard in this field before the epidemic broke out: all publications of this issue focus on the development of vaccines against viral infections, such as HIV by Kilpelainen et al. [1], Louis et al. [2], and Akulova et al. [3]; human hepatitis C virus by Masalova et al. [4]; Ebola virus by Bazhan et al. [5]; Zika virus [2]; influenza by Hinkula et al. [6] and Louis et al. [2]; and Epstein–Barr virus by Wojtak et al. [7].

The majority of studies presented in this issue used different forms of plasmid DNA: genes optimized for expression and/or consensus immunogens [2,3,7], polyepitope constructs [5], or plasmids with viral enhancers increasing protein expression and thus allowing one to reduce the DNA dose (Chapman & Rybicki [8]). A still more efficient way to ensure high-level expression of the immunogen is to use RNA/DNA layered alphavirus vectors, which provide a superior expression of immunogens in comparison with conventional plasmid DNA technology (Lundstrom [9]). Besides, immunization with alphavirus DNA vectors elicits an immune response compared with the conventional plasmid at a 1000-fold lower DNA dose, allowing for considerable vaccine sparing [9].

In most of the studies presented in this Special Issue, plasmid DNA was introduced by intramuscular or intradermal injections, with or without subsequent electroporation. Two more sophisticated ways of indirect delivery of DNA encoding immunogens presented include immunization with recombinant BCG as a vehicle to express HIV-1 and SIV antigens [1] and by mesenchymal stem cells made to express nonstructural proteins of hepatitis C virus [4]. In both cases, delivery using bacterial or eukaryotic cells as a vehicle allowed the researchers to significantly increase the cellular response against viral antigens as compared with immunization with naked plasmid DNA.

A recent development is the use of plasmid DNA to encode an adjuvant; for instance, a cytokine or another noncytokine immunomodulator with the power to enhance and shape the immune response. In this Special Issue, we see demonstrations of the efficient use of an immunomodulatory plasmid DNA encoding IL-36 gamma, giving a boost to an immune response against HIV, Zika virus, and influenza in mice [2]. The review by Shrestha & Grubor-Bauk gives an excellent example of the use of a novel cytolytic platform of DNA immunization based on truncated mouse perforin [10], whereas Hinkula et al. [6] use a plasmid DNA encoding the TLR5 ligand flagellin as an immunomodulator which, if administered together with formalin-inactivated whole influenza A vaccine, increases the antibody response 200-fold, hemagglutination inhibition (HAI) titer by 100-fold, and the cellular response against flu by 40-fold.

An overview of the experimental papers in this Special Issue reveals that DNA vaccines of the pre-COVID-19 era were not yet mature enough to be an instrument of human vaccination, as six out of seven experimental papers describe the immunization of mice; only one, by Akulova et al., describes the results of the Phase II clinical trial of a HIV DNA vaccine candidate [3]. However, today, the situation is rapidly changing.

The spread of the SARS-CoV-2 virus and the COVID-19 disease has triggered an unprecedented surge in vaccine research and development, as well as attracting an unsurpassed amount of funding in a very limited time—and for good reasons. Worldwide infections with SARS-CoV-2 are increasing rapidly and, at the time of writing this editorial, approach 40 million diagnosed cases; the actual number of infections is much higher. Over one million deaths have resulted from a disease that did not exist for us a year ago. This new virus disseminates in a way that has been impossible to predict; traditional countermeasures such as hygiene, physical distancing, various levels of public lockdowns, and quarantines have proven to be insufficient, highlighting the urgent need for prophylactic vaccine(s) to be applied worldwide as the only way to stop viral spread.

The ongoing COVID-19 crisis has led to a very rapid development of vaccine candidates from academia and small and medium-sized biotech companies, as well as pharmaceutical giants. Now, nine months down the road, several candidates have already gone through discovery, preclinical testing demonstrating immunogenicity, and, in some cases, efficacy, process development, toxicity testing, production and recruitment for and completion of Phase 1 safety and immunogenicity studies. The most advanced candidates have already proceeded into Phase 2 and 3 testing and scaling up; preparation for large-scale production is well under way. It is hard to comprehend what an achievement this really is and it is important to recognize that a lot of the progress has been made through performing multiple steps in the vaccine (Research & Development) R&D process in parallel and at great financial risk: in the case where a vaccine candidate does not show the expected immunogenicity or safety, for instance, the resources invested in that candidate will be lost. In a traditional stepwise approach to vaccine development, unsuccessful candidates would have been deselected at an earlier stage and the financial risks would have been mitigated.

It is important to emphasize that this approach is only made possible through numerous initiatives both from states, not-for-profit organizations such as the Coalition for Epidemic Preparedness Innovations (CEPI) and the Bill and Melinda Gates Foundation, and private equity alike. One such initiative is Operation Warp Speed, to which the US Congress has directed almost 10 billion USD. Operation Warp Speed aims to deliver 300 million doses of a safe, effective vaccine for COVID-19 by January 2021 as part of a broader strategy to accelerate the development, manufacturing, and distribution of COVID-19 vaccines, therapeutics, and diagnostics (https://www.hhs.gov/about/news/2020/06/16/fact-sheet-explaining-operation-warp-speed.html).

At no time in history has biomedical research moved forward at such a high pace. The research community, the pharmaceutical sector, and funding agencies have responded to the threat with dedication. Moreover, the dissemination of data has never been faster. Rapid publication of data has been a key factor in the battle against the virus and the role of preprint servers such as biorxiv and biomedrxiv cannot be underestimated. For instance, the genome sequence of SARS-CoV-2 was published online less than two weeks after the Wuhan Municipal Health Commission in Wuhan City, China, reported a cluster of 27 pneumonia cases of unknown etiology, and only one day after the Chinese CDC reported that a novel coronavirus had been detected as the causative agent of COVID-19 (https://virological.org/t/novel-2019-coronavirus-genome/319/26). Since then, COVID-19 research has exploded; never before have studies on a previously undescribed disease and disease-causing agent provided so much knowledge in such a short time. The remarkable progress in synthetic biology and manufacturing of DNA sequences, based on the availability of sequences, not biological materials, enabled the rapid development of vaccine candidates against COVID-19. We see this as an argument in favor of the synthetic nucleic acid-based vaccines.

Thus, it is not surprising that some of the most advanced vaccine candidates against COVID-19 represent novel previously unlicensed technology platforms exploiting synthetic genes, such as adenovirus vector platforms (e.g., Astra Zeneca, CanSino Biologics, Sputnik-V; https://clinicaltrials.gov/ct2/show/NCT04437875), mRNA (e.g., Moderna, Sanofi, Curevac, Pfizer/BioNTech), and, of course, DNA, such as INO-4800 by Inovio, thought to be the furthest ahead among four DNA-based vaccines that have started human testing for COVID-19 (https://clinicaltrials.gov/ct2/show/NCT04336410). A concise review by Liu in this Special Issue underpins pre-COVID-19 era efforts to make DNA vaccines more efficient, comparing them with similar efforts made for mRNA vaccines [11]. At the moment, the reader may get an impression that the mRNA vaccines have the upper hand, specifically referring to the many advanced mRNA COVID-19 vaccine candidates in clinical trials. However, the INO-4800 DNA vaccine also showed promise in a Phase 1 trial: INO-4800 was safe and well-tolerated and induced immune responses in a majority of participants (https://www.fdanews.com/articles/199278-inovios-covid-19-vaccine-trial-placed-on-partial-hold). Taking this stand, we are far from expressing DNA vaccine pessimism. It is likely that the emergence of RNA vaccines as a viable vaccine modality and the technological developments that are driven by this field may also impact the development of new DNA vaccine and related technologies. Given the tremendous need for: (i) high speed in vaccine development relying on the availability of sequence information, (ii) the ease and speed of vaccine production using already established platforms, and (iii) no cold chain to allow for worldwide distribution, which are provided by DNA vaccines, one can be sure that the first vaccines of this type will soon see licensure for human use and find clinical application abroad.

When the smoke of the battle against COVID-19 and the race for an effective vaccine settles, we will face a new normal where the dissemination of SARS-CoV-2 is hopefully controlled, although the way we interact with each other and the way we work would be changed once and forever. People would gradually forget the times of hardship that we are currently facing. It may happen that our collective memory will be shorter than the T cell memory. Nevertheless, we hope that the insights gained and lessons learned in vaccinology will prevail and that investments will continue to be made in this domain to further advance vaccinology and prevention of infectious diseases in all corners of the world, since every dollar invested in vaccinology has an enormous potential return in saving lives and improving peoples' health. As scientists and vaccine advocates, we have to act to preserve this momentum. One day, we will be out of the COVID-19 pandemic, but we can be sure that new challenges will appear on the horizon. We have to keep up the pace to be prepared.

Author Contributions: Conceptualization, M.I.; original draft preparation, K.L., M.I.; revisions and editing K.L., M.I.; funding acquisition, M.I. All authors have read and agreed to the published version of the manuscript.

Funding: This research was funded by LZP-2018/2-0308 and RFBR 17-54-30002 to M.I., and by COST action ENOVA CA1623.

Conflicts of Interest: The authors declare no conflict of interest.

References

1. Kilpeläinen, A.; Saubi, N.; Guitart, N.; Olvera, A.; Hanke, T.; Brander, C.; Joseph, J. Recombinant BCG Expressing HTI Prime and Recombinant ChAdOx1 Boost Is Safe and Elicits HIV-1-Specific T-Cell Responses in BALB/c Mice. *Vaccines* **2019**, *7*, 78. [CrossRef] [PubMed]
2. Louis, L.; Wise, M.C.; Choi, H.; Villarreal, D.O.; Muthumani, K.; Weiner, D.B. Designed DNA-Encoded IL-36 Gamma Acts as a Potent Molecular Adjuvant Enhancing Zika Synthetic DNA Vaccine-Induced Immunity and Protection in a Lethal Challenge Model. *Vaccines* **2019**, *7*, 42. [CrossRef] [PubMed]
3. Akulova, E.; Murashev, B.; Verevochkin, S.; Masharsky, A.; Al-Shekhadat, R.; Poddubnyy, V.; Zozulya, O.; Vostokova, N.; Kozlov, A.P. The Increase of the Magnitude of Spontaneous Viral Blips in Some Participants of Phase II Clinical Trial of Therapeutic Optimized HIV DNA Vaccine Candidate. *Vaccines* **2019**, *7*, 92. [CrossRef] [PubMed]
4. Masalova, O.V.; Lesnova, E.I.; Klimova, R.R.; Momotyuk, E.D.; Kozlov, V.V.; Ivanova, A.M.; Payushina, O.V.; Butorina, N.N.; Zakirova, N.F.; Narovlyansky, A.N.; et al. Genetically Modified Mouse Mesenchymal Stem Cells Expressing Non-Structural Proteins of Hepatitis C Virus Induce Effective Immune Response. *Vaccines* **2020**, *8*, 62. [CrossRef] [PubMed]
5. Bazhan, S.I.; Antonets, D.V.; Karpenko, L.I.; Oreshkova, S.F.; Kaplina, O.N.; Starostina, E.V.; Dudko, S.G.; Fedotova, S.A.; Ilyichev, A.A. In silico Designed Ebola Virus T-Cell Multi-Epitope DNA Vaccine Constructions Are Immunogenic in Mice. *Vaccines* **2019**, *7*, 34. [CrossRef]
6. Hinkula, J.; Nyström, S.; Devito, C.; Bråve, A.; Applequist, S.E. Long-Lasting Mucosal and Systemic Immunity against Influenza A Virus Is Significantly Prolonged and Protective by Nasal Whole Influenza Immunization with Mucosal Adjuvant N3 and DNA-Plasmid Expressing Flagellin in Aging In- and Outbred Mice. *Vaccines* **2019**, *7*, 64. [CrossRef]
7. Wojtak, K.; Perales-Puchalt, A.; Weiner, D.B. Novel Synthetic DNA Immunogens Targeting Latent Expressed Antigens of Epstein-Barr Virus Elicit Potent Cellular Responses and Inhibit Tumor Growth. *Vaccines* **2019**, *7*, 44. [CrossRef]
8. Chapman, R.; Rybicki, E.P. Use of a Novel Enhanced DNA Vaccine Vector for Preclinical Virus Vaccine Investigation. *Vaccines* **2019**, *7*, 50. [CrossRef]
9. Lundstrom, K. Plasmid DNA-based Alphavirus Vaccines. *Vaccines* **2019**, *7*, 29. [CrossRef]

10. Shrestha, A.C.; Wijesundara, D.K.; Masavuli, M.G.; Mekonnen, Z.A.; Gowans, E.J.; Grubor-Bauk, B. Cytolytic Perforin as an Adjuvant to Enhance the Immunogenicity of DNA Vaccines. *Vaccines* **2019**, *7*, 38. [CrossRef] [PubMed]
11. Liu, M.A. A Comparison of Plasmid DNA and mRNA as Vaccine Technologies. *Vaccines* **2019**, *7*, 37. [CrossRef]

vaccines

MDPI

Review

Use of a Novel Enhanced DNA Vaccine Vector for Preclinical Virus Vaccine Investigation

Rosamund Chapman [1] and Edward P. Rybicki [1,2,*]

1 Institute of Infectious Disease and Molecular Medicine, Faculty of Health Sciences, University of Cape Town, Observatory, Cape Town 7925, South Africa; ros.chapman@uct.ac.za

2 Biopharming Research Unit, Department of Molecular & Cell Biology, University of Cape Town, PB X3 Rondebosch, Cape Town 7701, South Africa; ed.rybicki@uct.ac.za

* Correspondence: ed.rybicki@uct.ac.za; Tel.: +27-21-650-3265

Received: 17 April 2019; Accepted: 11 June 2019; Published: 13 June 2019

Abstract: DNA vaccines are stable, safe, and cost effective to produce and relatively quick and easy to manufacture. However, to date, DNA vaccines have shown relatively poor immunogenicity in humans despite promising preclinical results. Consequently, a number of different approaches have been investigated to improve the immunogenicity of DNA vaccines. These include the use of improved delivery methods, adjuvants, stronger promoters and enhancer elements to increase antigen expression, and codon optimization of the gene of interest. This review describes the creation and use of a DNA vaccine vector containing a porcine circovirus (PCV-1) enhancer element that significantly increases recombinant antigen expression and immunogenicity and allows for dose sparing. A 172 bp region containing the PCV-1 capsid protein promoter (Pcap) and a smaller element (PC; 70 bp) within this were found to be equally effective. DNA vaccines containing the Pcap region expressing various HIV-1 antigens were found to be highly immunogenic in mice, rabbits, and macaques at 4–10-fold lower doses than normally used and to be highly effective in heterologous prime-boost regimens. By lowering the amount of DNA used for immunization, safety concerns over injecting large amounts of DNA into humans can be overcome.

Keywords: DNA vaccine; HIV-1; enhancer element; circovirus; immunogenicity

---

1. Introduction

DNA vaccines were hailed as long ago as the 1990s as the next best thing in vaccines: Plasmid-based DNA vaccines are relatively easy and affordable to produce, sharing a common production method for all vaccines; they are thermostable and safe with no risk of virulence or apparently of anti-vector immunity, can be administered to immunocompromised individuals, and multiple plasmids can be mixed and used as a broad spectrum combination vaccine. DNA vaccines elicit mainly cell-mediated immune responses due to presentation of expressed antigens via major histocompatibility complex class I (MHC-I) presentation, which is similar to viral pathogens and a desirable feature of a vaccine [1]. One important drawback to DNA vaccines, however, is their lack of immunogenicity compared to protein-based or whole virus vaccines: Humoral responses are generally weak if not lacking altogether, and high, repeated doses of DNA are needed in order to obtain reasonable response rates in animal models. Additionally, results in small experimental animals have not translated well into human clinical trial results, and there are concerns over the safety of injecting large amounts of DNA (milligrams) into humans [2].

2. A Novel Enhancer Sequence for DNA Vaccine Antigen Expression

Our group therefore previously investigated the potential of short enhancer sequences derived from a mammalian single-stranded DNA virus—porcine circovirus type I (PCV-1)—for dose-sparing potential and immunogenicity enhancement in a clinically trialed HIV-1 subtype C DNA vaccine [3]. The plasmid vector (pTH) has been well used in preclinical and clinical studies [4–6] and is regarded as being a high-potency vaccine antigen vector for HIV and other agents. It relies on the human cytomegalovirus immediate/early promoter (CMV I/E) enhancer element constituting the promoter Pcmv [7], one of the strongest known promoters in mammalian expression systems, driving in vivo antigen expression with the help of the CMV intron A and the bovine growth hormone polyadenylation signal. It has been used to vector the synthetic HIV-1 subtype C vaccine antigen GrttnC, a polyprotein incorporating Gag, reverse transcriptase (RT), Tat, and Nef sequences, in studies in mice, guinea pigs, monkeys, and humans [8–12].

PCV-1, like all circoviruses, has a compact, genetically dense, bi-directionally transcribed genome of 1759 bp that encodes only a viral capsid protein (*cap* gene) and the replication-associated proteins Rep and Rep′, which derive by alternative splicing from one open reading frame (ORF) (*rep*) (Figure 1). Bidirectional transcription of the two genes originates in the origin of replication (Ori) for *rep*, and in an intron within *rep* for *cap* [13]. In vitro expression studies in human embryonic kidney 293 (HEK293) cells with various constructs derived from the PCV-1 genomes showed that enhancement activity resided in a 70 base pair "core sequence" (C) of the 172 base pair (bp) capsid promoter, Pcap, that includes a putative composite transcription factor binding site comprising CCAAT/enhancer-binding protein beta (C/EBPb), GATA-1, and cAMP response element-binding protein (CREB) sites, as well as a 47 bp conserved late element, or CLE. Inclusion of the 70 bp sequence in the reverse orientation immediately upstream of the Pcmv sequence in pTHgrttnC (yielding pTHCRgrttnC) resulted in 2.4-fold enhancement of polyprotein expression level in vitro following transfection of HEK293 cells, as assessed by Gag p24 ELISA. The cognate sequence from the related PCV-2 was equally effective. The 172 bp Pcap sequence also enhanced luciferase expression in HEK293 cells three-fold when inserted in reverse orientation upstream of the simian virus 40 (SV40) promoter in the commercial pGL vector [3]. Accordingly, we tested the enhancement of immunogenicity in vivo by intramuscular injection of mice with a variety of pTHgrttnC constructs with additives from PCV-1 (Figure 1C): The best enhancement over pTHgrttnC, as assayed by interferon-gamma enzyme-linked immune absorbent spot (IFN-γ ELISPOT) responses to a RT $CD8^+$ peptide, was obtained using the Pcap (172 bp) insert, after two intramuscular inoculations of 100 µg of pTHPcapRgrttnC DNA (five-fold increase in spot forming units (sfu)/10^6 splenocytes). Moreover, two inoculations of 10 µg of pTHPcapgrttnC DNA was significantly more immunogenic (3.5-fold) than pTHgrttnC and boosting with 10^4 plaque forming units (pfu) of modified vaccinia Ankara (MVA) vectoring Grttn showed the same trend (Figure 2). The response to the 10 µg of pTHPcapgrttnC DNA alone was also equivalent to or higher than to 100 µg of pTHgrttnC, indicating that significant dose sparing (10-fold) was possible for the same priming effect for a vaccine-relevant antigen. This proof that a simple enhancement could dramatically improve the functionality of a DNA vaccine vector led to its being employed in subsequent studies in our HIV vaccine research program.

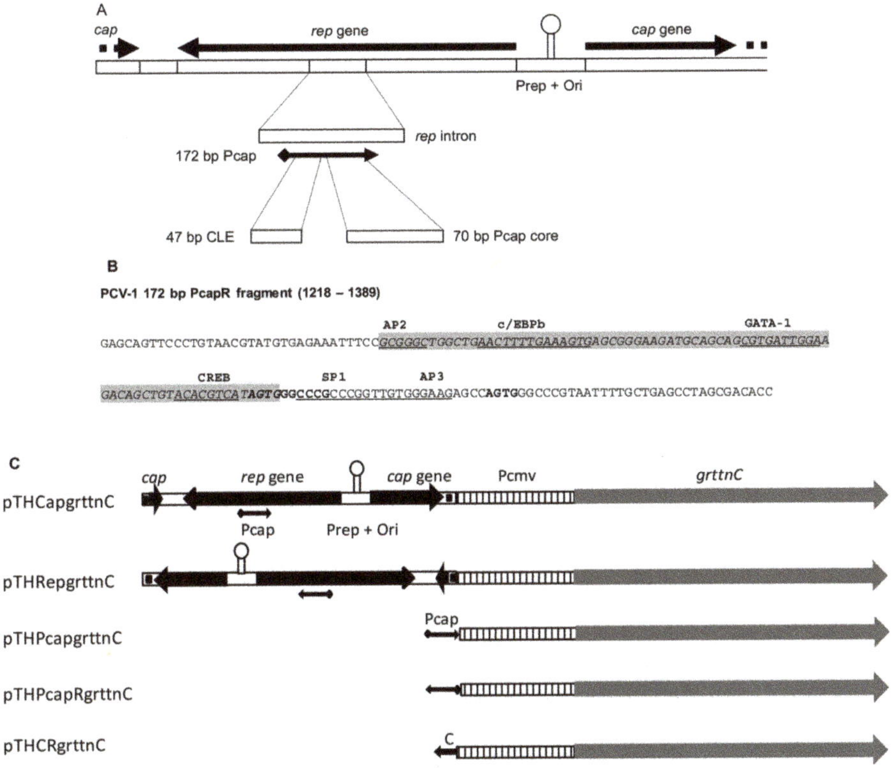

Figure 1. Porcine circovirus type-1 (PCV-1) genome arrangement. (**A**) Diagram of the linearized PCV-1 genome, depicted in the orientation cloned into pTHCapgrttnC. The *rep* intron is enlarged and the capsid gene promoter (Pcap) indicated. The core and conserved late elements (CLE) components of Pcap are shown. *rep* = replication associated protein gene, *cap* = capsid protein gene, Prep = *rep* gene promoter, Ori = origin of replication, core = composite host transcription factor binding site. (**B**) DNA sequence of 172 bp PcapR fragment. Putative host transcription factor binding sites are indicated and underlined, CLE motifs are in bold and the minimal PcapR sequence (1252–1238; as identified by Mankertz and Hillenbrand [13]) is highlighted in gray. PCV-1 accession number Y09921. (**C**) Schematic diagrams of plasmids showing assembly of PCV elements. Pcmv = Cytomegalovirus (CMV) promoter, *grttnC* = gene encoding polyprotein of HIV-1 Gag, reverse transcriptase (RT), Tat and Nef, C = 70 bp Pcap core. Figure reproduced from Tanzer et al. [3] under the Creative Commons Attribution (CC-BY) license as specified by BioMed Central.

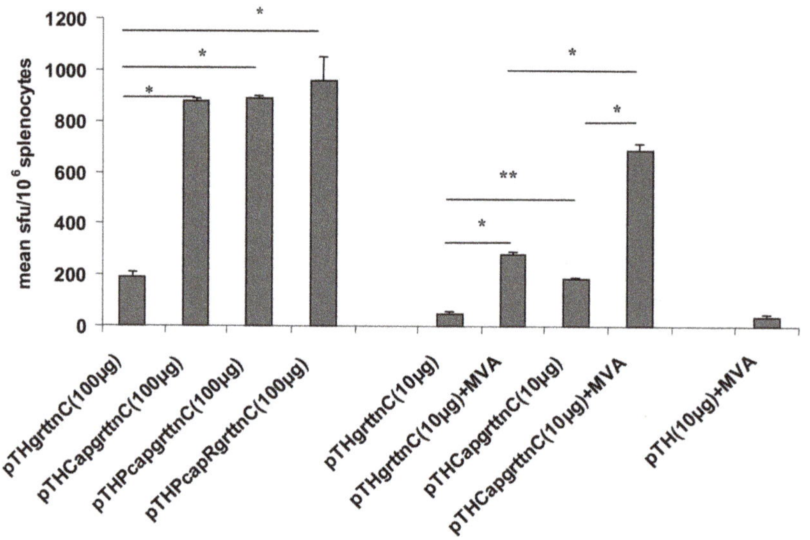

Figure 2. HIV-1 specific IFN-γ ELISPOT responses to pTHgrttnC DNA vaccines containing portions of the PCV-1 genome. Groups of mice were vaccinated intramuscularly with DNA vaccines on days 0 and 28. Two groups of mice were subsequently boosted with 10^4 pfu of modified vaccinia Ankara (MVA) on day 56. A separate group of mice was vaccinated with 10 µg pTH (empty vector) on days 0 and 28 and subsequently boosted with 10^4 pfu of MVA on day 56. * $p < 0.001$; ** $p < 0.05$ Student *t*-test. Figure reproduced from Tanzer et al. [3] under the Creative Commons Attribution (CC-BY) license as specified by BioMed Central.

3. Testing the Enhanced DNA Vector with HIV-1 Subtype C pr55Gag

Strong polyfunctional $CD8^+$ T cell responses to HIV-1 Gag or Gag-derived antigens have been found to be important for controlling viremia in HIV+ people who are termed "elite controllers." Accordingly, Gag should be and often is included in candidate HIV vaccination regimes, so as to allow early clearance of infected cells at the initial sites of infection, as well as control of spread from these sites and later control of viremia [14]. A subtype C mosaic Gag sequence was chosen to increase the coverage of both $CD8^+$ and $CD4^+$ T cell epitopes from that of natural sequences with the hope of reducing the HIV-1 escape pathways [15–18]. Subtype C (HIV-1C) was chosen as it is the most prevalent subtype in the world, accounting for over 50% of all global infections and is the dominant subtype in southern Africa. In a study carried out by our group, the pTHPcapR plasmid backbone [3] was used to construct a DNA vaccine containing an HIV-1 subtype C mosaic *gag* gene, DNA-Gag^M [19,20].

HEK293T cells transfected with DNA-Gag^M expressed high levels of Gag (up to 26 ng/mL in the media). The immune responses to the DNA vaccine were evaluated in mice using homologous and heterologous prime boosts with MVA vaccine expressing the matching HIV-1 subtype C mosaic Gag antigen (MVA-Gag^M). To confirm that the DNA vaccine was immunogenic at a low dose, mice were vaccinated with 10 µg of the DNA vaccine. Mice vaccinated with two doses of DNA-Gag^M had mean cumulative Gag-specific IFN-γ ELISPOT responses of 882 sfu/10^6 splenocytes (Figure 3). These responses were higher for $CD8^+$ rather than for $CD4^+$ Gag peptides (604 and 278 sfu/10^6, respectively). Mice that received a heterologous prime boost consisting of two doses of DNA-Gag^M followed by a single dose of MVA-Gag^M had mean cumulative Gag-specific IFN-γ ELISPOT responses of 2675 sfu/10^6, that were evenly balanced for both Gag $CD4^+$ and $CD8^+$ peptides. Both the homologous and heterologous vaccination regimen elicited a higher proportion of $CD8^+$ T cells expressing cytokines than $CD4^+$ T cells. All the cytokine-positive $CD8^+$ T cells had an effector–memory phenotype. This study confirmed that the pTHPcapR DNA vector backbone containing the porcine circovirus enhancer elicits high-magnitude, Gag-specific T cell responses in BALB/c mice at a low dose.

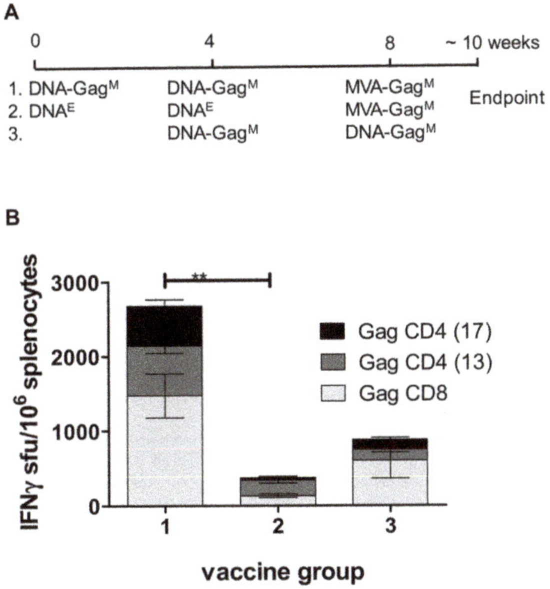

Figure 3. DNA vaccine elicits high Gag-specific IFN-γ ELISPOT responses both alone and in a heterologous prime boost with MVA. (**A**) Vaccination schedule. DNA-Gag^M = pTHPcapR containing mosaic *gag*; DNA^E = pTHPcapR empty vector; MVA-Gag^M = MVA containing mosaic *gag*. (**B**) Cumulative IFN-γ ELISPOT CD8$^+$ and CD4$^+$ responses of vaccinated mice to HIV-1 Gag peptides. ** $p < 0.01$ Student *t*-test of unpaired data.

4. Testing the Enhanced DNA Vector with HIV-1 Subtype C Env Immunogens

The kinds of immune responses that an effective HIV-1 vaccine would need to elicit include non-neutralizing antibody responses as well as broadly neutralizing antibody responses, together with polyfunctional cytotoxic T cell responses to a variety of epitopes from the HIV-1 proteome [21–23]. One of the main targets of recent HIV-1 vaccine candidates is broadly neutralizing antibody (bNAb) responses: bNAbs that can neutralize diverse primary HIV-1 subtype isolates protect against viral challenge in nonhuman primates (NHP) with Env-pseudotyped simian–human immunodeficiency viruses (SHIVs), suggesting that infection in humans could be similarly prevented [24,25]. Ranking of HIV-1 isolates according to their sensitivities to neutralizing antibodies allows identification of viruses as Tier 1 (sensitive), Tier 2 (moderately resistant), and Tier 3 (resistant) [26]. The circulating viruses that vaccines will need to protect against are largely Tier 2 type: Accordingly, HIV vaccines should elicit responses that neutralize laboratory Tier 2 virus isolates. We showed previously that using a DNA prime/MVA boost immunization regime in mice with vaccines expressing HIV-1 subtype C mosaic Gag resulted in strong cellular immune responses directed against Gag [19]. We wished to extend these results by improving the vaccine regimen to allow the elicitation of Env-specific neutralizing antibodies in a rabbit model.

The pTHPcapR vector was used to construct a DNA vaccine expressing a HIV-1 envelope (DNA Env). The envelope sequence (CAP256SU) used in this study was selected as it elicited broadly neutralizing antibodies (bNAbs) in the patient [27] and was sensitive to several prototype broadly neutralizing monoclonal antibodies [28]. Several modifications were made to the envelope sequence, these included replacing the native leader sequence with the tissue plasminogen activator leader sequence, replacing the furin cleavage site with a flexible linker, introducing an I548P mutation equivalent to the I559P in the SOSIP trimers to improve the trimerization of gp41 [29] and truncating the sequence from gp160 to gp150 [30]. A second plasmid expressing the soluble envelope protein (gp140) with the same modifications was also constructed using the pTHPcapR backbone [31]. This plasmid was used to generate a stable cell line expressing high levels of the soluble HIV-1 envelope protein, which was subsequently purified and utilized as a protein boost in rabbit immunogenicity studies. MVA vaccines expressing the matching gp150 Env and Env plus mosaic Gag were also constructed.

Rabbits were inoculated with different combinations of vaccines in different regimens, in order to ascertain the overall effects on immunogenicity of the Env component. The first test group was injected with 100 µg of each of DNA Env- and DNA-Gag^{M}-encoding plasmids at weeks 0 and 4, boosted with doses of 10^8 pfu of rMVA Env + Gag^{M} at weeks 8 and 12, and further boosted with gp140Env protein at weeks 20 and 28 (regime designated as DDMMPP). The other group received 10^8 pfu of rMVA Env + Gag^{M} intramuscularly at weeks 0 and 4, followed by three protein boosts at weeks 12, 20, and 28 (MMPPP) (Figure 4).

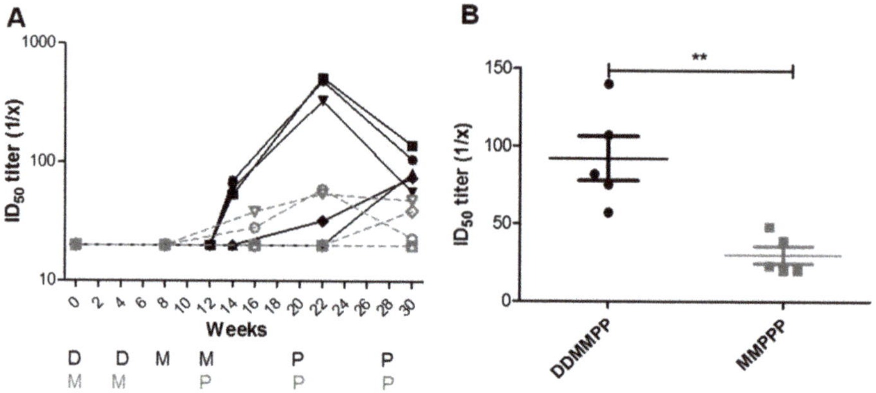

Figure 4. Rabbits primed with DNA produce higher autologous Tier 2 neutralizing antibodies than those receiving MVA and protein alone. (**A**) Longitudinal, Tier 2 neutralizing antibody responses to autologous CAP256SU pseudovirion from the serum of individual rabbits. (**B**) Neutralizing antibody titers at week 30. ** $p < 0.01$ Mann–Whitney U test, median of $N = 5$.

Both the DDMMPP and MMPPP vaccination regimens elicited NAbs to the autologous Tier 2 CAP256SU pseudovirion. Moreover, high titers of antibodies that bound to the homologous CAP256 Env and a CAP256 V1V2 loop scaffold were also elicited [30]. It was noticeable that the DDMMPP regimen elicited higher mean peak titers of Tier 2 NAbs than did the MMPPP regimen: This suggests that priming with a DNA vaccine (DDMMPP) gives a better, wider anti-Env immune response than the MMPPP regime (Figure 4). The DDMMPP regimen rabbits also apparently developed a slight increase in breadth of the response as they had low levels of NAbs to clade A pseudovirus 398F1. Our findings that DNA primes a good humoral response agree with others: For example, adding DNA-C priming in the EV01 phase-I trial resulted in increased anti-Env IgG responses (from 27% for attenuated vaccinia virus strain NYVAC alone to 75% for DNA + NYVAC [32]). Priming with DNA also resulted in significantly boosted T cell responses.

5. Comparison of DNA Vaccines between Two Initiatives in South Africa

In 2000, a University of Cape Town (UCT)-based consortium headed by Prof. Anna-Lise Williamson was awarded funds by the South African AIDS Vaccine Initiative (SAAVI) for the development of HIV-1C vaccines for South Africa. Two vaccines—designated SAAVI DNA-C2 and SAAVI MVA-C—were deemed suitable for human clinical trials [9,10]. The vaccines expressed a HIV-1 subtype C truncated envelope protein Du151 (gp150) and the polyprotein designated Grttn described above, consisting of translational fusions of HIV-1 subtype C Gag Du422, and modified reverse transcriptase (RT), Tat-, and Nef-encoding ORFs. The vector backbone utilized for the DNA vaccines contained the regulatory R region from the 5′ long terminal repeat (LTR) of human T-cell leukemia virus type 1, which acts as a transcriptional and post-transcriptional enhancer [33]. Rhesus macaques were inoculated at weeks 0, 4, and 8 with 4 mg of SAAVI DNA-C2. No HIV-specific ELISPOT responses were detected following the DNA vaccinations (unpublished data). In a more recent study funded by the South African Medical Research Council Strategic Health Innovation Partnerships (SHIP), DNA vaccines expressing the SIV Gag and HIV-1 subtype C truncated envelope ZM109F.PB4 were constructed utilizing the pTHPcapR vector backbone (unpublished data). Rhesus macaques were inoculated, at weeks 0 and 4 with 1 mg of the DNA vaccines (four-fold lower dose). Four out of five macaques developed IFN-γ ELISPOT responses following stimulation with SIV Gag and HIV-1 subtype Env peptides. It should be noted that the antigens used in the SHIP vaccines have been designed to be more immunogenic than those used in the SAAVI vaccines and thus the improvement in the immune response cannot be solely attributed to the increased expression of the Gag and Env due to the inclusion of the porcine circovirus in the DNA vaccines. However, the SHIP DNA vaccines elicited a HIV-specific T cell response despite being administered at a four-fold lower dose than the SAAVI DNA-C2 vaccine.

6. Future Possibilities for Enhanced DNA Vaccine or Expression Vectors Based on Circoviruses

Our group has recently published an investigation of the possibility of using circovirus-derived replication control elements to create replicons, or replicating dsDNA plasmid-like molecules, in plants and in mammalian cells [34]. This followed our extensive success with use of a plant ssDNA geminivirus-derived expression vector in plants as an enhanced expression vector [35]: Geminiviruses are very similar to circoviruses in having small circular ssDNA genomes that replicate via a Rep-mediated rolling circle mechanism, and very similar sequences for their non-nucleotide origins of replication (TAATATT/AC vs. TAGTATT/AC). In this study, we used a synthetic, partially dimeric clone of the genome of beak and feather disease virus (BFDV), a circovirus generically related to PCV, to investigate cross-potentiation of replication between the plant and animal viruses in plants and replication of the BFDV genome alone in HEK293TT cells.

Initial experiments where both the geminivirus-derived vector bean yellow dwarf virus (BeYDV) and BFDV genome were introduced into *Nicotiana benthamiana* plants via *Agrobacterium tumefaciens*-mediated DNA transfer showed that replication of BeYDV facilitated the co-replication of BFDV, albeit to levels only 100× less than for BeYDV replicons. More importantly, however, transfection of HEK293TT cells with the BFDV construct resulted in a ten-fold increase in genome copy number after three days. This was the first time that BFDV genomes had been shown to replicate in any animal-derived cell culture, in contrast to PCVs which readily infect a variety of cells [36]. Improvement in replicon copy number could be achieved by expressing BFDV in trans from another co-transfected vector with a strong promoter: This is not surprising, considering the native *rep* promoter is quite weak and is probably not well recognized in mammalian cells, meaning expression in trans could mean a far higher availability of Rep.

These results open up a number of fascinating possibilities for using BFDV-derived sequences as replication-competent DNA expression and vaccine vectors, several of which we are currently investigating (W. de Moor, G. Regnard, A.-L. Williamson, E.P. Rybicki, unpublished results and ongoing work). There are currently no small DNA virus-derived vectors in use in vaccinology, other than recombinant adeno-associated viruses (rAAV), and AAV2 has recently been implicated in insertional mutagenesis in human hepatocellular carcinomas [37]. Papilloma- and polyomaviruses are also known to be associated with cancers, which may preclude their use as replicating vectors. The essentially ubiquitous ssDNA torque teno viruses are potentially associated with some human disease conditions, although causation is not proven [38,39].

Circoviruses have never been implicated in any human disease: Although PCV-1 and PCV-2 were famously discovered in live rotavirus vaccines given to millions of children [40], and PCV-1 was shown to be able to infect a human hepatocellular carcinoma cell line [41], there was no evidence that PCV-1 infected the infants given the contaminated rotavirus vaccine [42]. There have been concerns, however, over ssDNA viruses of pigs associated with xenotransplantation in humans [43], and swine–human contacts are frequent and worldwide in agriculture. Thus, use of a circovirus such as BFDV as the source of elements for a replicating DNA expression vector, when the virus is host-restricted to one type of birds and has never been associated with human disease, is probably more likely to be regarded as safe. Our preliminary investigations have revealed considerable promise in this regard; however, these will be reported elsewhere (W. de Moor, G. Regnard, A.-L. Williamson, E.P. Rybicki, unpublished results).

7. Conclusions

It has been over 25 years since DNA vaccines were first introduced and many advances have been made in the field. However, despite showing promise in small animals, with some DNA vaccines being licensed for veterinary use [44,45], no DNA vaccines have been licensed for human use as immunogenicity is still relatively poor. Thus, a great deal of research has gone into improving the immunogenicity of DNA vaccines. Some of the strategies that have been shown to be effective are: (i) RNA optimization to remove mRNA structures that inhibit ribosomal loading and sequences that inhibit nuclear export of mRNA [46,47]; (ii) codon optimization [46,48,49]; (iii) use of Kozak sequences [50]; (iv) use of leader sequences to improve stability, translation, and secretion [46]; (v) use of 3′ untranslated regions (UTR) such as polyadenylation signals and post-transcriptional response elements which are important for nuclear export, translation, and mRNA stability [51]; (vi) use of different promoters and enhancers [52–54]; (vii) the inclusion of genes expressing immunomodulatory molecules in the plasmid vector such as GM-CSF or IL-2 [55,56]; (viii) formulation of DNA vaccines in lipids and polymers [57]; (ix) use of better delivery systems [58–60]; and (x) use of suitable adjuvants [58,59].

In this review, we have only focused on a single method of improving DNA vaccine immunogenicity. This was the use of a short enhancer sequence derived from the circovirus PCV-1 capsid gene promoter to increase recombinant antigen expression. This enhancer element led to increased antigen expression and immunogenicity of HIV-1 subtype C candidate DNA vaccines and allowed for the use of 10-fold lower doses. The improved performance of the DNA vaccines with these candidates, compared to non-enhanced vectors that went into human clinical trial, has prompted the inclusion of the enhancer into all DNA vaccines under investigation in our research group, with excellent results. Future use of replicating circovirus-derived DNA expression and vaccine vectors may yet open up even more exciting possibilities.

Author Contributions: Both authors contributed equally to the review article.

Funding: This work is based upon research supported by the South African Medical Research Council with funds received from the South African Department of Science and Technology and the South African Research Chairs Initiative of the Department of Science and Technology and National Research Foundation.

Acknowledgments: We acknowledge the pioneering work of Dr. Fiona Tanzer, and the gift of the original PCV-1 genome by Kenneth Palmer.

Conflicts of Interest: The authors declare no conflict of interest. The funders had no role in the design of the study; in the collection, analyses, or interpretation of data; in the writing of the manuscript or in the decision to publish the results.

References

1. Doria-Rose, N.A.; Haigwood, N.L. DNA vaccine strategies: Candidates for immune modulation and immunization regimens. *Methods* **2003**, *31*, 207–216. [CrossRef]
2. Forde, G.M. Rapid-response vaccines—Does DNA offer a solution? *Nat. Biotechnol.* **2005**, *23*, 1059–1062. [CrossRef] [PubMed]

3. Tanzer, F.L.; Shephard, E.G.; Palmer, K.E.; Burger, M.; Williamson, A.L.; Rybicki, E.P. The porcine circovirus type 1 capsid gene promoter improves antigen expression and immunogenicity in a HIV-1 plasmid vaccine. *Virol. J.* **2011**, *8*, 51. [CrossRef] [PubMed]
4. Hanke, T.; Schneider, J.; Gilbert, S.C.; Hill, A.V.; McMichael, A. DNA multi-CTL epitope vaccines for HIV and Plasmodium falciparum: Immunogenicity in mice. *Vaccine* **1998**, *16*, 426–435. [CrossRef]
5. Im, E.J.; Nkolola, J.P.; di Gleria, K.; McMichael, A.J.; Hanke, T. Induction of long-lasting multi-specific CD8+ T cells by a four-component DNA-MVA/HIVA-RENTA candidate HIV-1 vaccine in rhesus macaques. *Eur. J. Immunol.* **2006**, *36*, 2574–2584. [CrossRef] [PubMed]
6. Sharpe, S.; Hanke, T.; Tinsley-Bown, A.; Dennis, M.; Dowall, S.; McMichael, A.; Cranage, M. Mucosal immunization with PLGA-microencapsulated DNA primes a SIV-specific CTL response revealed by boosting with cognate recombinant modified vaccinia virus Ankara. *Virology* **2003**, *313*, 13–21. [CrossRef]
7. Stinski, M.F.; Isomura, H. Role of the cytomegalovirus major immediate early enhancer in acute infection and reactivation from latency. *Med. Microbiol. Immunol.* **2008**, *197*, 223–231. [CrossRef]
8. Chege, G.K.; Burgers, W.A.; Muller, T.L.; Gray, C.M.; Shephard, E.G.; Barnett, S.W.; Ferrari, G.; Montefiori, D.; Williamson, C.; Williamson, A.-L. DNA-MVA-protein vaccination of rhesus macaques induces HIV-specific immunity in mucosal-associated lymph nodes and functional antibodies. *Vaccine* **2017**, *35*, 929–937. [CrossRef]
9. Churchyard, G.; Mlisana, K.; Karuna, S.; Williamson, A.L.; Williamson, C.; Morris, L.; Tomaras, G.D.; De Rosa, S.C.; Gilbert, P.B.; Gu, N.; et al. Sequential Immunization with gp140 Boosts Immune Responses Primed by Modified Vaccinia Ankara or DNA in HIV-Uninfected South African Participants. *PLoS ONE* **2016**, *11*, e0161753. [CrossRef]
10. Gray, G.E.; Mayer, K.H.; Elizaga, M.L.; Bekker, L.G.; Allen, M.; Morris, L.; Montefiori, D.; De Rosa, S.C.; Sato, A.; Gu, N.; et al. Subtype C gp140 Vaccine Boosts Immune Responses Primed by the South African AIDS Vaccine Initiative DNA-C2 and MVA-C HIV Vaccines after More than a 2-Year Gap. *Clin. Vaccine Immunol.* **2016**, *23*, 496–506. [CrossRef]
11. Shephard, E.; Burgers, W.A.; Van Harmelen, J.H.; Monroe, J.E.; Greenhalgh, T.; Williamson, C.; Williamson, A.L. A multigene HIV type 1 subtype C modified vaccinia Ankara (MVA) vaccine efficiently boosts immune responses to a DNA vaccine in mice. *AIDS Res. Hum. Retrovir.* **2008**, *24*, 207–217. [CrossRef] [PubMed]
12. Williamson, A.L.; Rybicki, E.; Shephard, E.; Gray, G.; Bekker, L.G.; Downing, K.; Williamson, C. South African HIV-1 vaccine candidates—The journey from the bench to clinical trials. *S. Afr. Med. J.* **2012**, *102*, 452–455. [CrossRef] [PubMed]
13. Mankertz, A.; Hillenbrand, B. Analysis of transcription of Porcine circovirus type 1. *J. Gen. Virol.* **2002**, *83*, 2743–2751. [CrossRef]
14. Williamson, A.L.; Rybicki, E.P. Justification for the inclusion of Gag in HIV vaccine candidates. *Expert Rev. Vaccines* **2016**, *15*, 585–598. [CrossRef] [PubMed]
15. Abdul-Jawad, S.; Ondondo, B.; van Hateren, A.; Gardner, A.; Elliott, T.; Korber, B.; Hanke, T. Increased Valency of Conserved-mosaic Vaccines Enhances the Breadth and Depth of Epitope Recognition. *Mol. Ther.* **2016**, *24*, 375–384. [CrossRef]
16. Barouch, D.H.; O'Brien, K.L.; Simmons, N.L.; King, S.L.; Abbink, P.; Maxfield, L.F.; et al. Mosaic HIV-1 vaccines expand the breadth and depth of cellular immune responses in rhesus monkeys. *Nat. Med.* **2010**, *16*, 319–323. [CrossRef]
17. Barouch, D.H.; Stephenson, K.E.; Borducchi, E.N.; Smith, K.; Stanley, K.; McNally, A.G.; Liu, J.; Abbink, P.; Maxfield, L.F.; Seaman, M.S.; et al. Protective efficacy of a global HIV-1 mosaic vaccine against heterologous SHIV challenges in rhesus monkeys. *Cell* **2013**, *155*, 531–539. [CrossRef]
18. Santra, S.; Liao, H.X.; Zhang, R.; Muldoon, M.; Watson, S.; Fischer, W.; Theiler, J.; Szinger, J.; Balachandran, H.; Buzby, A.; et al. Mosaic vaccines elicit CD8+ T lymphocyte responses that confer enhanced immune coverage of diverse HIV strains in monkeys. *Nat. Med.* **2010**, *16*, 324–328. [CrossRef]
19. Chapman, R.; Jongwe, T.I.; Douglass, N.; Chege, G.; Williamson, A.L. Heterologous prime-boost vaccination with DNA and MVA vaccines, expressing HIV-1 subtype C mosaic Gag virus-like particles, is highly immunogenic in mice. *PLoS ONE* **2017**, *12*, e0173352. [CrossRef]
20. Fischer, W.; Perkins, S.; Theiler, J.; Bhattacharya, T.; Yusim, K.; Funkhouser, R.; Kuiken, C.; Haynes, B.; Letvin, N.L.; Walker, B.D.; et al. Polyvalent vaccines for optimal coverage of potential T-cell epitopes in global HIV-1 variants. *Nat. Med.* **2007**, *13*, 100–106. [CrossRef]

21. Bricault, C.A.; Kovacs, J.M.; Badamchi-Zadeh, A.; McKee, K.; Shields, J.L.; Gunn, B.M.; Neubauer, G.H.; Ghantous, F.; Jennings, J.; Gillis, L.; et al. Neutralizing Antibody Responses following Long-Term Vaccination with HIV-1 Env gp140 in Guinea Pigs. *J. Virol.* **2018**, *92*, e00369-18. [CrossRef] [PubMed]
22. Cohen, K.W.; Frahm, N. Current views on the potential for development of a HIV vaccine. *Expert Opin. Biol. Ther.* **2017**, *17*, 295–303. [CrossRef] [PubMed]
23. Plotkin, S.A. Complex correlates of protection after vaccination. *Clin. Infect. Dis.* **2013**, *56*, 1458–1465. [CrossRef] [PubMed]
24. Hessell, A.J.; Poignard, P.; Hunter, M.; Hangartner, L.; Tehrani, D.M.; Bleeker, W.K.; Parren, P.W.; Marx, P.A.; Burton, D.R. Effective, low-titer antibody protection against low-dose repeated mucosal SHIV challenge in macaques. *Nat. Med.* **2009**, *15*, 951–954. [CrossRef] [PubMed]
25. Julg, B.; Sok, D.; Schmidt, S.D.; Abbink, P.; Newman, R.M.; Broge, T.; Linde, C.; Nkolola, J.; Le, K.; Su, D.; et al. Protective Efficacy of Broadly Neutralizing Antibodies with Incomplete Neutralization Activity against Simian-Human Immunodeficiency Virus in Rhesus Monkeys. *J. Virol.* **2017**, *91*, e01187-17. [CrossRef] [PubMed]
26. Kim, M.; Qiao, Z.S.; Montefiori, D.C.; Haynes, B.F.; Reinherz, E.L.; Liao, H.X. Comparison of HIV Type 1 ADA gp120 monomers versus gp140 trimers as immunogens for the induction of neutralizing antibodies. *AIDS Res. Hum. Retrovir.* **2005**, *21*, 58–67. [CrossRef] [PubMed]
27. Bhiman, J.N.; Anthony, C.; Doria-Rose, N.A.; Karimanzira, O.; Schramm, C.A.; Khoza, T.; Kitchin, D.; Botha, G.; Gorman, J.; Garrett, N.J.; et al. Viral variants that initiate and drive maturation of V1V2-directed HIV-1 broadly neutralizing antibodies. *Nat. Med.* **2015**, *21*, 1332–1336. [CrossRef] [PubMed]
28. Moore, P.L.; Sheward, D.; Nonyane, M.; Ranchobe, N.; Hermanus, T.; Gray, E.S.; Abdool Karim, S.S.; Williamson, C.; Morris, L. Multiple pathways of escape from HIV broadly cross-neutralizing V2-dependent antibodies. *J. Virol.* **2013**, *87*, 4882–4894. [CrossRef] [PubMed]
29. Sanders, R.W.; Vesanen, M.; Schuelke, N.; Master, A.; Schiffner, L.; Kalyanaraman, R.; Paluch, M.; Berkhout, B.; Maddon, P.J.; Olson, W.C.; et al. Stabilization of the soluble, cleaved, trimeric form of the envelope glycoprotein complex of human immunodeficiency virus type 1. *J. Virol.* **2002**, *76*, 8875–8889. [CrossRef]
30. Van Diepen, M.T.; Chapman, R.; Douglass, N.; Galant, S.; Moore, P.L.; Margolin, E.; Ximba, P.; Morris, L.; Rybicki, E.P.; Williamson, A.L. Prime boost immunisations with DNA, MVA and protein-based vaccines elicit robust HIV-1, Tier 2 neutralizing antibodies against the CAP256 superinfecting virus. *J. Virol.* **2019**. [CrossRef]
31. Van Diepen, M.T.; Chapman, R.; Moore, P.L.; Margolin, E.; Hermanus, T.; Morris, L.; Ximba, P.; Rybicki, E.P.; Williamson, A.L. The adjuvant AlhydroGel elicits higher antibody titres than AddaVax when combined with HIV-1 subtype C gp140 from CAP256. *PLoS ONE* **2018**, *13*, e0208310. [CrossRef] [PubMed]
32. Asbach, B.; Kliche, A.; Kostler, J.; Perdiguero, B.; Esteban, M.; Jacobs, B.L.; Montefiori, D.C.; LaBranche, C.C.; Yates, N.L.; Tomaras, G.D.; et al. Potential To Streamline Heterologous DNA Prime and NYVAC/Protein Boost HIV Vaccine Regimens in Rhesus Macaques by Employing Improved Antigens. *J. Virol.* **2016**, *90*, 4133–4149. [CrossRef] [PubMed]
33. Barouch, D.H.; Yang, Z.Y.; Kong, W.P.; Korioth-Schmitz, B.; Sumida, S.M.; Truitt, D.M.; Kishko, M.G.; Arthur, J.C.; Miura, A.; Mascola, J.R.; et al. A human T-cell leukemia virus type 1 regulatory element enhances the immunogenicity of human immunodeficiency virus type 1 DNA vaccines in mice and nonhuman primates. *J. Virol.* **2005**, *79*, 8828–8834. [CrossRef] [PubMed]
34. Regnard, G.L.; de Moor, W.R.J.; Hitzeroth, I.I.; Williamson, A.L.; Rybicki, E.P. Xenogenic rolling-circle replication of a synthetic beak and feather disease virus genomic clone in 293TT mammalian cells and Nicotiana benthamiana. *J. Gen. Virol.* **2017**, *98*, 2329–2338. [CrossRef] [PubMed]
35. Regnard, G.L.; Halley-Stott, R.P.; Tanzer, F.L.; Hitzeroth, I.I.; Rybicki, E.P. High level protein expression in plants through the use of a novel autonomously replicating geminivirus shuttle vector. *Plant Biotechnol. J.* **2010**, *8*, 38–46. [CrossRef] [PubMed]
36. Karuppannan, A.K.; Kwang, J. ORF3 of porcine circovirus 2 enhances the in vitro and in vivo spread of the of the virus. *Virology* **2011**, *410*, 248–256. [CrossRef]
37. Nault, J.C.; Datta, S.; Imbeaud, S.; Franconi, A.; Mallet, M.; Couchy, G.; Letouzé, E.; Pilati, C.; Verret, B.; Blanc, J.F.; et al. Recurrent AAV2-related insertional mutagenesis in human hepatocellular carcinomas. *Nat. Genet.* **2015**, *47*, 1187–1193. [CrossRef]

38. Eibach, D.; Hogan, B.; Sarpong, N.; Winter, D.; Struck, N.S.; Adu-Sarkodie, Y.; Owusu-Dabo, E.; Schmidt-Chanasit, J.; May, J.; Cadar, D. Viral metagenomics revealed novel betatorquevirus species in pediatric inpatients with encephalitis/meningoencephalitis from Ghana. *Sci. Rep.* **2019**, *9*, 2360. [CrossRef]
39. Herrmann, A.; Sandmann, L.; Adams, O.; Herrmann, D.; Dirks, M.; Widera, M.; Westhaus, S.; Kaiser, R.; di Cristanziano, V.; Manns, M.P.; et al. Role of BK polyomavirus (BKV) and Torque teno virus (TTV) in liver transplant recipients with renal impairment. *J. Med. Microbiol.* **2018**, *67*, 1496–1508. [CrossRef]
40. Gilliland, S.M.; Forrest, L.; Carre, H.; Jenkins, A.; Berry, N.; Martin, J.; Minor, P.; Schepelmann, S. Investigation of porcine circovirus contamination in human vaccines. *Biologicals* **2012**, *40*, 270–277. [CrossRef]
41. Beach, N.M.; Cordoba, L.; Kenney, S.P.; Meng, X.J. Productive infection of human hepatocellular carcinoma cells by porcine circovirus type 1. *Vaccine* **2011**, *29*, 7303–7306. [CrossRef] [PubMed]
42. Dubin, G.; Toussaint, J.F.; Cassart, J.P.; Howe, B.; Boyce, D.; Friedland, L.; Abu-Elyazeed, R.; Poncelet, S.; Han, H.H.; Debrus, S. Investigation of a regulatory agency enquiry into potential porcine circovirus type 1 contamination of the human rotavirus vaccine, Rotarix: Approach and outcome. *Hum. Vaccines Immunother.* **2013**, *9*, 2398–2408. [CrossRef] [PubMed]
43. Karuppannan, A.K.; Opriessnig, T. Possible risks posed by single-stranded DNA viruses of pigs associated with xenotransplantation. *Xenotransplantation* **2018**, *25*, e12453. [CrossRef]
44. Anderson, E.D.; Mourich, D.V.; Fahrenkrug, S.C.; LaPatra, S.; Shepherd, J.; Leong, J.A. Genetic immunization of rainbow trout (*Oncorhynchus mykiss*) against infectious hematopoietic necrosis virus. *Mol. Mar. Biol. Biotechnol.* **1996**, *5*, 114–122. [PubMed]
45. Davis, B.S.; Chang, G.J.; Cropp, B.; Roehrig, J.T.; Martin, D.A.; Mitchell, C.J.; Bowen, R.; Bunning, M.L. West Nile virus recombinant DNA vaccine protects mouse and horse from virus challenge and expresses in vitro a noninfectious recombinant antigen that can be used in enzyme-linked immunosorbent assays. *J. Virol.* **2001**, *75*, 4040–4047. [CrossRef] [PubMed]
46. Megati, S.; Garcia-Hand, D.; Cappello, S.; Roopchand, V.; Masood, A.; Xu, R.; Luckay, A.; Chong, S.Y.; Rosati, M.; Sackitey, S.; et al. Modifying the HIV-1 env gp160 gene to improve pDNA vaccine-elicited cell-mediated immune responses. *Vaccine* **2008**, *26*, 5083–5094. [CrossRef] [PubMed]
47. Zhou, W.; Cook, R.F.; Cook, S.J.; Hammond, S.A.; Rushlow, K.; Ghabrial, N.N.; Berger, S.L.; Montelaro, R.C.; Issel, C.J. Multiple RNA splicing and the presence of cryptic RNA splice donor and acceptor sites may contribute to low expression levels and poor immunogenicity of potential DNA vaccines containing the env gene of equine infectious anemia virus (EIAV). *Vet. Microbiol.* **2002**, *88*, 127–151. [CrossRef]
48. Fath, S.; Bauer, A.P.; Liss, M.; Spriestersbach, A.; Maertens, B.; Hahn, P.; Ludwig, C.; Schäfer, F.; Graf, M.; Wagner, R. Multiparameter RNA and codon optimization: A standardized tool to assess and enhance autologous mammalian gene expression. *PLoS ONE* **2011**, *6*, e17596. [CrossRef]
49. Ko, H.J.; Ko, S.Y.; Kim, Y.J.; Lee, E.G.; Cho, S.N.; Kang, C.Y. Optimization of codon usage enhances the immunogenicity of a DNA vaccine encoding mycobacterial antigen Ag85B. *Infect. Immun.* **2005**, *73*, 5666–5674. [CrossRef] [PubMed]
50. Kozak, M. Point mutations define a sequence flanking the AUG initiator codon that modulates translation by eukaryotic ribosomes. *Cell* **1986**, *44*, 283–292. [CrossRef]
51. Barrett, L.W.; Fletcher, S.; Wilton, S.D. Regulation of eukaryotic gene expression by the untranslated gene regions and other non-coding elements. *Cell. Mol. Life Sci.* **2012**, *69*, 3613–3634. [CrossRef] [PubMed]
52. Garg, S.; Oran, A.E.; Hon, H.; Jacob, J. The hybrid cytomegalovirus enhancer/chicken beta-actin promoter along with woodchuck hepatitis virus posttranscriptional regulatory element enhances the protective efficacy of DNA vaccines. *J. Immunol.* **2004**, *173*, 550–558. [CrossRef] [PubMed]
53. Vanniasinkam, T.; Reddy, S.T.; Ertl, H.C. DNA immunization using a non-viral promoter. *Virology* **2006**, *344*, 412–420. [CrossRef] [PubMed]
54. Wang, S.; Farfan-Arribas, D.J.; Shen, S.; Chou, T.H.; Hirsch, A.; He, F.; Lu, S. Relative contributions of codon usage, promoter efficiency and leader sequence to the antigen expression and immunogenicity of HIV-1 Env DNA vaccine. *Vaccine* **2006**, *24*, 4531–4540. [CrossRef] [PubMed]
55. Hellerstein, M.; Xu, Y.; Marino, T.; Lu, S.; Yi, H.; Wright, E.R.; Robinson, H.L. Co-expression of HIV-1 virus-like particles and granulocyte-macrophage colony stimulating factor by GEO-D03 DNA vaccine. *Hum. Vaccines Immunother.* **2012**, *8*, 1654–1658. [CrossRef] [PubMed]

56. Henke, A.; Rohland, N.; Zell, R.; Wutzler, P. Co-expression of interleukin-2 by a bicistronic plasmid increases the efficacy of DNA immunization to prevent influenza virus infections. *Intervirology* **2006**, *49*, 249–252. [CrossRef]
57. O'Hagan, D.T.; Singh, M.; Ulmer, J.B. Microparticle-based technologies for vaccines. *Methods* **2006**, *40*, 10–19. [CrossRef]
58. Burton, S.; Spicer, L.M.; Charles, T.P.; Gangadhara, S.; Reddy, P.B.J.; Styles, T.M.; Velu, V.; Kasturi, S.P.; Legere, T.; Hunter, E.; et al. Clade C HIV-1 Envelope Vaccination Regimens Differ in Their Ability To Elicit Antibodies with Moderate Neutralization Breadth against Genetically Diverse Tier 2 HIV-1 Envelope Variants. *J. Virol.* **2019**, *93*, e01846-18. [CrossRef]
59. Li, L.; Petrovsky, N. Molecular Adjuvants for DNA Vaccines. *Curr. Issues Mol. Biol.* **2017**, *22*, 17–40. [CrossRef]
60. Porter, K.R.; Raviprakash, K. DNA Vaccine Delivery and Improved Immunogenicity. *Curr. Issues Mol. Biol.* **2017**, *22*, 129–138. [CrossRef]

vaccines

MDPI

Review

A Comparison of Plasmid DNA and mRNA as Vaccine Technologies

Margaret A. Liu

ProTherImmune, 3656 Happy Valley Road, Lafayette, CA 94549, USA; Liu@ProTherImmune.com

Received: 7 March 2019; Accepted: 19 April 2019; Published: 24 April 2019

Abstract: This review provides a comparison of the theoretical issues and experimental findings for plasmid DNA and mRNA vaccine technologies. While both have been under development since the 1990s, in recent years, significant excitement has turned to mRNA despite the licensure of several veterinary DNA vaccines. Both have required efforts to increase their potency either via manipulating the plasmid DNA and the mRNA directly or through the addition of adjuvants or immunomodulators as well as delivery systems and formulations. The greater inherent inflammatory nature of the mRNA vaccines is discussed for both its potential immunological utility for vaccines and for the potential toxicity. The status of the clinical trials of mRNA vaccines is described along with a comparison to DNA vaccines, specifically the immunogenicity of both licensed veterinary DNA vaccines and select DNA vaccine candidates in human clinical trials.

Keywords: DNA vaccine; mRNA vaccine; plasmid DNA; in vitro transcribed mRNA; immune responses; formulations; Cytolytic T Lymphocytes; antibodies; innate immunity

1. Introduction

Plasmid DNA [1] and now mRNA [2] vaccines have generated significant interest and efforts because of their potential as platform technologies that could be used for a variety of applications ranging from prophylaxis to therapy and from personalized medicine to global health solutions. Both can be quickly made with fairly generic manufacturing processes and can be constructed directly from the genetic sequence of the desired protein, whether the origin of the protein is human or from a pathogen. For vaccines, making a gene construct coding for the antigen instead of inactivating or attenuating the pathogen, or instead of making a recombinant protein, is vastly easier, more rapid, and avoids potential risks of working with live pathogens. Likewise, the vaccine construct can encode only the key antigen without including other proteins that may be either deleterious (such as toxins) or that may be irrelevant for protection yet immunodominant.

The ease and speed of making the constructs also means that these are considered potential gamechangers for targeting epidemic or emerging diseases where rapidly designing, constructing, and manufacturing the vaccine are crucial. For cancer, rather than relying on tumor-associated antigens that are common to many tumors, it would require little more effort to make the vaccines specific for that individual's exact tumor antigens, now referred to as personalized vaccines. The concept was demonstrated pre-clinically in the mid-1990s with DNA vaccines targeting lymphoma, where the idiotype of a tumor could be rapidly sequenced, and a DNA vaccine made much more quickly than a recombinant protein version [3,4]. Alternatively, as is being tested now for mRNA [2,5], libraries of gene-based constructs encoding various antigens could be made. Then, based on a patient's individual tumor antigens, a combination of constructs could be easily combined from this pre-made library.

At a time when many scientists are turning from plasmid DNA to explore mRNA technology while remaining uncertain about when or whether DNA vaccines will be licensed for human diseases, it is useful to compare the two technologies by analyzing both the theoretical issues and the experimental data and progress for both.

2. Background

In 1990, Felgner and colleagues published, in Science [6], their demonstration that so-called "naked DNA", that is, plasmid DNA that was not formulated in transfecting agents, could be directly injected into muscle with resultant expression of the encoded protein by myocytes. The observation was important because up until then, significant effort had been devoted to formulations to deliver DNA in vivo, and many such compounds were used for in vitro transfection. The surprising simplicity of the approach generated significant interest, and when it was soon shown (in 1993) that plasmid DNA coding for a conserved internal influenza protein could generate protection in a pre-clinical mouse model against influenza challenge with a very different influenza strain than the strain from which the protein antigen was sequenced [7], many groups began developing plasmid DNA for vaccines, cancer immunotherapies, and immune interventions for autoimmune and allergic diseases.

The same 1990 publication also demonstrated that naked RNA could similarly result in the in vivo expression of encoded protein. However, more attention focused on utilizing plasmid DNA, rather than mRNA, likely because of concerns about the instability of mRNA. In 1992, Bloom and colleagues [8] demonstrated the efficacy of mRNA to express protein in vivo by showing that mRNA encoding a hormone could correct a disease following direct injection into rat brains. In the same year (1993) that the first demonstration of the ability of DNA plasmid to protect mice from heterosubtypic challenge with influenza was published [7], liposome-formulated mRNA was also shown to generate influenza-specific cytolytic T cells in mice [9] (although protection from infectious challenge, as was shown for plasmid DNA, was not tested, perhaps explaining part of the difference in excitement about the technologies). Nevertheless, for both entities, a key issue was how to optimally deliver the DNA plasmid or the mRNA into the desired cells, either for optimal expression of the desired therapeutic protein as a drug or for gene therapy (to supply a missing or defective protein), or to generate the desired immune response against the protein if it were an antigen. For gene therapy, the encoded protein needs to not stimulate an immune response. For a vaccine, which cell produces the protein encoded by the mRNA or the plasmid DNA can be a key issue because, although for antibodies [10] where the protein would likely need to be secreted, for cellular immune responses of the Cytolytic T Lymphocyte variety [11], the type of cell producing the protein (and hence the cell type transduced by the plasmid DNA or the mRNA) is relevant, as is discussed later.

Why was there relatively less interest in mRNA compared to plasmid DNA as a platform technology for over a decade? What led to the recent explosion of interest and progress for mRNA? The transient nature of messenger RNA, possibly an asset for the process whereby organisms control the production of desired proteins, is due to RNAses that are widely present [12]. This instability of mRNA has been a significant reason for the lack of interest in mRNA as a drug. In addition, RNA has long been known to be an immunologically active molecule. For example, poly (I:C) (polyinosine-polycytidylic acid) is a synthetic analog of dsRNA (double-stranded RNA) that is an agonist of TLR3 and has long been used as an immunostimulatory mimic of viral infection and tested as an adjuvant to increase immune responses for experimental vaccines [13–15]. mRNA has a number of immunostimulatory mechanisms, which may be useful—or detrimental—for mRNA used for vaccines or cancer immunotherapeutics (discussed below). However, these properties contributed to the lower degree of interest in mRNA versus plasmid DNA for gene therapy applications when provision of a missing or defective protein with no immune responses against either the protein or the vector delivery system was the goal.

Two developments were important for changing the perception and reality of mRNA. These were the demonstration by Weissman and Kariko that the use of modified nucleosides made in vitro-transcribed mRNA less immunogenic [16]. In follow-up work, they showed that using pseudouridine instead of uridine resulted in mRNA that was more stable and had increased translational capacity [17]. This use of modified nucleosides thus addressed key issues for mRNA—stability of the mRNA, increased production of the encoded protein, and some decrease of the innate immunogenicity.

Additional work explored the use of other nucleosides, such as substituting 5-methylcytidine for cytidine with further improvement [2,11].

3. mRNA Structure and Implications for Use as a Vaccine

At this stage, it is perhaps useful to review the structure of the mRNA as designed for drug and vaccine delivery, which incorporates elements to improve both stability and protein expression. The mRNA comprises a 5′ cap, a 5′ untranslated region (UTR) (also called leader RNA), the coding sequence with a stop signal, a 3′ UTR, and a poly(A) tail. This molecule provides the template in the cytoplasm of a cell for translation by the ribosome and tRNA into the encoded protein, making multiple copies of the protein from each mRNA template. This amplification provides a quantitative advantage per molecule compared to providing individual proteins. However, offsetting that numeric advantage is that, in addition to the instability of the mRNA, it is thought that only one out of 10,000 molecules of mRNA will escape an endosome into the cytoplasm [5]. The amplification by translation of the mRNA into protein has to overcome the losses and the inefficiencies of degradation and the transduction process. Another obvious implication for this is that, compared to plasmid DNA, which must enter the nucleus of a cell, the mRNA only needs to be present in the cytoplasm, which eliminates the additional cellular (i.e., nuclear) membrane that plasmid DNA needs to cross. On the other hand, plasmid DNA is more stable than mRNA, and each DNA molecule results in the production of multiple mRNA molecules, thus the theoretical advantages of one over the other boil down to the realities of the net stability of plasmid DNA versus mRNA in their final formulation, as well as the efficiencies of targeting to the desired cell, the transduction to the cytoplasm or nucleus followed by the efficiencies of transcription of the plasmid DNA (resulting in amplification from DNA to mRNA), and the translation of mRNA, whether transcribed from DNA or in vitro-transcribed mRNA, to protein (also resulting in amplification).

Lower quantities of the (antigenic) protein are presumably needed for vaccines (due to amplification of the immune response against the antigen) compared to amounts of protein that might be needed for therapeutic disease targets. Additionally, whereas for gene therapy, where long-lasting or even permanent production of the therapeutic protein is desired, vaccines likely benefit from the transient nature of the antigen (followed by boosting). This is because, for example, the development of high affinity antibodies occurs as antigen becomes scarcer. Subsequent boosts with antigen then expand the production of these high affinity antibodies. The relatively temporary nature and presumably small amounts of protein produced by mRNA would fit with this paradigm if the mRNA is present in great enough quantities, persists, and is active long enough to produce sufficient amounts of protein antigen to stimulate the desired immune responses. DNA vaccines likewise have been demonstrated to produce the encoded protein for a limited period of time, although this is likely longer than mRNA constructs given the greater inherent stability of plasmid DNA compared to mRNA. Plasmid DNA has been shown to persist in muscle up to six months in a non-integrated fashion [18].

As noted above, the ability to make either a plasmid DNA or an mRNA construct quickly by simply knowing the genetic sequence of a desired antigen makes plasmid DNA or mRNA much faster technologies (compared to current approaches) to produce a vaccine, if needed, for an epidemic or an emerging disease. Five characteristics—rapidity of making constructs, relatively temporary presence in vivo of the encoded protein, amplification by the immune system responding to even small amounts of expressed protein, the manufacturing advantages (generic and rapid processes compared to drugs or recombinant proteins), and the intrinsic immunostimulatory properties of both plasmid DNA and mRNA—combine to make a compelling rationale for vaccines to be viewed as the best initial targets for widespread development efforts for both technologies.

4. Manufacture

The manufacture of plasmid DNA has been considered to be one of its strengths, making it a platform technology where the same process could essentially be used regardless of the gene that was encoded [19]. Moreover, the process of bacterial fermentation is fairly simple, since the product is a plasmid grown in bacteria, such as *Escherichia coli*, and the plasmid DNA is relatively stable, making purification straightforward. This is in contrast to the time-consuming process of earlier generation vaccines, which required finding ways to grow the pathogen such as making it weaker or inactivating it. Historically, the process to develop vaccines, including the manufacturing process, has been long and could reach up to decades (e.g., the chicken pox vaccine). The advent of recombinant proteins provided a simpler means of making vaccine antigens, and one that eliminated the need to work with a virulent pathogen during manufacture. However, this still had drawbacks, such as ensuring that the antigen had any crucial antigenically correct post-translational modifications (such as glycosylations), which can differ between host cells (such as yeast or baculovirus compared to humans), that the antigen was properly folded, and so on. Recombinant proteins generally also need to be soluble, providing a challenge for proteins with a transmembrane domain that is needed either antigenically or for any necessary oligomerization [e.g., HIV envelope]. Recombinant proteins administered exogenously (e.g., given in an immunization) also have an inherent limitation of not stimulating Major Histocompatibility Complex (MHC) Class I-restricted Cytolytic T Lymphocytes (CTLs), as is discussed later.

mRNA is made by in vitro transcription starting from a linearized DNA template, performing in vitro transcription, then getting rid of the template by digestion with DNAses, at which point the mRNA can be purified. Manufacturing mRNA by in vitro transcription is thus even more appealing than manufacturing plasmid DNA because while it is also a generic process, (i.e., independent of the gene insert), it is essentially a chemical process with no animal or cellular components (although the cost is potentially greater [20]). A graphic detailing the various steps and suggested possible improved processes can be seen in the reference [21]. The manufacturing process might be guided by pharmaceutical product Good Manufacturing Practice (GMP) guidelines [22,23] rather than those for biologicals [24], a likely advantage. Of course, any formulations or the addition of immunomodulators, adjuvants, or delivery systems may increase the complexity and cost of the manufacture for either mRNA or plasmid DNA.

5. Stability as a Product

DNA vaccines as a manufactured entity are noted for their stability [25], particularly when supercoiled. As noted above, this stability is reflected even in vivo, since plasmid has been detected in a non-integrated form in muscle up to six months following injection [18]. Although the ubiquity of RNAses with the resulting instability of native mRNA has been a significant reason for the delay in development of mRNA, the actual manufactured mRNA is stable in liquid or lyophilized form, (reported to be stable up to two years at room temperature [26]) with an inverse relationship of stability to temperature. It has been reported that a rabies mRNA vaccine was still effective for pre-clinical protection after several months at temperatures ranging from −80 °C to as high as +70 °C [26]. The stability of mRNA as a vialed product (i.e., protected from RNAses) is a separate consideration from the stability in vivo, and any formulations or delivery devices (which may cause shearing during delivery) are key factors in the final stability as a delivered product.

6. Cellular Targets for mRNA and Plasmid DNA Vaccine Delivery

For many vaccines, antibodies play a key role in protection. The cell that is transfected by the plasmid DNA or the mRNA vaccine does not have to be a professional antigen presenting cell (APC) in order to produce the antigenic protein that stimulates B cells. Cellular immune responses, notably CTLs, are thought to be important for tumor immunotherapy as well as to potentially play a role in protection against certain infectious diseases, e.g., tuberculosis (Tb), HIV, and malaria, or for vaccines effective against multiple strains of a virus, such as influenza, even though CTLs alone would not provide sterilizing immunity. In order for a vaccine to generate MHC Class I-restricted CTLs, the antigen either needs to be produced inside a professional APC or by a cell from which antigen can be cross-presented by an APC to then stimulate CTLs. The most direct way to ensure delivery of the gene encoding an antigen to a professional APC is to transfect the cells in vitro prior to administering the transfected cells back to the patient. Indeed, the largest number of mRNA clinical trials currently underway, notably for cancer immunotherapy, involve the ex vivo transfection of cells with mRNA encoding tumor antigens followed by re-infusion of the transfected cells into the patient. Because this is a more cumbersome process for making a product than having a non-personalized product in a vial, direct administration of the plasmid DNA or the mRNA to a patient is preferable for convenience, cost, and time.

Plasmid DNA was shown to be effective for stimulating CTLs that were capable of protecting mice against influenza caused by a strain different from the strain from which the encoded antigen was derived [7,27,28]. Because the plasmid DNA, when injected intramuscularly (i.m.), primarily transduced muscle cells rather than professional Antigen Presenting Cells (APCs), the mechanism whereby MHC Class I-restricted CTLs were generated needed explaining. It was found that cross-priming appeared to be a key mechanism for generating CTLs following DNA vaccine immunization, as directly demonstrated by experiments with chimeric mice using bone-marrow derived dendritic cells [27], and because muscle cells were the only cells observed to translate the protein encoded by directly-injected plasmid DNA [6,29]. The efficacy in pre-clinical models raised the hopes that such plasmid DNA-based CTL-inducing vaccines could be developed that would be protective against multiple strains of HIV or influenza [7,30] (so as to produce a "universal" flu vaccine). Currently, existing influenza vaccines depend upon strain-specific antibodies, which result in strain-specific or strain-limited protection. Similarly, mRNA delivered in liposomes was shown early on to be capable of inducing CTLs [9]. The uptake of the mRNA is also mainly by non-immune cells, including muscle cells [31].

Both plasmid DNA and mRNA are also being developed for indications other than vaccines, such as for gene therapy. The delivery of plasmid DNA and mRNA to specific tissues or cells may thus be intentionally directed (in part) by the mode of delivery, the injection route, the formulation, and so on. Both entities are anionic due to the negative charges of the phosphate groups, and various formulations have utilized polycations. Thus, the biodistribution of each molecule depends not simply on the inherent charge and the size of the plasmid or mRNA, but the net charge of all the components of the formulation and the effect of any lipids.

7. Increasing the Potency of DNA and mRNA Vaccines

For DNA vaccines, despite the ease with which preclinical studies demonstrated efficacy for a variety of disease models, the potency in humans proved generally disappointing. This led to a number of approaches to increasing the potency by increasing the amount of protein produced through redesigns of the plasmid. Additionally, adjuvants and other immunostimulants were included (such as cytokines and co-stimulatory molecules) either as recombinant proteins or encoded by plasmid DNA, by various formulations and delivery devices, and by strategies such as prime-boost combinations (generally using plasmid DNA as a prime followed by a heterologous boost with a viral vector or protein). The DNA plasmids themselves were optimized by trying different promoters, adding CpG motifs, (cytosine connected via a phosphodiester bond to guanine-such CpG motifs are pathogen-associated molecular patterns) (see below), codon optimization, etc. As noted above, the initial work by Felgner [6] demonstrated that the expression of protein encoded by plasmid DNA was highest in muscle following intramuscular injection versus expression in other tissues after intravenous or subcutaneous injection. Likewise, immune responses were highest with direct i.m. syringe injection of naked plasmid DNA rather than via intravenous (i.v.), intradermal (i.d.), or subcutaneous (s.c.) injections [7]. Early delivery devices for plasmid DNA included a biolistics gene gun that propelled DNA-coated gold particles into cells [32]. In addition to simple i.m. injection, approaches now include pressurized devices (such as the Biojector® or Stratis®), or electroporation, which supplies an electric current to cause temporary fenestration of membranes to increase the passage of plasmid into the cells and the nuclei.

For mRNA, the areas of continued Research and Development (R&D) efforts for improving the potency of mRNA vaccines are shown in Table 1, which describes efforts similar to those for DNA vaccines. These focus on augmenting delivery of the mRNA and increasing potency via increased stability and greater expression of the protein. Alterations of the mRNA itself include changing the codon usage and the GC (guanine-cytosine) content [5], along with modifications of the other regions, such as the 5′ cap, the UTRs, and the poly-A tails. A more detailed description of the efforts to increase the mRNA potency and of delivery formulations that include lipids, nanoparticles, polymers, polycations, and various proprietary entities are presented and reviewed elsewhere with tabular and chemical descriptions [2,11,33,34]. Cells generally take up mRNA by endocytosis, thus efforts are also being made to design delivery systems that increase the endosomal release of the mRNA into the cytoplasm [35]. Certain formulations, such as delivery of a particular encapsulated lipoplex mRNA vaccine, were found to specifically be taken up by dendritic cells via micropinocytosis [36]. As with DNA vaccines, possible immunomodulators added as recombinant proteins or encoded by mRNA are being evaluated [37]. Various routes of injection of mRNA are being explored, including i.m., i.d., s.c., i.v., and intranodal [2], in addition to the ex vivo approach described. Delivery devices such as the gene gun (where mRNA is put onto gold particles) [38] and electroporation are also being explored.

Table 1. Continued Research and Development (R&D) Focus for mRNA Vaccines.

- Stabilize/protect mRNA
- Target mRNA to desired cells (e.g., professional antigen presenting cells, APCs)
- Increase escape of mRNA from endosome
- Deliver mRNA directly to dendritic cells
- Increase amount of protein translated
- Increase duration of protein production (may not be needed for vaccines versus therapeutic protein applications)
- Optimize immune responses for the antigen (e.g., type of T helper response, subclass of antibody)
- Decrease or select desired inflammatory effects of mRNA
- Optimize the above for potency, safety, complexity of formulation, cost of manufacture, product stability

Circular RNAs (circRNA) are endogenously expressed and are thought to play roles mainly for gene regulation, with potential activity as tumor antigens [39]. They can be exogenously constructed to produce proteins in cells [40]. These engineered circRNA molecules appear to be more stable and to result in more potent production of protein than linear mRNA. However, the mechanisms for their effects upon gene regulation and other activities are still being explored [41].

7.1. Self-Amplifying Systems for Both mRNA and DNA Vaccines

Significant efforts have been expended to take advantage of a system employed by certain viruses, notably alpha viruses, which utilize a strategy of self-amplification of key viral proteins. Such self-amplifying replicon systems have been developed for viral vectors, plasmid DNA, and now mRNA [42–45]. These constructs encode viral proteins that result in the transduced cell producing many copies of mRNA encoding the protein of interest (i.e., the antigen) without making a whole viral particle. Thus, for a given DNA or mRNA vector, significantly more mRNA encoding the antigen and hence antigen protein, are made. In pre-clinical models, this has resulted in increased potency for these vectors on a per molecule of vector basis. The reason for the increased efficacy may be more than simply the increased amount of antigen produced, as the dsRNA intermediaries result in increased production of interferon and subsequently other immunologic effects, although the dsRNA can also have other possibly deleterious effects (see below).

8. Inflammatory Responses and Toxicities

8.1. Immune Activation

While both DNA and mRNA vaccines are often thought of as simply an expression system for the desired protein, neither is immunologically inert. Both DNA vectors (which are based on bacterial plasmids) and in vitro transcribed mRNA activate the innate immune system. DNA plasmids do so via their CpG motifs, which stimulate TLR9. While CpG was successfully used as an adjuvant [46] for a recombinant protein-based Hepatitis B vaccine licensed in 2018, the impact on the immunogenicity of DNA vaccines by increasing the number of CpG motifs in the plasmid has been less clear. In fact, for certain DNA vaccine efforts, notably those of Steinman's group, as therapies for autoimmune diseases, they specifically switched CpG motifs for GpG motifs (guanine connected via a phosphodiester bond to another guanine; these compete with CpG motifs for binding to TLR9 receptors) in an effort to specifically decrease the Th1 help for their human clinical studies (see below) [47]. The double-stranded structure of the DNA plasmid is also thought to be an immune stimulant [48] through non-TLR mechanisms. In fact, plasmid DNA also acts on the TBK1-STING pathway through cytosolic receptors [49,50]. This results in the generation of Type 1 interferons, which then act as adjuvants for the generation of immune responses against the antigen(s) encoded by the plasmid DNA vaccine.

As noted above, the use of modified nucleosides for the construction of mRNA is one method of decreasing the reactogenicity of the in vitro transcribed mRNA. However, mRNA acts via multiple pathways, including the innate system (via TLR3, TLR 7, and TLR8) and via cytoplasmic proteins (PKR, OAS, RIG-I, and MDA5) [11,51]. The multiple routes of activation result in several effects in addition to inflammation and include inhibition of mRNA replication (both via TLR7 through an MYD88 pathway affecting interferon, and via TLR3 through TRIF), stalled translation, and RNA degradation [5]. Some of these various activities could decrease the potency of the mRNA by a net decreased protein production, as was seen pre-clinically for an HIV mRNA vaccine complexed in cationic lipids [52]. This also raises the issue of how effective repeat dosing of mRNA will be if previous injections result in an environment with decreased translation or increased RNA degradation, although simply changing an injection site may potentially circumvent this particular issue.

Other molecular entities that are introduced or generated during the manufacture of the in vitro-transcribed mRNA and then remain (left-over contaminating nucleoside triphosphates, DNA templates, and dsRNA) are also quite immunostimulatory and therefore need to be purified following production of the mRNA [53].

The potential issues due to the various inflammatory effects of mRNA vaccines upon clinical efficacy and safety are summarized in Table 2 and are discussed below. The possible utility of RNA-induced inflammation for vaccines is demonstrated by the fact that one of the first uses of RNA for vaccines was to include non-coding RNA in human clinical trials as an adjuvant for a rabies vaccine (composed of an inactivated virus) [54], although this effort has been replaced by a rabies vaccine that utilizes mRNA that itself encodes the rabies antigen [55], as is discussed below. The continued evaluation of non-coding RNA as an adjuvant is ongoing in clinical testing for various cancers without the provision of an antigen (see below).

Table 2. Issues to be addressed for clinical efficacy and safety of mRNA related to inflammation.

- Potency: Impact of mRNA innate immune responses (e.g., induction of interferon alpha which slows translation)
- Potency: Impact of other drugs (antibiotics and anti-cancer drugs) on mRNA metabolism and extent of translation into proteins.
- Potential toxicity of mRNA due to inherent mRNA inflammatory activity, use of unnatural modified nucleoside, and the formulations;
    - Several pathways of RNA-induced inflammation: TLR 3, 7, 8, plus cytoplasmic pathways
    - Known toxicities of drugs containing unnatural modified nucleosides
    - Potential mitigation or enhancement due to formulation of the mRNA
- Formulation itself also apparently can affect immune activation and types of immunity (see below, Crigler-Najjar discussion)
- Will anti-self RNA antibodies be generated and play any role in autoimmune diseases?
- Design of clinical trials to detect inflammation/toxicity due to mRNA

8.2. Toxicities of mRNA

The flip side of the possibly beneficial adjuvant inflammation, however, is potential toxicity of the mRNA vaccines. Toxicities are seen with antivirals and anti-cancer drugs that contain unnatural nucleoside analogues [56–58]. Such toxicities, not predicted by pre-clinical studies due to species differences between humans and the animals used for pre-clinical safety testing, have been seen with drugs that contain unnatural modified nucleosides. The clinical adverse effects have included myopathy (caused by mitochondrial toxicity), lactic acidosis, pancreatitis, lipodystrophy, liver steatosis, and nerve damage; certain ones have been fatal.

Indeed, some toxicity has been reported for mRNA pre-clinically along with limited human adverse events. Liver toxicity was observed in pre-clinical studies with one potential mRNA therapeutic delivered in lipid nanoparticles for Crigler-Najjar syndrome, selected as a "lowest-hanging fruit" target because very low doses of protein were needed. These were serious enough to apparently halt the work with this particular entity, or at least that formulation [59]. The formulation of the mRNA was thought to potentially play a role in the toxicity [60], and repeat doses were used. Nevertheless, this observed toxicity may be concerning for vaccines as well, since even live replicating viruses and viral vector vaccines (which generally are more immunogenic than subunit vaccines) need repeat dosing. In addition, most of the mRNA vaccines in clinical trials appear to need formulation. The mRNA vaccines in clinical trials against infectious diseases from this same company are described as formulated in lipid nanoparticles, but whether they are the same formulations as those used for the Crigler-Najjar study is not publicly known.

Self-limited local and systemic adverse events (AEs) seen in a human clinical trial for an mRNA rabies vaccine, although summarized as still indicating the vaccine was generally safe (described below in the clinical trials section), may also reflect the inflammatory nature of the mRNA [55]. These results highlight the potential toxicity downside of the inflammatory activity of mRNA vaccines, adverse effects not seen to this extent with plasmid DNA. Also note that, for providing monoclonal antibodies [61] (whether for preventing or for treating infectious diseases for other therapeutic applications), this would likely require repeat administration of mRNA, which might not only increase the potential for toxicities, but may also have an impact upon potency due to effects of the mRNA upon decreasing translation, etc., via the other inflammatory effects.

Thus, it may still be a work in progress to find the best balance of inflammation and any deleterious toxicities via harnessing adjuvant activities of mRNA while limiting or suppressing inherent toxicities for vaccines and immunotherapeutics. This will involve optimizing nucleoside substitutions, the design of other elements of the mRNA construct, any included immunostimulants, and/or specific formulations, delivery devices, and routes of administration. The mechanisms of mRNA inflammation that are relevant to their potential efficacy and safety as vaccines are also reviewed elsewhere [34], where they are aptly referred to as the "yin and yang of innate immunity".

9. Other Potential Safety Issues

When DNA vaccines initially entered into human clinical trials, concern was raised about the theoretical possibility of them causing autoimmunity or that the DNA would integrate into the genome. The rationale for concerns about autoimmunity was that anti-DNA antibodies are a hallmark of various autoimmune diseases. To date, both pre-clinical testing and careful clinical monitoring have shown DNA vaccines to not induce or to worsen auto-immunity, and in fact, human clinical trials employing DNA vaccines for therapy of two autoimmune diseases (diabetes mellitus and multiple sclerosis) gave encouraging results in human clinical trials for a therapeutic benefit of the DNA vaccines [47,62]. For mRNA, a proposed mechanism for possible autoimmune responses is via the induction of type I interferon [63], which may result in both inflammation and possibly autoimmune responses [64]. This includes work showing that the responses seen in mice were similar to those seen in humans for an influenza mRNA vaccine construct via TLR7 and TLR8 in humans and via cytoplasmic RNA sensors in both mice and humans [65].

DNA vaccines did not need to be evaluated by the US National Institutes of Health (NIH) Recombinant Advisory Committee prior to human clinical trials, unlike viral vectors for gene therapy. Nevertheless, significant safety studies were initially required to evaluate the possibility of integration of the plasmid DNA into the host genome. As a result of these studies for both human vaccines [18,66] and for the licensed DNA vaccines for fish [67], as well as the many human studies with DNA vaccines that have demonstrated safety, little concern now exists regarding integration. Comparisons have stated that mRNA offers an advantage because RNA itself cannot integrate into genomic DNA without the presence of the viral elements in a retrovirus that enable such integration (reverse transcriptase and integrase). However, HERVs [68] (human endogenous retroviruses) whose remnants are now permanent parts of human genomes as retrovirus-like sequences comprise up to 8% of the human genome. In addition, some recipients of mRNA drugs or vaccines may be already infected with a retrovirus (e.g., HIV), thus providing a theoretical means for provision of the proteins needed for integration [69,70]. Nevertheless, the risk of integration remains, at this point, extremely unlikely for mRNA, even from a theoretical standpoint, nor is it any longer a significant concern for plasmid DNA. This means that mRNA does not offer any clear advantage compared to plasmid DNA in this regard. From a regulatory perspective, mRNA prophylactic vaccines appear to not be considered gene therapy products [71], similar to DNA vaccines before them.

10. Clinical Trials

10.1. DNA

10.1.1. Licensed Veterinary DNA Vaccines

Five plasmid DNA products (four of them vaccines) have received licensure for veterinary applications. These include a fish vaccine for infectious hematopoietic necrosis virus licensed in 2005, and a vaccine against salmon pancreas disease licensed in 2016 [72]. A dog cancer immunotherapeutic vaccine for melanoma was licensed originally based upon comparison with historic controls in the US in 2010. After submission to the European Medicines Agency, the application was withdrawn in 2014 by the company, stating that their priorities had changed such that they did not justify the investment in research and development to answer the remaining questions [73]. A vaccine for West Nile virus (WNV) prevention in horses was licensed in 2005 [74], although it is no longer used in favor of the previously licensed killed virus vaccine for unpublished reasons. Yet, a promising observation was that the equine WNV DNA vaccine was able to protect various species of birds from WNV [75–78], including the California condor, and has been credited by U.S. Center for Disease Control (CDC) scientists with saving this endangered species from potential extinction [79]. A fifth plasmid DNA product was licensed in 2008 for veterinary use; this plasmid encodes growth hormone releasing hormone (GHRH) and is given via electroporation to pregnant sows, resulting in litters with an increased number of surviving piglets and of higher birthweights [80,81].

10.1.2. Significance of Licensed Veterinary DNA Vaccines for Human DNA Vaccines

The licensure and the immunogenicity of the equine WNV vaccine are significant for human DNA vaccine efforts. The first reason is that scientists have often stated that DNA vaccines are not very good at inducing antibodies, yet this DNA vaccine induced neutralizing antibodies of sufficient titer for protection and licensure in horses. Also significant is that these antibodies were made in horses. Frequently, the lack of potency of DNA vaccines in human trials was considered to reflect the size of humans compared to the usual small pre-clinical animal models.

10.1.3. Select Human DNA Vaccine Clinical Trials Results

In related observations to the equine WNV DNA vaccine, in a human clinical trial of a WNV DNA vaccine in humans, all subjects generated titers of antibodies that were considered protective in the horses [82]. In a subsequent study using a construct with a stronger promoter, older adults (who generally are considered to have senescent immune systems and respond to licensed vaccines such as the influenza vaccine more poorly than younger persons) had neutralizing antibody responses as good as the younger adults [83]. In a clinical trial of a DNA vaccine for Ebola and Marburg viruses, the individuals likewise generated antibodies that were boostable [84]. These observations demonstrate that DNA vaccines are capable of inducing antibodies in humans of relevant titers, suggesting that it is not a limitation of the technology per se to generate effective antibodies, but rather the target and the optimized constructs are key elements (much as finding the right target for monoclonal antibodies (MAbs) was needed for MAbs to become such effective anti-cancer agents). Also of note is that the first two Zika vaccines brought to human clinical trial were DNA vaccines [85]. This underscores the point made earlier about how the ease of making both DNA and mRNA vaccines is considered a tremendous advantage for rapid responses to emergent or epidemic diseases.

10.1.4. Additional Categories of Disease Targets for DNA Vaccines and Methods to Increase Efficacy

In addition to the various diseases for which DNA vaccines used alone have resulted in promising human clinical immune responses, in a variety of clinical trials for several other diseases, such as HIV, plasmid DNA as a prime followed by a heterologous boost has resulted in significant potency for the generation of immune responses, including CTLs. Additionally, as mentioned above, phase II studies for the treatment of two autoimmune diseases, diabetes and multiple sclerosis, yielded encouraging clinical responses, which may mechanistically be due in part to the design of the vectors to avoid the Th1 cell responses that generally are seen with the plasmids utilized for other diseases [47]. Moreover, clinical trials of DNA vaccines for cancer therapy utilizing electroporation have provided encouraging results, including for CIN3 (cervical carcinoma in situ 3) [86] and CIN2/3 [87] as well as for head and neck cancer [88], which are all related to human papillomavirus (HPV) infection. Other clinical trials of DNA vaccines for cancer have included using DNA that encoded fusion proteins including a tumor CTL epitope(s) and a T helper stimulator(s) [89–91]. Therefore, even though no human DNA vaccines have been licensed, the existing data have provided evidence for immunogenicity and early stage evidence of clinical effect in humans for certain antigens/diseases as well as efficacy in animals ranging from fish to horses. The remainder of this special issue deals with these efforts and ongoing clinical trials, thus they are not elaborated upon here.

10.2. RNA

10.2.1. Prophylactic mRNA Vaccines for Infectious Diseases

Prophylactic vaccine human trials for infectious diseases utilizing mRNA encoding the antigen(s) are shown in Table 3. These are all Phase I trials. Any known formulations are listed, as are any described results and references, along with the clinical trials identifier numbers. The rabies vaccine effort utilizing a licensed vaccine with RNA as the adjuvant (discussed above, and listed in Table 4) was replaced by a vaccine using mRNA encoding the rabies virus glycoprotein. Following either i.d. or i.m. injection of this rabies mRNA vaccine, boostable antibodies were obtained. However, 78% of each group had "solicited systemic adverse events" including ten patients (~10% of all injected patients) with grade three (i.e., serious but not life-threatening) adverse events, although the conclusion was that the vaccine was "generally safe with a reasonable tolerability profile" [55]. A second construct for rabies is now in clinical testing.

As noted earlier, one company initially highlighted a focus on therapeutic disease areas but reprioritized vaccines, possibly due to the recognition of the low amount of antigen actually produced by the mRNA coupled with the low amounts of protein needed for vaccines because of the amplification by the immune system, possibly as a response to emerging diseases such as the Zika epidemic, and possibly influenced by the liver toxicity seen in their pre-clinical studies [59] for delivering even the low amounts of mRNA needed for the disease (Crigler-Najjar, see above). Lipid nanoparticles are also used for that company's vaccine formulations, although it is not known how these relate to the formulation used for Crigler-Najjar (the company has published relatively little in the peer-reviewed scientific literature related to their clinical trials). References, when available, are provided within the table, although in some cases, the assumption is made that the pre-clinical construct in the reference is the same construct (antigen) as the one in the clinical trial.

10.2.2. Additional Clinical Trials of RNA

Table 4 lists clinical trials of mRNA for additional applications. Data are taken from clinicaltrials.gov in addition to the citations listed. Table 4 excludes studies that employ cells transfected ex vivo prior to re-administration to patients and excludes those that supply mRNA encoding immunomodulators without a specific antigen also being provided.

RNA as an Adjuvant

Trials utilizing non-coding RNA as an adjuvant are listed. These studies include using non-coding RNA as an adjuvant for a licensed rabies vaccine resulting in improved immunogenicity with mainly mild AEs, but with two of the 14 patients having severe but limited influenza-like symptoms [54]. Studies are ongoing for using this non-coding RNA adjuvant for cancer applications (not using any co-administered mRNA-encoded antigen).

Immunotherapeutic Vaccine

mRNA as a therapy for HIV infection was tested in two clinical trials where it was administered intranodally. Although immunogenicity in the Phase I trial appeared promising [92], the second, a phase 2 trial, was terminated after the interim analysis due to lack of immunogenicity above that seen with the placebo.

Immunoprophylaxis via Provision of mRNA Encoding a Monoclonal Antibody

One company recently announced in a press release [93] (no citations found on PubMed for the entity) that a clinical trial has been initiated with mRNA encoding a monoclonal antibody for use in prevention of Chikungunya virus infection.

Table 3. Clinical trials for mRNA prophylactic vaccines for infectious diseases.

Product, Company/Institution	Indication (disease)	Antigen	Formulation	Phase	Status	Results	National Clinical Trial Identifier
RNActive® CureVac	Rabies	Rabies virus glycoprotein [55]	None	1	Active, Not Recruiting	Generally safe, but some significant adverse events (AEs); boostable functional antibodies	NCT02241135
RNActive® CureVac	Rabies	Rabies virus glycoprotein	None	1	Recruiting	New construct versus prior trial	NCT03713086
mRNA-1851 Moderna	Influenza H7N9	Influenza Hemagglutinin H7N9 A/Anhui/1/2013 [94]	Lipid Nano-particles	1	Active, Not Recruiting	Moderna website says 1° and 2° endpoints met, but no published data	NCT03345043
mRNA-1440 Moderna	Influenza H10N8	Influenza Hemagglutinin H10N8 (A/Jiangxi-Donghu/346/2013) [94]	Lipid Nano-particles	1	Active, Not Recruiting	Interim: AEs: Majority mild moderate; A few: severe; Seroconversion rates high	NCT03076385
mRNA-1653 Moderna	Human Metapneumo-virus + Parainfluenza virus 3	Fusion proteins of each virus	Lipid Nano-particle	1	Active, Not Recruiting	Announced via press release safe and immunogenic; no publications found	NCT03392389
mRNA-1388 Moderna/DARPA	Chikungunya	Not Disclosed (ND)	ND	1	Active, Not Recruiting	Primary Completion: March 2019; no results posted at time of publication	NCT03325075
RNA-1325 Moderna/BARDA	Zika	prM and E [95,96]	Lipid Nano-particles	1	Active, Not Recruiting	Primary Completion: February 2019; no results posted at time of publication	NCT03014089
mRNA-1647 and mRNA-1443 Moderna	Cytomegalovirus	mRNA-1647 is gB, pentameric complex, and mRNA-1443 is pp65 [97]	Lipid Nano-particles	1	Recruiting	Primary Completion: February 2020	NCT03382405
mRNA-1777 Moderna/Merck-V171	Respiratory Syncytial Virus	ND	ND	1	ND	Moderna press release says 1° and 2° endpoints met, but no published data	Not listed on clinicaltrials.gov

Table 4. Clinical Phase I and II trials of mRNA excluding prophylactic infectious diseases (see Table 3) and ex vivo-transduced cells. Information is taken from https://clinicaltrials.gov.

RNA-based Adjuvant: long-chain non-coding RNA complexed with a short cationic peptide (ssRNA adjuvant); no mRNA-encoded antigen

- Rabies: Phase 1, Completed, ssRNA adjuvant plus licensed rabies vaccine; NCT02238756 [54]
- Melanoma, squamous cell carcinoma of the skin, squamous cell carcinoma of the head and neck, or adenoid cystic carcinoma: Phase 1, Recruiting, ssRNA adjuvant plus anti-PD-1 therapy; NCT03291002
- Hepatocellular carcinoma (HCC): Phase 1/2, Recruiting, ssRNA adjuvant plus multi-peptide-based HCC vaccine; NCT03203005

Therapeutic mRNA Vaccines for Infectious Disease Targets

- HIV-therapeutic:

  a. Phase 1, Completed; NCT02413645 [92]
  b. Phase 2, Terminated due to no immunogenicity above placebo at interim analysis; NCT02888756

mRNA Monoclonal Antibody Prophylaxis for Infectious Disease Targets

- Chikungunya: Monoclonal antibody prophylaxis, Phase 1, Recruiting; NCT03829384

mRNA Vaccines for Cancer (excluding studies where cells are transfected ex vivo, and excluding when no antigen-encoding mRNA is given); multiple groups/companies are sponsors

- Prostate [98,99]: multiple
- Solid tumors: including personalized tumor-associated antigens
- Melanoma and epithelial tumors: multiple trials, personalized, tumor-derived antigens
- Gastronintestinal cancers
- Non-small cell lung cancer
- Breast cancer
- Various personalized tumor vaccines

Cancer

For cancer therapy, four completed studies (two each per different mRNA constructs) have been terminated or completed for prostate cancer. Those failed to demonstrate efficacy [98,99], but new trials, including those for other cancers, have been initiated by a variety of groups with various mRNA constructs. Another approach being developed is steering towards personalized cancer immunotherapeutic vaccine products via a library of mRNAs coding for different antigens that can be combined to be personalized for an individual.

As mentioned earlier, a much larger number of trials for cancer utilize mRNA for ex vivo transfection of dendritic cells that are then re-infused into the patient. These are reviewed elsewhere [2,11].

11. Summary and Conclusions

In summary, despite all the excitement over pre-clinical efficacy of mRNA, it should be remembered that in many ways, the mRNA field is recapitulating what occurred with plasmid DNA 20+ years ago, when seemingly almost any disease could be prevented or treated in pre-clinical animal disease models with the administration of an unformulated plasmid encoding a key antigen [1]. Therefore, one must keep in mind that pre-clinical immunogenicity or even protection/therapy, and human immunogenicity are low hurdles and are not predictive of human efficacy. One reason this is so challenging is that, for many of the diseases under evaluation, scientists do not know which immune response or combination of immune responses and which antigen targets are the crucial elements for efficacy; the vaccine technology alone is not the only piece of the puzzle. Table 5 summarizes the main advantages and disadvantages of mRNA vaccines with a comparison to DNA vaccines.

Table 5. Advantages and Disadvantages of mRNA Vaccines (and comparison to DNA vaccines).

Advantages:

1) Rapid vaccine construction (as with DNA vaccines)
2) Generic manufacturing process (as with DNA vaccines)
3) Manufacturing does not require cells or animal substrates (an advantage from a regulatory perspective compared to DNA vaccines)
4) mRNA does not need to enter the nucleus (an advantage compared to DNA vaccines)
5) Amplification—number of protein antigen molecules produced per molecule of mRNA delivered, compared to no expansion of antigen for traditional antigens (proteins, inactivated virus particles), however, less amplification per molecule of plasmid DNA in the nucleus and likely less amplification than live virus vaccines)
6) Immunostimulatory effects may benefit desired vaccine responses (plasmid DNA also has immunostimulatory effects, but fewer and better defined)
7) Theoretically should not integrate if no endogenous retroviruses or retroviruses due to infection are present. (DNA vaccines have been extensively studied pre-clinically and clinically, easing regulatory concerns about integration for DNA vaccines.)

Disadvantages:

1) Amplification to protein antigen per molecule of mRNA is less than that per molecule of plasmid DNA (although the entry into the cytosol is one membrane fewer than needs to be traversed for plasmid DNA)
2) mRNA needs to escape the endosome (but does not need entry into the nucleus, whereas plasmid DNA does)
3) Immunostimulatory effects may decrease potency via multiple pathways:
    a. Decreased stability of mRNA
    b. Decreased translation into protein
    c. Effects upon desired type of immunity
4) Formulation may still be needed (this observation is based upon the use of formulations by the majority of mRNA entities in clinical trials)
    a. Finding the optimal delivery formulation/device for humans may be challenging given the unknown predictability of animal models (as with DNA vaccines, although DNA vaccines are much further advanced in clinical trials with different formulations and delivery devices for a number of different diseases)
5) Known toxicity of RNA-based drugs using unnatural modified nucleoside analogues; will this occur with mRNA vaccines?
6) In vitro-transcribed mRNA vaccines may be expensive based on current processes
7) Concomitant administration of other drugs may impact mRNA metabolism and thus may decrease potency of mRNA vaccine

Reported Phase I clinical trial results for mRNA vaccines are encouraging, although only the results of the first rabies mRNA vaccine have been published in the peer reviewed literature. The results for the human Metapneumovirus + Parainfluenza virus 3, and the Respiratory syncytial virus (RSV) phase I studies were announced via press release, thus details are not available. The target for the RSV vaccine mRNA was not publicly disclosed at the time the Phase I study was initiated, and to this date, the study appears to not be listed on clinicaltrials.gov. Whether the immune responses are at sufficient levels or have the types of needed immune responses and the necessary duration to result in protective efficacy is unknown and is not necessarily predicted by the Phase I studies.

One should also not ignore the reported toxicities seen with the rabies mRNA vaccine [55] that included limited systemic AEs for the majority of patients (78%) and even grade three AEs in ~10% of patients following doses of 80–400 µg mRNA via different routes, although the conclusions were that the vaccine was generally safe. It is not known whether the pre-clinical hepatic toxicity that proved to be a "no go" result for a particular Crigler-Najjar mRNA candidate is relevant to the mRNA vaccine studies from the same company, because, despite the low doses used, the doses and mRNA formulation for vaccine studies may be different. This is in comparison to DNA vaccine clinical trials where 4 mg doses of DNA i.m. with boosts have been used in a variety of clinical trials with limited systemic symptoms [83–85] while generating good immune responses.

Just as DNA vaccines, after more than 25 years since the first publication of preclinical protective efficacy, are still a work in progress in improving potency and finding the right antigens and targets, there remain challenges for mRNA to become clinical products. For both DNA and mRNA vaccines (and monoclonal antibodies and bi-specific antibodies before them), a simple concept may have a challenging path to reality, and the technology may not be totally generic. mRNA may be even more complex than plasmid DNA because of the modifications (modified nucleosides) plus the formulations needed for stability, delivery, and the need to control the innate immunostimulatory activity of the mRNA. However, it also offers advantages in terms of manufacture that avoids the need for any animal or cellular products. The hope is that once the fundamental key challenges are solved for both plasmid DNA and mRNA, the clinical successes will come rapidly, although that has not occurred for moving from the veterinary licensed products for DNA vaccines into humans, demonstrating how much still needs to be understood, not just about the technologies but about the diseases that are being treated or prevented.

Funding: None relevant to this review.

Conflicts of Interest: The author declares no conflict of interest.

References

1. Liu, M.A. DNA vaccines: An historical perspective and view to the future. *Immunol. Rev.* **2011**, *239*, 62–84. [CrossRef] [PubMed]
2. Pardi, N.; Hogan, M.J.; Porter, F.W.; Weissman, D. mRNA vaccines—A new era in vaccinology. *Nat. Rev. Drug Discov.* **2018**, *17*, 261–279. [CrossRef] [PubMed]
3. Stevenson, F.K.; Zhu, D.; King, C.A.; Ashworth, L.J.; Kumar, S.; Hawkins, R.E. Idiotypic DNA vaccines against B-cell lymphoma. *Immunol. Rev.* **1995**, *145*, 211–228. [CrossRef] [PubMed]
4. Syrengelas, A.D.; Chen, T.T.; Levy, R. DNA immunization induces protective immunity against B-cell lymphoma. *Nat. Med.* **1996**, *2*, 1038–1041. [CrossRef] [PubMed]
5. Sahin, U.; Karikó, K.; Türeci, Ö. mRNA-based therapeutics—Developing a new class of drugs. *Nat. Rev. Drug Discov.* **2014**, *13*, 759–780. [CrossRef] [PubMed]
6. Wolff, J.A.; Malone, R.W.; Williams, P.; Chong, W.; Acsadi, G.; Jani, A.; Felgner, P.L. Direct gene transfer into mouse muscle in vivo. *Science* **1990**, *247*, 1465–1468. [CrossRef] [PubMed]
7. Ulmer, J.B.; Donnelly, J.J.; Parker, S.E.; Rhodes, G.H.; Felgner, P.L.; Dwarki, V.J.; Gromkowski, S.H.; Deck, R.R.; DeWitt, C.M.; Friedman, A.; et al. Heterologous protection against influenza by injection of DNA encoding a viral protein. *Science* **1993**, *259*, 1745–1749. [CrossRef]
8. Jirikowski, G.F.; Sanna, P.P.; Maciejewski-Lenoir, D.; Bloom, F.E. Reversal of diabetes insipidus in Brattleboro rats: Intrahypothalamic injection of vasopressin mRNA. *Science* **1992**, *255*, 996–998. [CrossRef] [PubMed]
9. Martinon, F.; Krishnan, S.; Lenzen, G.; Magné, R.; Gomard, E.; Guillet, J.G.; Lévy, J.P.; Meulien, P. Induction of virus-specific cytotoxic T lymphocytes in vivo by liposome-entrapped mRNA. *Eur. J. Immunol.* **1993**, *23*, 1719–1722. [CrossRef]
10. Deck, R.R.; DeWitt, C.M.; Donnelly, J.J.; Liu, M.A.; Ulmer, J.B. Characterization of humoral immune responses induced by an influenza hemagglutinin DNA vaccine. *Vaccine* **1997**, *15*, 71–78. [CrossRef]
11. Hajj, K.A.; Whitehead, K.A. Tools for translation: Non-viral materials for therapeutic mRNA delivery. *Nat. Rev. Mater.* **2017**, *2*, 17056. [CrossRef]
12. Houseley, J.; Tollervey, D. The many pathways of RNA degradation. *Cell* **2009**, *136*, 763–776. [CrossRef]
13. Quinn, K.M.; Yamamoto, A.; Costa, A.; Darrah, P.A.; Lindsay, R.W.; Hegde, S.T.; Johnson, T.R.; Flynn, B.J.; Loré, K.; Seder, R.A. Coadministration of polyinosinic:polycytidylic acid and immunostimulatory complexes modifies antigen processing in dendritic cell subsets and enhances HIV gag-specific T cell immunity. *J. Immunol.* **2013**, *191*, 5085–5096. [CrossRef]

14. Domingos-Pereira, S.; Decrausaz, L.; Derré, L.; Bobst, M.; Romero, P.; Schiller, J.T.; Jichlinski, P.; Nardelli-Haefliger, D. Intravaginal TLR agonists increase local vaccine-specific CD8 T cells and human papillomavirus-associated genital-tumor regression in mice. *Mucosal Immunol.* **2013**, *6*, 393–404. [CrossRef]
15. Zhang, L.; Bai, J.; Liu, J.; Wang, X.; Li, Y.; Jiang, P. Toll-like receptor ligands enhance the protective effects of vaccination against porcine reproductive and respiratory syndrome virus in swine. *Vet. Microbiol.* **2013**, *164*, 253–260. [CrossRef]
16. Karikó, K.; Buckstein, M.; Ni, H.; Weissman, D. Suppression of RNA recognition by Toll-like receptors: The impact of nucleoside modification and the evolutionary origin of RNA. *Immunity* **2005**, *23*, 165–175. [CrossRef]
17. Karikó, K.; Muramatsu, H.; Welsh, F.A.; Ludwig, J.; Kato, H.; Akira, S.; Weissman, D. Incorporation of pseudouridine into mRNA yields superior nonimmunogenic vector with increased translational capacity and biological stability. *Mol. Ther.* **2008**, *16*, 1833–1840. [CrossRef]
18. Ledwith, B.J.; Manam, S.; Troilo, P.J.; Barnum, A.B.; Pauley, C.J.; Griffiths, T.G., 2nd.; Harper, L.B.; Beare, C.M.; Bagdon, W.J.; Nichols, W.W. Plasmid DNA vaccines: Investigation of integration into host cellular DNA following intramuscular injection in mice. *Intervirology* **2000**, *43*, 258–272. [CrossRef]
19. Schmeer, M.; Buchholz, T.; Schleef, M. Plasmid DNA Manufacturing for Indirect and Direct Clinical Applications. *Hum. Gene Ther.* **2017**, *28*, 856–861. [CrossRef]
20. Reautschnig, P.; Vogel, P.; Stafforst, T. The notorious R.N.A. in the spotlight—Drug or target for the treatment of disease. *RNA Biol.* **2017**, *14*, 651–668. [CrossRef]
21. Whisenand, J.M.; Azizian, K.T.; Henderson, J.M.; Shore, S.; Shin, D.; Lebedev, A.; McCaffrey, A.P.; Hogrefe, R.I. Considerations for the Design and cGMP Manufacturing of mRNA Therapeutics. Available online: https://www.trilinkbiotech.com/work/mRNA_OTS1.pdf (accessed on 21 February 2019).
22. Schmid, A. Considerations for Producing mRNA Vaccines for Clinical Trials. *Methods Mol. Biol.* **2017**, *1499*, 237–251.
23. WHO Expert Committee on Specifications for Pharmaceutical Preparations. WHO Technical Report Series, No. 908. Thirty-Seventh Report: Annex 4 Good Manufacturing Practices for Pharmaceutical Products: Main Principles. Available online: http://apps.who.int/medicinedocs/en/d/Js5517e/20.html (accessed on 21 February 2019).
24. Good Manufacturing Practices for Biological Products. In WHO Expert Committee on Biological Standardization. Forty-Second Report. Geneva, World Health Organization, 1992, Annex 1.WHO Technical Report Series, No. 822. Available online: http://apps.who.int/medicinedocs/documents/s16114e/s16114e.pdf (accessed on 21 February 2019).
25. Middaugh, C.R.; Evans, R.K.; Montgomery, D.L.; Casimiro, D.R. Analysis of plasmid DNA from a pharmaceutical perspective. *J. Pharm. Sci.* **1998**, *87*, 130–146. [CrossRef]
26. Stitz, L.; Vogel, A.; Schnee, M.; Voss, D.; Rauch, S.; Mutzke, T.; Ketterer, T.; Kramps, T.; Petsch, B. A thermostable messenger RNA based vaccine against rabies. *PLoS Negl. Trop. Dis.* **2017**, *11*, e0006108. [CrossRef]
27. Fu, T.M.; Ulmer, J.B.; Caulfield, M.J.; Deck, R.R.; Friedman, A.; Wang, S.; Liu, X.; Donnelly, J.J.; Liu, M.A. Priming of cytotoxic T lymphocytes by DNA vaccinequirement for professional antigen presenting cells and evidence for antigen transfer from myocytes. *Mol. Med.* **1997**, *3*, 362–371. [CrossRef]
28. Fu, T.M.; Friedman, A.; Ulmer, J.B.; Liu, M.A.; Donnelly, J.J. Protective cellular immunity: Cytotoxic T-lymphocyte responses against dominant and recessive epitopes of influenza virus nucleoprotein induced by DNA immunization. *J. Virol.* **1997**, *71*, 2715–2721.
29. Dupuis, M.; Denis-Mize, K.; Woo, C.; Goldbeck, C.; Selby, M.J.; Chen, M.; Otten, G.R.; Ulmer, J.B.; Donnelly, J.J.; Ott, G.; et al. Distribution of DNA vaccines determines their immunogenicity after intramuscular injection in mice. *J. Immunol.* **2000**, *165*, 2850–2858. [CrossRef]
30. Donnelly, J.J.; Friedman, A.; Ulmer, J.B.; Liu, M.A. Further protection against antigenic drift of influenza virus in a ferret model by DNA vaccination. *Vaccine* **1997**, *15*, 865–868. [CrossRef]
31. Probst, J.; Weide, B.; Scheel, B.; Pichler, B.J.; Hoerr, I.; Rammensee, H.G.; Pascolo, S. Spontaneous cellular uptake of exogenous messenger RNA in vivo is nucleic acid-specific, saturable and ion dependent. *Gene Ther.* **2007**, *14*, 1175–1180. [CrossRef]
32. Tang, D.C.; DeVit, M.; Johnston, S.A. Genetic immunization is a simple method for eliciting an immune response. *Nature* **1992**, *356*, 152–154. [CrossRef]

33. Hajj, K.A.; Ball, R.L.; Deluty, S.B.; Singh, S.R.; Strelkova, D.; Knapp, C.M.; Whitehead, K.A. Branched-Tail Lipid Nanoparticles Potently Deliver mRNA In Vivo due to Enhanced Ionization at Endosomal pH. *Small* **2019**, *15*, e1805097. [CrossRef]
34. Iavarone, C.; O'Hagan, D.T.; Yu, D.; Delahaye, N.F.; Ulmer, J.B. Mechanism of action of mRNA-based vaccines. *Expert Rev. Vaccines* **2017**, *16*, 871–881. [CrossRef]
35. Kaczmarek, J.C.; Kowalski, P.S.; Anderson, D.G. Advances in the delivery of RNA therapeutics: From concept to clinical reality. *Genome Med.* **2017**, *9*, 60. [CrossRef]
36. Persano, S.; Guevara, M.L.; Li, Z.; Mai, J.; Ferrari, M.; Pompa, P.P.; Shen, H. Lipopolyplex potentiates anti-tumor immunity of mRNA-based vaccination. *Biomaterials* **2017**, *125*, 81–89. [CrossRef]
37. Rauch, S.; Jasny, E.; Schmidt, K.E.; Petsch, B. New Vaccine Technologies to Combat Outbreak Situations. *Front. Immunol.* **2018**, *9*, 1963. [CrossRef]
38. Pascolo, S. Vaccination with messenger RNA. *Methods Mol. Med.* **2006**, *127*, 23–40.
39. Xu, Z.; Li, P.; Fan, L.; Wu, M. The Potential Role of circRNA in Tumor Immunity Regulation and Immunotherapy. *Front Immunol.* **2018**. [CrossRef]
40. Wesselhoeft, R.A.; Kowalski, P.S.; Anderson, D.G. Engineering circular RNA for potent and stable translation in eukaryotic cells. *Nat. Commun.* **2018**, *9*. [CrossRef]
41. Holdt, L.M.; Kohlmaier, A.; Teupser, D. *Circular RNAs as Therapeutic Agents and Targets. Front. Physiol.* **2018**. [CrossRef]
42. Ljungberg, K.; Liljeström, P. Self-replicating alphavirus RNA vaccines. *Expert Rev. Vaccines* **2015**, *14*, 177–194. [CrossRef]
43. Brazzoli, M.; Magini, D.; Bonci, A.; Buccato, S.; Giovani, C.; Kratzer, R.; Zurli, V.; Mangiavacchi, S.; Casini, D.; Brito, L.M.; et al. Induction of Broad-Based Immunity and Protective Efficacy by Self-amplifying mRNA Vaccines Encoding Influenza Virus Hemagglutinin. *J. Virol.* **2016**, *90*, 332–344. [CrossRef] [PubMed]
44. Brito, L.A.; Kommareddy, S.; Maione, D.; Uematsu, Y.; Giovani, C.; Berlanda Scorza, F.; Otten, G.R.; Yu, D.; Mandl, C.W.; Mason, P.W.; et al. Self-amplifying mRNA vaccines. *Adv. Genet.* **2015**, *89*, 179–233.
45. Samsa, M.M.; Dupuy, L.C.; Beard, C.W.; Six, C.M.; Schmaljohn, C.S.; Mason, P.W.; Geall, A.J.; Ulmer, J.B.; Yu, D. Self-Amplifying RNA Vaccines for Venezuelan Equine Encephalitis Virus Induce Robust Protective Immunogenicity in Mice. *Mol Ther.* **2019**, *27*, 850–865. [CrossRef] [PubMed]
46. Campbell, J.D. Development of the CpG Adjuvant 1018: A Case Study. *Methods Mol. Biol.* **2017**, *1494*, 15–27. [PubMed]
47. Gottlieb, P.; Utz, P.J.; Robinson, W.; Steinman, L. Clinical optimization of antigen specific modulation of type 1 diabetes with the plasmid DNA platform. *Clin. Immunol.* **2013**, *149*, 297–306. [CrossRef] [PubMed]
48. Coban, C.; Kobiyama, K.; Aoshi, T.; Takeshita, F.; Horii, T.; Akira, S.; Ishii, K.J. Novel strategies to improve DNA vaccine immunogenicity. *Curr. Gene Ther.* **2011**, *11*, 479–484. [CrossRef]
49. Coban, C.; Kobiyama, K.; Jounai, N.; Tozuka, M.; Ishii, K.J. DNA vaccines—-A simple DNA sensing matter? *Hum. Vaccin. Immunother.* **2013**, *9*. [CrossRef] [PubMed]
50. Allen, A.; Wang, C.; Caproni, L.J.; Sugiyarto, G.; Harden, E.; Douglas, L.R.; Duriez, P.J.; Karbowniczek, K.; Extance, J.; Rothwell, P.J.; et al. Linear doggybone DNA vaccine induces similar immunological responses to conventional plasmid DNA independently of immune recognition by TLR9 in a pre-clinical model. *Cancer Immunol. Immunother.* **2018**, *67*, 627–638. [CrossRef]
51. Chen, N.; Xia, P.; Li, S.; Zhang, T.; Wang, T.T.; Zhu, J. RNA sensors of the innate immune system and their detection of pathogens. *IUBMB Life* **2017**, *69*, 297–304. [CrossRef]
52. Pollard, C.; Rejman, J.; De Haes, W.; Verrier, B.; Van Gulck, E.; Naessens, T.; De Smedt, S.; Bogaert, P.; Grooten, J.; Vanham, G.; et al. Type I IFN counteracts the induction of antigen-specific immune responses by lipid-based delivery of mRNA vaccines. *Mol. Ther.* **2013**, *21*, 251–259. [CrossRef] [PubMed]
53. Karikó, K.; Muramatsu, H.; Ludwig, J.; Weissman, D. Generating the optimal mRNA for therapy: HPLC purification eliminates immune activation and improves translation of nucleoside-modified, protein-encoding mRNA. *Nucleic Acids Res.* **2011**, *39*, e142. [CrossRef]
54. Doener, F.; Hong, H.S.; Meyer, I.; Tadjalli-Mehr, K.; Daehling, A.; Heidenreich, R.; Koch, S.D.; Fotin-Mleczek, M.; Gnad-Vogt, U. RNA-based adjuvant CV8102 enhances the immunogenicity of a licensed rabies vaccine in a first-in-human trial. *Vaccine* **2019**. [CrossRef]

55. Alberer, M.; Gnad-Vogt, U.; Hong, H.S.; Mehr, K.T.; Backert, L.; Finak, G.; Gottardo, R.; Bica, M.A.; Garofano, A.; Koch, S.D.; et al. Safety and immunogenicity of a mRNA rabies vaccine in healthy adults: An open-label, non-randomised, prospective, first-in-human phase 1 clinical trial. *Lancet* **2017**, *390*, 1511–1520. [CrossRef]
56. Feng, J.Y.; Johnson, A.A.; Johnson, K.A.; Anderson, K.S. Insights into the Molecular Mechanism of Mitochondrial Toxicity by AIDS Drugs. *J. Biol. Chem.* **2001**, *276*, 23832–23837. [CrossRef]
57. Johnson, A.A.; Ray, A.S.; Hanes, J.; Suo, Z.; Colacino, J.M.; Anderson, K.S.; Johnson, K.A. Toxicity of Antiviral Nucleoside Analogs and the Human Mitochondrial DNA Polymerase. *J. Biol. Chem.* **2001**, *276*, 40847–40857. [CrossRef]
58. Moyle, G. Toxicity of antiretroviral nucleoside and nucleotide analogues: Is mitochondrial toxicity the only mechanism? *Drug Saf.* **2000**, *23*, 467–481. [CrossRef]
59. Moderna Hits Safety Problems in Bold Bid to Reinvent Medicine. STAT (2017). Available online: https://www.statnews.com/2017/01/10/moderna-trouble-mrna/ (accessed on 27 February 2019).
60. Apgar, J.F.; Tang, J.P.; Singh, P.; Balasubramanian, N.; Burke, J.; Hodges, M.R.; Lasaro, M.A.; Lin, L.; Miliard, B.L.; Moore, K.; et al. Quantitative Systems Pharmacology Model of hUGT1A1-modRNA Encoding for the UGT1A1 Enzyme to Treat Crigler-Najjar Syndrome Type 1. *CPT Pharmacomet. Syst. Pharmacol.* **2018**, *7*, 404–412. [CrossRef]
61. Schlake, T.; Thess, A.; Thran, M.; Jordan, I. mRNA as novel technology for passive immunotherapy. *Cell. Mol. Life Sci.* **2019**, *76*, 301–328. [CrossRef]
62. Garren, H.; Robinson, W.H.; Krasulová, E.; Havrdová, E.; Nadj, C.; Selmaj, K.; Losy, J.; Nadj, I.; Radue, E.W.; Kidd, B.A.; et al. Phase 2 trial of a DNA vaccine encoding myelin basic protein for multiple sclerosis. *Ann. Neurol.* **2008**, *63*, 611–620. [CrossRef]
63. Pepini, T.; Pulichino, A.M.; Carsillo, T.; Carlson, A.L.; Sari-Sarraf, F.; Ramsauer, K.; Debasitis, J.C.; Maruggi, G.; Otten, G.R.; Geall, A.J.; et al. Induction of an IFN-Mediated Antiviral Response by a Self-Amplifying RNA Vaccine: Implications for Vaccine Design. *J. Immunol.* **2017**, *198*, 4012–4024. [CrossRef]
64. Theofilopoulos, A.N.; Baccala, R.; Beutler, B.; Kono, D.H. Type I interferons (alpha/beta) in immunity and autoimmunity. *Annu. Rev. Immunol.* **2005**, *23*, 307–336. [CrossRef]
65. Edwards, D.K.; Jasny, E.; Yoon, H.; Horscroft, N.; Schanen, B.; Geter, T.; Fotin-Mleczek, M.; Petsch, B.; Wittman, V.; et al. Adjuvant effects of a sequence-engineered mRNA vaccine: Translational profiling demonstrates similar human and murine innate response. *J. Transl. Med.* **2017**, *15*, 1. [CrossRef] [PubMed]
66. Sheets, R.L.; Stein, J.; Manetz, T.S.; Duffy, C.; Nason, M.; Andrews, C.; Kong, W.P.; Nabel, G.J.; Gomez, P.L. Biodistribution of DNA Plasmid Vaccines against HIV-1, Ebola, Severe Acute Respiratory Syndrome, or West Nile Virus Is Similar, without Integration, despite Differing Plasmid Backbones or Gene Inserts. *Toxicol. Sci.* **2006**, *91*, 610–619. [CrossRef]
67. European Food Safety Authority (EFSA); Houston, R.; Moxon, S.; Nogué, F.; Papadopoulou, N.; Ramon, M.; Waigmann, E. Assessment of the potential integration of the DNA plasmid vaccine CLYNAV into the salmon genome. *EFSA J.* **2017**, *15*, e04689.
68. Griffiths, D.J. Endogenous retroviruses in the human genome sequence. *Genome Biol.* **2001**, *2*, PMC138943. [CrossRef]
69. Honda, T.; Tomonaga, K. Endogenous non-retroviral RNA virus elements evidence a novel type of antiviral immunity. *Mob. Genet. Elem.* **2016**, *6*, e1165785. [CrossRef]
70. Douville, R.N.; Nath, A. Human endogenous retroviruses and the nervous system. *Handb. Clin. Neurol.* **2014**, *123*, 465–485.
71. Hinz, T.; Kallen, K.; Britten, C.M.; Flamion, B.; Granzer, U.; Hoos, A.; Huber, C.; Khleif, S.; Kreiter, S.; Rammensee, H.G.; et al. The European Regulatory Environment of RNA-Based Vaccines. *Methods Mol. Biol.* **2017**, *1499*, 203–222. [PubMed]
72. Dalmo, R.A. DNA vaccines for fish: Review and perspectives on correlates of protection. *J. Fish Dis.* **2018**, *41*, 1–9. [CrossRef]
73. Anonymous. Oncept Melanoma: Withdrawn Application. European Medicines Agency—Commission (2018). Available online: https://www.ema.europa.eu/en/medicines/veterinary/withdrawn-applications/oncept-melanoma (accessed on 21 February 2019).
74. CDC-Media Relations-Press Release-July 18 2005. Available online: https://www.cdc.gov/media/pressrel/r050718.htm (accessed on 21 February 2019).

75. Wheeler, S.S.; Langevin, S.; Woods, L.; Carroll, B.D.; Vickers, W.; Morrison, S.A.; Chang, G.-J.J.; Reisen, W.K.; Boyce, W.M. Efficacy of three vaccines in protecting Western Scrub-Jays (*Aphelocoma californica*) from experimental infection with West Nile virus: implications for vaccination of Island Scrub-Jays (Aphelocoma insularis). *Vector Borne Zoonotic Dis.* **2011**, *11*, 1069–1080. [CrossRef]
76. Kilpatrick, A.M.; Dupuis, A.P.; Chang, G.-J.J.; Kramer, L.D. DNA vaccination of American robins (Turdus migratorius) against West Nile virus. *Vector Borne Zoonotic Dis.* **2010**, *10*, 377–380. [CrossRef]
77. Bunning, M.L.; Fox, P.E.; Bowen, R.A.; Komar, N.; Chang, G.J.; Speaker, T.J.; Stephens, M.R.; Nemeth, N.; Panella, N.A.; Langevin, S.A.; et al. DNA vaccination of the American crow (*Corvus brachyrhynchos*) provides partial protection against lethal challenge with West Nile virus. *Avian Dis.* **2007**, *51*, 573–577. [CrossRef]
78. Turell, M.J.; Bunning, M.; Ludwig, G.V.; Ortman, B.; Chang, J.; Speaker, T.; Spielman, A.; McLean, R.; Komar, N.; Gates, R.; et al. DNA vaccine for West Nile virus infection in fish crows (*Corvus ossifragus*). *Emerg. Infect. Dis.* **2003**, *9*, 1077–1081. [CrossRef] [PubMed]
79. Chang, G.-J.J.; Davis, B.S.; Stringfield, C.; Lutz, C. Prospective immunization of the endangered California condors (Gymnogyps californianus) protects this species from lethal West Nile virus infection. *Vaccine* **2007**, *25*, 2325–2330. [CrossRef]
80. Draghia-Akli, R.; Ellis, K.M.; Hill, L.-A.; Malone, P.B.; Fiorotto, M.L. High-efficiency growth hormone-releasing hormone plasmid vector administration into skeletal muscle mediated by electroporation in pigs. *FASEB J.* **2003**, *17*, 526–528. [CrossRef]
81. VGX Animal Health Announces Approval of LifeTideTM SW 5-World's First and Only Approved DNA Therapy for Food Animals. Available online: http://ir.inovio.com/news-and-media/news/press-release-details/2008/VGX-Animal-Health-announces-approval-of-LifeTideTM-SW-5---Worlds-First-and-Only-Approved-DNA-Therapy-for-Food-Animals/default.aspx (accessed on 21 February 2019).
82. Martin, J.E.; Pierson, T.C.; Hubka, S.; Rucker, S.; Gordon, I.J.; Enama, M.E.; Andrews, C.A.; Xu, Q.; Davis, B.S.; Nason, M.; et al. A West Nile virus DNA vaccine induces neutralizing antibody in healthy adults during a phase 1 clinical trial. *J. Infect. Dis.* **2007**, *196*, 1732–1740. [CrossRef]
83. Ledgerwood, J.E.; Pierson, T.C.; Hubka, S.A.; Desai, N.; Rucker, S.; Gordon, I.J.; Enama, M.E.; Nelson, S.; Nason, M.; Gu, W.; et al. A West Nile virus DNA vaccine utilizing a modified promoter induces neutralizing antibody in younger and older healthy adults in a phase I clinical trial. *J. Infect. Dis.* **2011**, *203*, 1396–1404. [CrossRef]
84. Sarwar, U.N.; Costner, P.; Enama, M.E.; Berkowitz, N.; Hu, Z.; Hendel, C.S.; Sitar, S.; Plummer, S.; Mulangu, S.; Bailer, R.T.; et al. Safety and immunogenicity of DNA vaccines encoding Ebolavirus and Marburgvirus wild-type glycoproteins in a phase I clinical trial. *J. Infect. Dis.* **2015**, *211*, 549–557. [CrossRef]
85. Gaudinski, M.R.; Houser, K.V.; Morabito, K.M.; Hu, Z.; Yamshchikov, G.; Rothwell, R.S.; Berkowitz, N.; Mendoza, F.; Saunders, J.G.; Novik, L.; et al. Safety, tolerability, and immunogenicity of two Zika virus DNA vaccine candidates in healthy adults: Randomised, open-label, phase 1 clinical trials. *Lancet* **2018**, *391*, 552–562. [CrossRef]
86. Kim, T.J.; Jin, H.T.; Hur, S.Y.; Yang, H.G.; Seo, Y.B.; Hong, S.R.; Lee, C.W.; Kim, S.; Woo, J.W.; Park, K.S.; et al. Clearance of persistent HPV infection and cervical lesion by therapeutic DNA vaccine in CIN3 patients. *Nat. Commun.* **2014**, *5*, 5317. [CrossRef]
87. Trimble, C.L.; Morrow, M.P.; Kraynyak, K.A.; Shen, X.; Dallas, M.; Yan, J.; Edwards, L.; Parker, R.L.; Denny, L.; Giffear, M.; Brown, A.S.; et al. Safety, efficacy, and immunogenicity of VGX-3100, a therapeutic synthetic DNA vaccine targeting human papillomavirus 16 and 18 E6 and E7 proteins for cervical intraepithelial neoplasia 2/3: A randomised, double-blind, placebo-controlled phase 2b trial. *Lancet* **2015**, *386*, 2078–2088. [CrossRef]
88. Aggarwal, C.; Cohen, R.B.; Morrow, M.P.; Kraynak, K.A.; Sylvester, A.J.; Knoblock, D.M.; Bauml, J.; Weinstein, G.S.; Lin, A.; Boyer, J.; et al. Immunotherapy targeting HPV 16/18 generates potent immune responses in HPV-Associated Head and Neck Cancer. *Clin. Cancer Res.* **2018**. [CrossRef]
89. Chudley, L.; McCann, K.; Mander, A.; Tjelle, T.; Campos-Perez, J.; Godeseth, R.; Creak, A.; Dobbyn, J.; Johnson, B.; Bass, P.; et al. DNA fusion-gene vaccination in patients with prostate cancer induces high-frequency CD8+ T-cell responses and increases PSA doubling time. *Cancer Immunol. Immunother.* **2012**, *61*, 2161–2170. [CrossRef] [PubMed]

90. McCann, K.J.; Mander, A.; Cazaly, A.; Chudley, L.; Stasakova, J.; Thirdborough, S.M.; King, A.; Lloyd-Evans, P.; Buxton, E.; Edwards, C.; et al. Targeting Carcinoembryonic Antigen with DNA Vaccination: On-Target Adverse Events Link with Immunologic and Clinical Outcomes. *Clin. Cancer Res.* **2016**. [CrossRef] [PubMed]
91. Patel, P.M.; Ottensmeier, C.H.; Mulatero, C.; Lorigan, P.; Plummer, R.; Pandha, H.; Elsheikh, S.; Hadjimichael, E.; Villasanti, N.; Adams, S.E.; et al. Targeting gp100 and TRP-2 with a DNA vaccine: Incorporating T cell epitopes with a human IgG1 antibody induces potent T cell responses that are associated with favourable clinical outcome in a phase I/II trial. *Oncoimmunology* **2018**, *7*, e1433516. [CrossRef]
92. Leal, L.; Guardo, A.C.; Morón-López, S.; Salgado, M.; Mothe, B.; Heirman, C.; Pannus, P.; Vanham, G.; van den Ham, H.J.; Gruters, R.; et al. Phase I clinical trial of an intranodally administered mRNA-based therapeutic vaccine against HIV-1 infection. *AIDS* **2018**, *32*, 2533–2545. [CrossRef] [PubMed]
93. Moderna Announces Dosing of the First Monoclonal Antibody Encoded by mRNA in a Clinical Trial. Moderna, Inc. Available online: https://investors.modernatx.com/news-releases/news-release-details/moderna-announces-dosing-first-monoclonal-antibody-encoded-mrna (accessed on 23 February 2019).
94. Bahl, K.; Senn, J.J.; Yuzhakov, O.; Bulychev, A.; Brito, L.A.; Hassett, K.J.; Laska, M.E.; Smith, M.; Almarsson, Ö.; Thompson, J.; et al. Preclinical and Clinical Demonstration of Immunogenicity by mRNA Vaccines against H10N8 and H7N9 Influenza Viruses. *Mol. Ther.* **2017**, *25*, 1316–1327. [CrossRef] [PubMed]
95. Richner, J.M.; Jagger, B.W.; Shan, C.; Fontes, C.R.; Dowd, K.A.; Cao, B.; Himansu, S.; Caine, E.A.; Nunes, B.T.D.; Medeiros, D.B.A.; et al. Vaccine Mediated Protection Against Zika Virus-Induced Congenital Disease. *Cell* **2017**, *170*, 273–283. [CrossRef]
96. Richner, J.M.; Himansu, S.; Dowd, K.A.; Butler, S.L.; Salazar, V.; Fox, J.M.; Julander, J.G.; Tang, W.W.; Shresta, S.; Pierson, T.C.; et al. Modified mRNA Vaccines Protect against Zika Virus Infection. *Cell* **2017**, *168*, 1114–1125. [CrossRef] [PubMed]
97. John, S.; Yuzhakov, O.; Woods, A.; Deterling, J.; Hassett, K.; Shaw, C.A.; Ciaramella, G. Multi-antigenic human cytomegalovirus mRNA vaccines that elicit potent humoral and cell-mediated immunity. *Vaccine* **2018**, *36*, 1689–1699. [CrossRef]
98. Rausch, S.; Schwentner, C.; Stenzl, A.; Bedke, J. mRNA vaccine CV9103 and CV9104 for the treatment of prostate cancer. *Hum. Vaccines Immunother.* **2014**, *10*, 3146–3152. [CrossRef] [PubMed]
99. Kübler, H.; Scheel, B.; Gnad-Vogt, U.; Miller, K.; Schultze-Seemann, W.; Vom Dorp, F.; Parmiani, G.; Hampel, C.; Wedel, S.; Trojan, L.; et al. Self-adjuvanted mRNA vaccination in advanced prostate cancer patients: A first-in-man phase I/IIa study. *J. Immunother. Cancer* **2015**, *3*, 26. [CrossRef]

vaccines

MDPI

Article

Novel Synthetic DNA Immunogens Targeting Latent Expressed Antigens of Epstein–Barr Virus Elicit Potent Cellular Responses and Inhibit Tumor Growth

Krzysztof Wojtak [1,2], Alfredo Perales-Puchalt [1] and David B. Weiner [1,*]

[1] Vaccine and Immunotherapy Center, The Wistar Institute, Philadelphia, PA 19104, USA; kwojtak@Wistar.org (K.W.); Alfredo.PeralesPuchalt@inovio.com (A.P.-P.)

[2] Cell and Molecular Biology Graduate Program, The University of Pennsylvania, Philadelphia, PA 19104, USA

* Correspondence: dweiner@wistar.org; Tel.: +1-215-495-6882; Fax: +1-610-631-7030

Received: 19 April 2019; Accepted: 22 May 2019; Published: 24 May 2019

Abstract: Infectious diseases are linked to 15%–20% of cancers worldwide. Among them, Epstein–Barr virus (EBV) is an oncogenic herpesvirus that chronically infects over 90% of the adult population, with over 200,000 cases of cancer and 150,000 cancer-related deaths attributed to it yearly. Acute EBV infection can present as infectious mononucleosis, and lead to the future onset of multiple cancers, including Burkitt lymphoma, Hodgkin lymphoma, nasopharyngeal carcinoma, and gastric carcinoma. Many of these cancers express latent viral genes, including Epstein–Barr virus nuclear antigen 1 (*EBNA1*) and latent membrane proteins 1 and 2 (LMP1 and LMP2). Previous attempts to create potent immunogens against EBV have been reported but generated mixed success. We designed novel Synthetic Consensus (SynCon) DNA vaccines against EBNA1, LMP1 and LMP2 to improve on the immune potency targeting important antigens expressed in latently infected cells. These EBV tumor antigens are hypothesized to be useful targets for potential immunotherapy of EBV-driven cancers. We optimized the genetic sequences for these three antigens, studied them for expression, and examined their immune profiles in vivo. We observed that these immunogens generated unique profiles based on which antigen was delivered as the vaccine target. EBNA1vax and LMP2Avax generated the most robust T cell immunity. Interestingly, LMP1vax was a very weak immunogen, generating very low levels of CD8 T cell immunity both as a standalone vaccine and as part of a trivalent vaccine cocktail. LMP2Avax was able to drive immunity that impacted EBV-antigen-positive tumor growth. These studies suggest that engineered EBV latent protein vaccines deserve additional study as potential agents for immunotherapy of EBV-driven cancers.

Keywords: Epstein-Barr virus; DNA vaccines; latent proteins; LMP2; EBNA1; LMP1

1. Introduction

Epstein–Barr virus (EBV) is a large double-stranded DNA gammaherpesvirus with about 170 kilobases in its genome, encoding over 100 open reading frames (ORFs). EBV accounts for about 1% of all cancer cases worldwide. This complex virus is ubiquitous in the human population, establishing a lifelong latent infection in 90% of people by adulthood [1,2]. The viral strains can be divided into two subgroups, type 1 and type 2, which are broadly similar and designated by differences in their nuclear antigens [3,4]. Primary infection is either asymptomatic, experienced as a non-specific infection, or the cause of infectious mononucleosis, with the latter more likely if exposure occurs during adolescence or later [5]. EBV targets human B cells after being transmitted through the oral epithelium via the saliva of an infected individual, establishing latency and allowing the viral genome to persist.

EBV is linked to the development of several human cancers. It was first identified in a Burkitt lymphoma sample [6], and is now known to be a cause of Hodgkin's lymphoma [7], nasopharyngeal carcinoma [8,9], and gastric carcinoma [10]. EBV infection is also linked to autoimmune disorders, such as multiple sclerosis [11] and systemic lupus erythematosus [12], which are likely tied to EBV-driven immune dysregulation [13]. The cancers associated with EBV are linked to their expression of EBV oncogenes, including Epstein–Barr virus nuclear antigen 1 (EBNA1) and latent membrane proteins 1 and 2 (LMP1 and LMP2) [14]. The latent viral oncoproteins of EBV are important cancer drivers and are implicated in directly contributing to EBV-associated malignancies [15–17].

EBNA1 is important in maintaining the viral genome and is required for EBV latency and associated transformation. LMP1 and LMP2 were discovered to colocalize in the membranes of latently infected lymphocytes [18], and these oncoproteins contribute to cancer progression via diverse signaling pathways [19]. LMP1 interacts with tumor necrosis factor receptor (TNFR)-associated factors (TRAFS) to drive nuclear factor-κB (NF-κB), mitogen-activated protein kinase (MAPK), and phosphatidylinositol 3-kinase (PI3K) pathways [20]. LMP2 mimics the B cell receptor, sending survival signals to B cells without the need for antigen stimulation [21]. The LMP2 gene produces LMP2A and LMP2B, of which LMP2A has an additional 119 amino acids at the N-terminus.

There are no approved vaccines available to prevent initial infection by EBV, and clinical trials of EBV vaccine candidates have had limited success. The target that progressed furthest along in the clinic was a recombinant subunit gp350 prophylactic vaccine adjuvanted with aluminum hydroxide and 3-O-desacyl-4′-monophosphoryl lipid A (AS04) which was tested in a phase 2 trial. The study reported that it statistically decreased the incidence of infectious mononucleosis, but this vaccine did not reduce infections by the virus, despite generating high-titer antibody responses in vaccine recipients [22]. Future vaccines against EBV can further explore the numerous other glycoproteins involved in EBV entry and the latent proteins essential for maintaining the virus [23].

EBV is a viable target for therapeutic approaches to treating cancer. Cellular immune responses are particularly important in targeting malignant cells, and they have been exploited in specific cancer immunotherapies [24,25]. It would be a major advantage for such approaches if they would drive both CD4 T cell responses and induce functional CD8 T cell responses that could clear EBV-infected targets. Prior vaccine approaches particularly lacked potent induction of CD8 cellular immunity.

Newer Synthetic Consensus (SynCon) DNA vaccines, combined with adaptive electroporation (EP), have demonstrated safety, as well as the potent induction of antibodies, T helper responses, and CD8 effector T cells, in multiple clinical trials. Clinical efficacy has been reported in the context of immunotherapy for human papillomavirus (HPV)-driven neoplasia, and clinical regressions with clearance have been described in early studies that use a combination approach involving engineered HPV nuclear gene targets and checkpoint inhibitor therapy with PD-1. Specifically, a therapeutic DNA vaccine targeting HPV E6/E7 antigens from the HPV 16 and 18 strains has shown a positive impact in patients when this vaccine was delivered by Cellectra adaptive EP in a phase 2b trial for the treatment of cervical intraepithelial neoplasia [26]. Importantly, this vaccine induced potent CD8 T cells that infiltrated the tumor and caused the lesions to regress, resulting in both histopathological regression and viral clearance in 40% of treated patients. Similar data has been reported impacting HPV-driven head and neck cancers in a preliminary report [27], where a similar genetically-adjuvanted HPV DNA vaccine has been shown to drive an increase in intratumoral T cell infiltration by CD8 cells, as well as result in complete clinical regression in metastatic head and neck cancer when the vaccine was followed by PD-1 immunotherapy (this outcome was observed in 2/4 patients).

These data support the importance of the synthetic DNA approach for the treatment of virally-driven cancers which rely on viral oncogenes for continued disease. This is the situation for EBV-driven cancer as well. Here we report on studies investigating the generation of a multiantigen immunotherapeutic vaccine for EBV infection. We focused on developing a vaccine cocktail consisting of the episome-maintaining EBNA1 antigen combined with the two important latency-related membrane antigens for EBV, LMP1 and LMP2. We report the immune potency and early impact of the combined immune responses to these constructs.

DNA vaccines have previously reported interesting responses against LMP1 [28] and LMP2 [29] in mouse models. This study furthers this research by exploring the immune responses to a combination of EBV latent proteins using newly designed synthetic DNA-encoded antigens studied in the context of facilitated in vivo local delivery. The results show potent and consistent induction of T cell immunity in targeted mouse models with an impact on antigen-positive tumor growth, suggesting further study of this approach for EBV immunotherapy is important.

2. Materials and Methods

2.1. DNA Vaccines

Latent protein vaccine consensus sequences for EBNA1vax, LMP1vax, and LMP2Avax were produced from sequences obtained from strains AG876, B95-8, and GD1. Codons corresponding to residues associated with cell signaling were modified. Repetitive sequences were deleted from the EBNA1vax consensus sequence to avoid their inhibition of translation and MHC class I presentation [30–32], and alanine mutations were made, affecting binding to USP7 [33]. Similarly, mutations were made to functional domains of LMP1vax and LMP2Avax to avoid signaling through potentially oncogenic pathways [34–39]. The sequences were codon optimized using SynCon technology and prepared for vaccination studies within modified pVAX1 plasmids, as previously described [40].

2.2. Western Blots

Proteins were extracted, denatured, and immunoblotted as previously described [41]. Detection antibodies used were anti-LMP2A clone 15F9 (Biorad, Hercules, CA, USA), anti-LMP1 clone CS 1-4 (Abcam, Cambridge, UK) and a polyclonal anti-EBNA1 antibody (Invitrogen, Carlsbad, CA, USA). Secondary anti-rat, -mouse, and -goat antibodies conjugated to horseradish peroxidase were used for visualization. Anti-β-actin (a5441, Sigma-Aldrich, St. Louis, MO, USA) was used as a loading control. Images were captured using an ImageQuantLAS 4000 (GE Healthcare Life Sciences, Marlborough, MA, USA).

2.3. Immunofluorescence

Cover slides coated in poly-L-lysine had 293T cells grow on them in 12-well plates and they were transfected with pVAX empty vector, EBNA1vax, LMP1vax, or LMP2Avax DNA vaccine plasmids using Lipofectamine 2000 per the manufacturer's protocol (Invitrogen, Carlsbad, CA, USA). After incubating for two days, the cells were washed with phosphate-buffered saline (PBS), fixed with 4% paraformaldehyde, and permeabilized using Triton X-100 in PBS, as previously described [42]. Commercial antibodies to EBNA1, LMP1, and LMP2A were used for primary staining as above and Invitrogen anti-mouse, anti-rat, and anti-goat secondary antibodies conjugated to AF488, AF647, and APC were used. Slides were imaged using a Leica TCS SP5 Confocal Laser Scanning Microscope and analyzed with Leica LAS AF software (Leica Microsystems, Wetzlar, Germany).

2.4. ELISPOT

Mouse splenocytes were incubated for 24 hours with peptide pools composed of 15mers overlapping by 11 amino acids and covering the full EBNA1, LMP1, and LMP2A proteins (PepTivator EBV, Miltenyi Biotec, Bergisch Gladbach, Germany). Peptides were resuspended at 5 µg/mL during stimulation. IFNγ ELISPOT was performed according to the manufacturer's instructions. Spots were counted using a Cellular Technology Limited ImmunoSpot Analyzer, as previously described [43].

2.5. Flow Cytometry

Two million splenocytes were cultured for 5–6 hours with the peptide pools used above, as previously described [44], and with eBioscience protein transport inhibitor cocktail (Invitrogen). Surface (for CD4 and CD8) and intracellular (for remaining markers) staining followed. Biolegend anti-mouse antibodies conjugated to fluorophores used in this experiment included CD3ε-PE/Cy5 (145-2C11), CD4-FITC (RM4-5), CD8a-APC/Cy7 (53-6.7), IFNγ-APC (XMG1.2), TNFα-BV605 (MP6-XT22), and IL-2-PE-Cy7 (JES6-5H4). Live-dead exclusion was performed using violet fluorescent reactive dye (Invitrogen). Data was collected using a BD Biosciences LSRII flow cytometer (BD Biosciences, Franklin Lakes, NJ, USA) and analyzed using FlowJo v10 (FlowJo LLC, Ashland, OR, USA).

2.6. Cell Lines

Retroviruses encoding B95-8 LMP2A and a green fluorescent protein (GFP) reporter were produced by transfecting Phoenix cells (ATCC) with LMP2A sequence in pBMN-I-GFP. The retrovirus-containing media harvested from these cells was used to infect TC-1 cells by spin-infection to generate a tumor cell line, as previously described [45], which stably expresses LMP2A. Cells expressing the GFP marker were isolated using FACS, and single-cell cloning was performed to obtain a clonal cell population.

2.7. Animal Studies

Female, 5-7-week-old C57BL/6 and BALB/c mice were purchased from Jackson Labs, and CD-1 mice were purchased from Charles River. The Wistar Institute Institutional Care and Use Committee approved all animal studies under protocol 112762.

Tumors were generated by injecting 2 million TC-1-LMP2A cells into the axillary region, with monitoring of tumor size thereafter. Tumor sizes were measured by taking their longest dimension as length and the perpendicular as width, with tumor volume being calculated using $\frac{1}{2} \times \text{length} \times \text{width}^2$. Multifocal tumors were separately measured, and their total volume was calculated as the sum of the individual volumes. Vaccinations introduced 25 μg of DNA delivered within 30 μL of deionized water by intramuscular injection into the tibialis anterior and were followed by EP with the Cellectra 3P device (Inovio Pharmaceuticals) under general anesthesia using inhaled isoflurane, as previously described [46,47]. Blood was collected through submandibular bleeding or post-mortem cardiac punctures.

2.8. Statistics

GraphPad Prism 7 and 8 were used to perform statistical analyses. The two-tailed unpaired Student's t test was used to calculate differences between means of experimental groups, with the Mann–Whitney test for non-parametric distributions. One-way analysis of variance (ANOVA) was used for comparisons between more than one group, with Kruskal-Wallis used in cases of nonparametric distributions. Error bars in all graphs show the standard error of the mean. The log-rank test was used to compare survival rates. $p < 0.05$ was considered statistically significant.

3. Results

3.1. Design of DNA Vaccines Targeting EBNA1, LMP1, and LMP2A

We designed consensus optimized DNA vaccines targeting the oncogenic EBV latent proteins commonly seen in malignancies, which are EBNA1, LMP1, and LMP2A. Consensus immunogens can focus the immune response towards conserved regions of important antigens, allowing for increased T cell cross reactivity as well as partially compensating for minor variability in the vaccine targeted antigens [48–50]. Consensus sequences using *GD1* (type 1), *B95-8* (type 1), and *AG876* (type 2) EBV genes were generated for all 3 antigens (Figure 1A) to optimize the ability of the vaccines to elicit immune responses against all common viral strains, which are phylogenetically similar [51]. Modifications were made to remove repetitive sequences and to ablate oncogenic properties inherent to the proteins while preserving the structures of the antigens (Figure 1B). EBNA1vax had repetitive sequence removed, and all three antigens had amino acids modified to abrogate functional regions and cell signaling pathways (Appendix A Figure A1). Phylogenetic trees show close relationships between the vaccine antigens and known sequences from viral isolates (Figure 1C). Large deletions were made to repetitive sequences when engineering EBNA1vax, leading to divergence from known EBNA1 sequences and the long branch away in the diagram, although the retained sequences are well-conserved. The LMP vaccines lie well within their phylogenetic trees, with LMP1 demonstrating roughly 10-fold more diversity than LMP2A. This conservation supports the likelihood that the targeted changes will elicit immune responses against native EBV antigens, as we have described in the clinic for HPV [26,27], Ebola [52], and Zika [53]. However, formal testing in animal models and evaluation in humans is important.

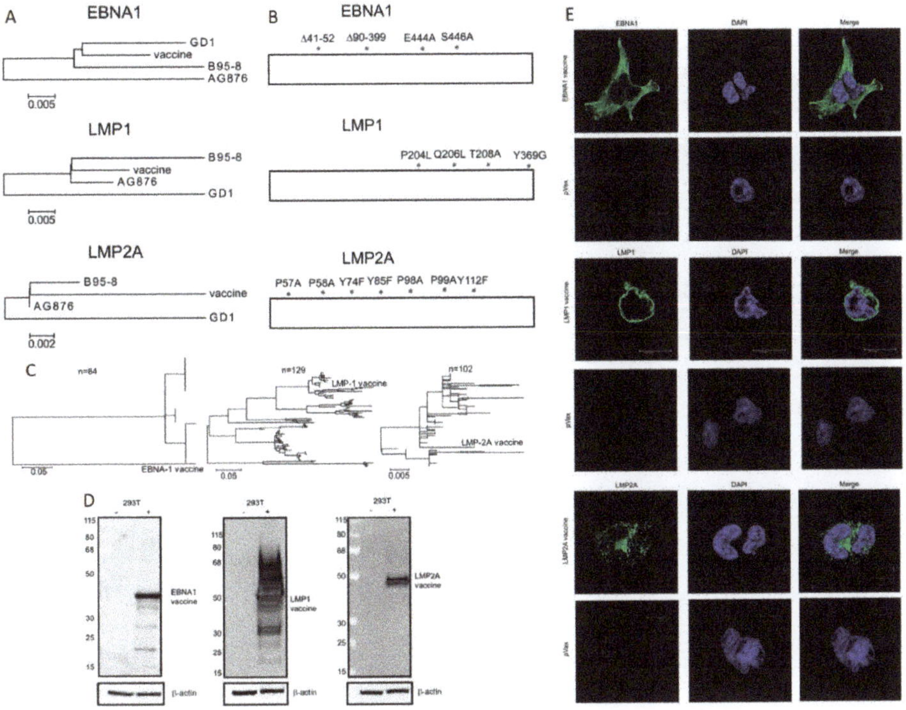

Figure 1. Design and expression of EBNA1vax, LMP1vax, and LMP2Avax vaccine antigens. (**A**) Diagram showing the similarity of the consensus sequence of the EBNA1, LMP1, and LMP2A vaccines, generated from the sequences of EBV strains B95-8, AG876, and GD1. The vaccine antigen designs use a SynCon sequence embedded in a pVAX plasmid. (**B**) Modifications were made to the consensus vaccine antigens to avoid potentially oncogenic properties and repetitive sequences. (**C**) Phylogenic trees showing relationship of vaccines to known EBV latent protein sequences. (**D**) Western blots showing the expression of vaccine antigens in untransfected cells (left columns) and cells transfected with the DNA vaccine (right columns). Beta-actin was used as a loading control. (**E**) Immunofluorescence images showing expression of the vaccine antigens in 293T cells, with cytoplasmic EBNA1vax, LMP1vax on the outer membrane, and LMP2Avax showing a vesicular localization. Antigens are labeled in green, and DAPI (4′,6-diamidino-2-phenylindole) shows the nucleus in blue. Scale bars are 10 μm.

3.2. In Vitro Expression of DNA Vaccines

293T cells were transfected with the vaccine DNA plasmids to test for expression of the designed synthetic DNA constructs. Western blots of lysates from the transfected cells showed bands for EBNA1vax, LMP1vax and LMP2Avax vaccines close to their predicted molecular weights (Figure 1D). We performed immunofluorescence on the transfected 293T cells to further evaluate the expression and localization of the constructs. These studies confirmed expression of all 3 proteins, with LMP2Avax showing its characteristic granular distribution and LMP1vax displaying membrane expression (Figure 1E). Interestingly, EBNA1vax was found in the cytoplasm instead of with the typical nuclear localization of EBNA1. This difference may be due to the changes to the consensus sequence aimed at avoiding sequence repeats and specific changes in the functional domains that affect the ability of EBNA1vax to bind to DNA, suggesting that the encoded changes result in attenuation.

3.3. *Inbred Mice Produced Significant Responses to Latent Protein DNA Vaccines*

In vivo immune responses to EBNA1vax, LMP1vax, and LMP2Avax were examined in BALB/c and C57BL/6 mice. The animals were vaccinated with either the empty vector, individual EBNA1vax, LMP1vax, or LMP2Avax vaccine antigens, or a combination vaccine incorporating all three plasmids. Groups of five mice received biweekly vaccinations, and a week after the second dose they were sacrificed to have their splenocytes collected for analysis (Figure 2A).

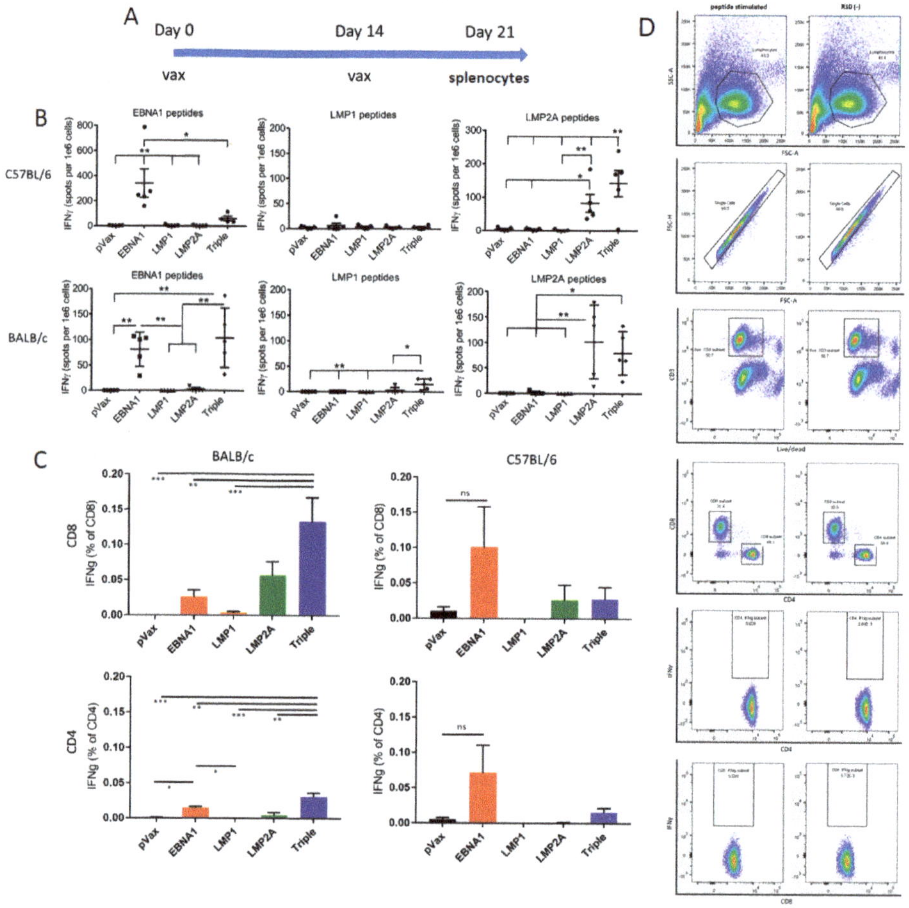

Figure 2. DNA vaccination produces strong cellular responses in inbred mice. (**A**) Vaccination schedule to test the immunogenicity of latent proteins in inbred mice. 2 doses of individual or combined latent protein vaccines (vax) were given to groups of 5 BALB/c or C57BL/6 mice two weeks apart, with mouse splenocytes being harvested one week after the final dose (sac). (**B**) Cellular responses of BALB/c and

C57BL/6 mice measured using IFNγ ELISPOT after overnight stimulation with peptide pools. Responses were minimal for LMP1vax, but much larger for EBNA1vax and LMP2Avax. (**C**) Cellular response measured by flow cytometry. IFNγ staining of cells was measured following their stimulation with latent protein peptides. Pooled EBNA1, LMP1, and LMP2A peptides were used for stimulation. (**D**) The gating of representative examples of the BALB/c CD8 data is shown. Peptide stimulated splenocytes from a mouse vaccinated with the combination vaccine are shown on the left, and control cells left in media are shown on the right. *$p < 0.05$, **$p < 0.01$, ns: not significant.

IFNγ responses to latent protein peptide pools were evaluated using an ELISPOT assay (Figure 2B). Splenocytes from mice vaccinated with EBNA1vax generated an average of 81 spot forming units (sfu) per million cells for the individual vaccine and 104 sfu for the combined triple vaccine in BALB/c mice, an insignificant difference. A more robust 340 sfu were observed for the same vaccine in C57BL/6 mice, whereas the combination vaccine was much less immunogenic, suggesting that other antigens in the mixture were more a focus of the immune response. LMP2Avax generated responses in both mouse strains as an individual vaccination and in combination with the other antigens. BALB/c mice showed 102 sfu for the individual vaccine and 80 sfu for the combined, and C57BL/6 mice exhibited 83 sfu for LMP2A vax alone and 178 sfu in combination. LMP1vax produced a more modest response of 15 sfu in BALB/c mice that was only notable in the combination vaccine and not observed in the C57BL/6 animals. The modifications that were made to LMP1vax may have limited its immunogenicity. Additional engineering was undertaken to enhance the immunity of the LMP1 antigen. Modified constructs involved the inclusion of an IgE leader sequence coincident with truncation of the N-terminal native sequence, as well as inclusion by gene fusion of tetanus toxoid fragments as part of the ORF. Two constructs were made, one with a short peptide fragment inserted at the C-terminus (LMP1tt30) and the other with a 256 amino acid fragment inserted after the leader sequence (LMP1ttDOM). This design improved the immunity generated by the fusion antigen vaccine (Appendix A Figure A2).

Evaluation of IFNγ by flow cytometry was showed that CD8 cells were driving the immune response (Figure 2C). The triple vaccine generated more robust CD4 and CD8 responses in BALB/c mice, with greater CD8 responses than in the C57BL/6 mice. Overall, the responses induced appeared to be more potent for the induction of CD8 T cell immunity, with a smaller percentage of CD4 T cell induction, suggesting the vaccine is CD8 T cell biased. Gating for the flow cytometry data is shown in Figure 2D.

3.4. CD8 Cellular Responses Were Robust in Outbred CD-1 Mice

To further study these immunogens in a more relevant outbred animal model, we next vaccinated CD-1 mice and compared their responses to control-vaccinated animals. These mice were vaccinated three times at two-week intervals, and immune studies were performed a week after the final vaccination (Figure 3A). Cellular responses were once again more robust for EBNA1 and LMP2A than for LMP1, as was again observed in the inbred mouse models. However, stimulation with each of the latent protein peptide pools produced some responses, as measured by IFNγ ELISPOT (Figure 3B). CD8 responses were dominant when the splenocytes were analyzed by flow cytometry, and CD4 responses were lower (Figure 3C). The CD-1 response supports the CD8 potency of this vaccine approach.

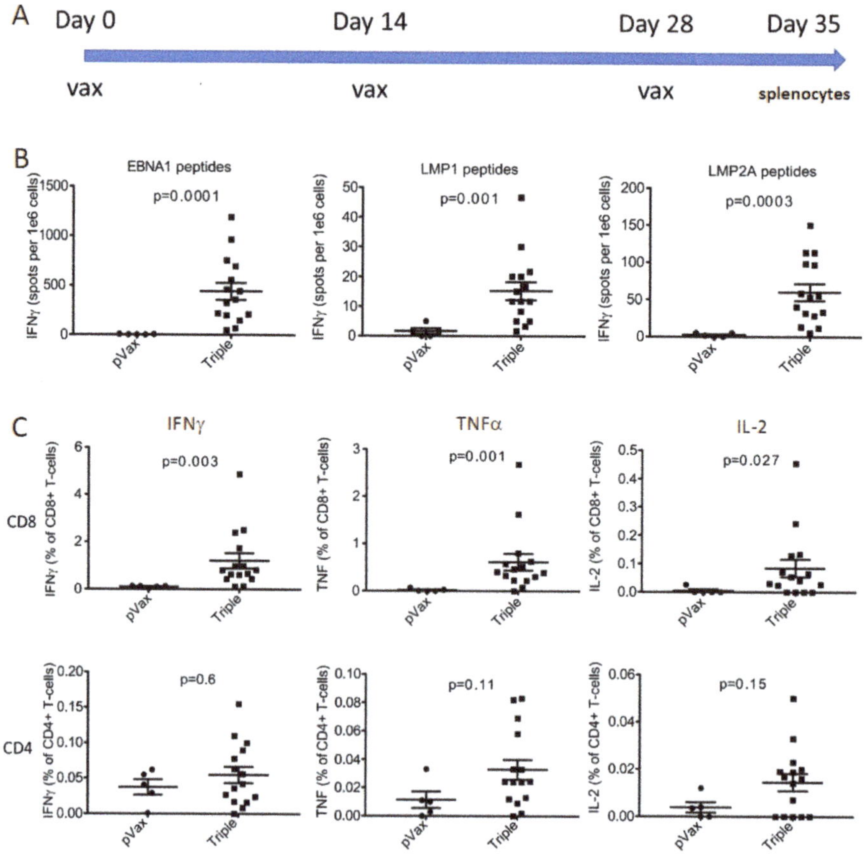

Figure 3. Cellular responses produced by combination vaccine in outbred CD-1 mice. (**A**) Vaccination schedule in outbred CD-1 mice. Mice were vaccinated with a combination of EBNA1vax, LMP1vax, and LMP2Avax three times at biweekly intervals, followed by harvesting of their splenocytes a week after the final vaccination. (**B**) Cellular responses to respective peptide pools, shown by IFNγ ELISPOT. (**C**) Plots showing CD4 or CD8 responses of CD-1 mice immunized with the triple vaccine or empty vector (pVax), stimulated with pooled peptides derived from EBNA1, LMP2A and LMP1. Cellular responses are driven by CD8+ cells, as shown by flow cytometry following stimulation of splenocytes.

3.5. LMP2Avax Delays Tumor Growth

In order to study the possible impact on an EBV+ tumor expressing a model LMP2A antigen, we next generated a murine epithelial tumor cell line using TC-1 cells that were constructed to express LMP2A using a retroviral transduction system. This may cause high expression of LMP2A relative to EBV-associated tumor cells, but LMP2A protein is expressed in the cancer cells of patients and its epitopes are recognized by T cells [54]. This cell line serves as a vaccine target for our LMP2A immunogens. We generated and selected the LMP2A line as shown in Figure 4A. Briefly, retroviral vectors produced by transfecting Phoenix cells with pBMN plasmids containing GFP and LMP2A were used to stably transduce TC-1 cells. These cells underwent selection via fluorescence-activated cell sorting (FACS) and single-cell cloning to produce a homogenous population expressing LMP2A, and this population was used to introduce tumors into mice.

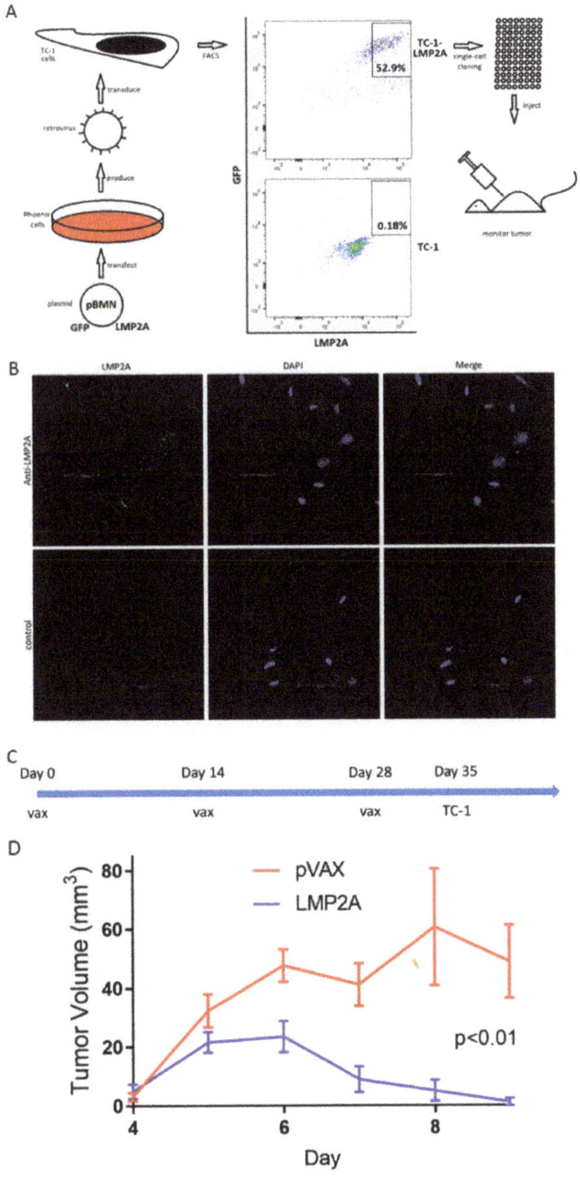

Figure 4. LMP2Avax inhibits tumor growth in mice. (**A**) Workflow to produce tumor cell lines expressing target antigen, in this case TC-1-LMP2A. (**B**) Immunofluorescence assay demonstrating LMP2A expression in TC-1-LMP2A cell line. DAPI is shown in blue, with LMP2A labeled in green. Anti-LMP2A antibodies were used as primary Abs (top), with secondary Abs conjugated to AF647. Anti-EBNA1 primary antibodies were used as a negative control (bottom). Scale bars are 50 μm. (**C**) Vaccination schedule prior to tumor introduction. Two groups of five C57BL/6 mice received three biweekly vaccinations followed by the subcutaneous axillary injection of 2 million TC-1 cells stably expressing LMP2A. The vaccines used 20 μg of DNA in 30 μL of water delivered by electroporation, with the vaccine group receiving plasmid encoding LMP2Avax and the control receiving the empty vector pVAX. Tumor sizes were monitored daily afterwards. (**D**) TC-1-LMP2A tumor volume over time in mice vaccinated with LMP2A or empty vector. Bars show scanning electron microscopy (SEM).

The expression of LMP2A in the derived TC-1-LMP2A tumor line was confirmed by antibody reactivity as demonstrated by immunofluorescence in Figure 4B. We next studied the use of this cell line as a tumor challenge antigen. C57BL/6 mice received either the LMP2Avax DNA vaccine or empty vector three times at biweekly intervals, followed by an axillary injection of 2 million tumor cells after the final vaccination (Figure 4C). LMP2Avax vaccinated mice showed a smaller tumor volume and more rapid tumor shrinkage than those vaccinated with the empty vector, demonstrating the anti-tumor immunogenic potential of the LMP2Avax vaccine (Figure 4D).

4. Discussion

EBV, formally known as human gammaherpesvirus 4, is responsible for infectious mononucleosis, multiple premalignant conditions, and various EBV-driven cancers. These cancers include Burkitt Lymphoma, Hodgkin's lymphoma, gastric cancer, nasopharyngeal carcinoma, HIV-associated oral hairy leukoplakia, and numerous other lymphoproliferative disorders. Additionally, EBV infection is associated with nonmalignant diseases and significant autoimmune disorders [55]. The worldwide burden of EBV-associated cancer is approximately 150,000 deaths per year, which represents almost 2% of all deaths from cancers. This burden continues to grow. EBV-associated gastric and nasopharyngeal carcinomas are each responsible for over 60,000 cancer deaths per year, and the incidence of the latter is increasing [56]. In light of this burden, additional approaches to EBV immunotherapy are important.

Here, we engineered synthetic consensus DNA vaccines of modified EBV latent proteins to generate immune responses which could impact tumor regression. Latent proteins are present in both lymphomas and carcinomas associated with EBV, and these have been studied as potential targets in various immunotherapeutic strategies. Currently there is no licensed approach for EBV immunotherapy. Cellular therapies have been studied in small trials and have shown some important effects [57,58]. However, these were early studies and additional approaches would be highly beneficial.

Along these lines, work in the HPV setting with SynCon DNA vaccines delivered by adaptive EP has evolved to be a robust approach for induction of antiviral cellular immunity, which can impact tumors and precancers in vivo [26,27]. We tested this approach here for a three-antigen synthetic DNA vaccine approach targeting the major EBV latent oncoproteins. We chose these antigen targets because they are present in EBV-associated cancers. Small trials of cellular therapies targeting EBNA1 [59] and LMPs [25,60,61] have shown improved outcomes against EBV-associated diseases. The high frequency of nasopharyngeal carcinoma concentrated in east Asia makes for a unique environment to test prophylactic and therapeutic approaches targeting the virus [62]. The frequency of Hodgkin's lymphoma in Europe and its temporal association with infectious mononucleosis offers another opportunity [7]. The growing burden of EBV in the US suggests immunotherapy for nasopharyngeal and gastric cancer as well as association of EBV with more common autoimmune disorders may also be important to consider as amenable to robust immunotherapy approaches [61].

Synthetic DNA vaccines can drive in vivo immune responses via MHC class I and II presentation through their delivery of and intracellular production of genetically encoded antigens. Newer delivery approaches have resulted in the generation of more consistent and robust immunity that can target cancer in the clinic [26,27]. Here we show that these designed latent antigen vaccines elicit significant cytotoxic T lymphocyte responses against the encoded vaccine targets EBNA1vax and LMP2Avax, which showed dominant CD8 T cell responses in vivo. These cellular responses are important in protecting mouse models from EBV antigen-expressing tumors in murine vaccine models, as recently shown in a novel heterologous prime-boost approach that impacted an EBNA1 tumor challenge [63]. Importantly, LMP2Avax-induced immunity protected against tumor growth in a TC-1 challenge model where LMP2A was targeted by the immunization. The immune responses produced by EBNA1vax and LMP2Avax merit further study. In addition, continued engineering may be interesting in this regard, as DNA delivery of LMP1 as an immunogen can clearly impact tumor growth as a standalone antigen in some models [28]. Combination development for this group of immunogens appears worthy of additional attention.

Recent developments in the DNA platform in formulation, engineering and delivery by adaptive EP have led to improved immune potency and improved consistency in clinical studies [26,27]. In these studies, we noted that the vaccines were biased towards driving highly desired CD8 immunity against the vaccine targets over CD4 immunity. This CD8 bias may be particularly relevant for clearing virally infected cells by cytotoxic T lymphocyte induction that would ultimately kill tumor cells. These latent antigen vaccines could be studied in the context of epithelial tumors, such as gastric and nasopharyngeal carcinomas, among others. The addition of checkpoint inhibitors in the context of these immunizations, as we have reported for HPV, might also be of interest for impacting EBV-related tumor progression [26,27,64].

5. Conclusions

There is a great need for new approaches targeting EBV, against which there are no licensed vaccines or immunotherapies available. Acute infection can lead to infectious mononucleosis, and the risk of autoimmune diseases such as multiple sclerosis is increased following symptomatic infection. Immunotherapy targeting conserved, expressed, and oncogenic viral genes has the potential to drive immunity that impacts EBV-associated cancers. Here we generated synthetic DNA immunogens targeting the EBV latent proteins EBNA1, LMP1, and LMP2. These engineered SynCon DNA vaccines were delivered by Cellectra EP into mice to study their immune responses. The combination of immunogens generated significant CD8 T cell responses. In addition, these responses impacted tumor growth in a mouse challenge model. Further study of this combination synthetic DNA approach in EBV-driven disease is warranted.

Author Contributions: Conceptualization, A.P.-P., D.B.W. and K.W.; methodology, A.P.-P. and K.W.; validation, A.P.-P. and K.W.; formal analysis, A.P.-P. and K.W.; investigation, A.P.-P. and K.W.; data curation, A.P.-P. and K.W.; Writing—Original Draft preparation, K.W.; Writing—Review and Editing, A.P.-P., D.B.W. and K.W.; visualization, A.P.-P. and K.W.; supervision, D.B.W.; project administration, A.P.-P. and K.W.; funding acquisition, D.B.W.

Funding: This work was supported by a University of Pennsylvania/Wistar Institute NIH Special Program of Research Excellence grant (P50 CA174523 to D.B.W.), the Wistar National Cancer Institute Cancer Center (P30 CA010815), the W.W. Smith Family Trust (to D.B.W.), a grant from Inovio Pharmaceuticals (to D.B.W.), and T32 CA 9171-41 (K.W.).

Acknowledgments: We would like to thank the Wistar Flow Cytometry Facility and Animal Facility for their technical assistance.

Conflicts of Interest: D.B.W. has received an SRA, has an ownership interest including IP, and performs Board service for Inovio, has received an SRA from and consulted for GeneOne; has received an SRA from and consulted with Geneos; and has served on advisory boards for AstraZeneca and Sanofi, among others. A.P.-P. is an employee at Inovio Pharmaceuticals. The other authors declare no conflicts of interest.

Appendix A

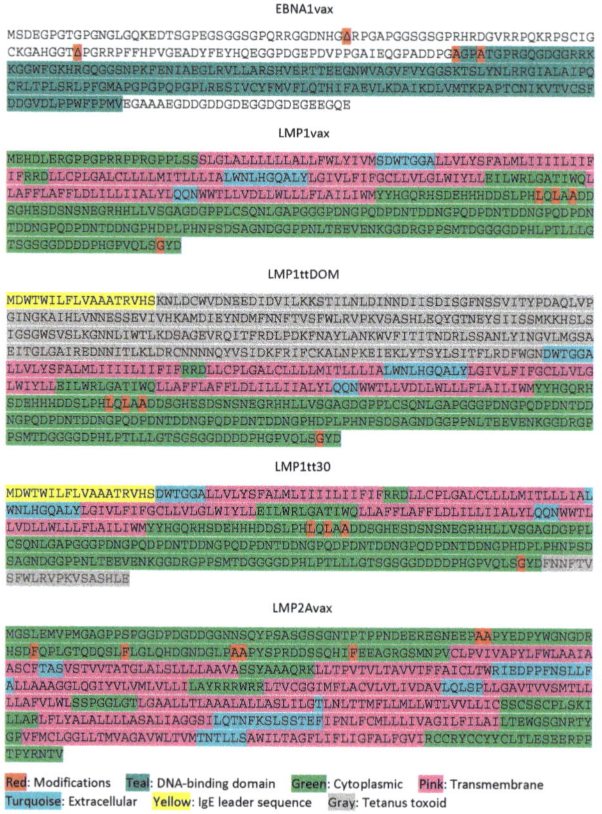

Figure A1. EBNA1vax contains deleted regions of glycine-arginine and glycine-alanine repeats marked by Δ (12 and 310 amino acid deletions) and has its DNA-binding domain highlighted. LMP1vax and LMP2Avax have their cytoplasmic, extracellular, and transmembrane regions indicated. Modifications to engineer LMP2Avax derivatives are labeled as well.

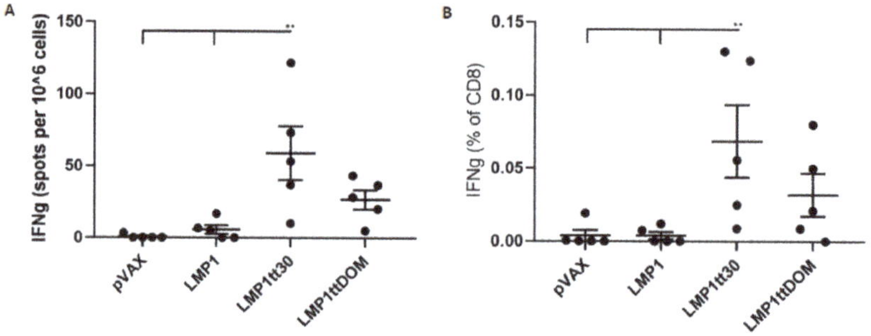

Figure A2. Engineered LMP1 vaccines enhance cellular immunity. The LMP1 antigen was truncated at the N-terminal, received an IgE leader sequence, and had tetanus toxoid added to its sequence. Splenocytes were stimulated with the 5 strongest MHC class I peptides to LMP1, as predicted in silico, after C57BL/6 mice were vaccinated. (**A**) IFNγ ELISPOT results showing an average of 59 sfu for LMP1tt30. (**B**) Flow cytometry data showing improved CD8 responses following plasmid engineering.

References

1. Balfour, H.H., Jr.; Sifakis, F.; Sliman, J.A.; Knight, J.A.; Schmeling, D.O.; Thomas, W. Age-Specific Prevalence of Epstein-Barr Virus Infection Among Individuals Aged 6-19 Years in the United States and Factors Affecting Its Acquisition. *J. Infect. Dis.* **2013**, *208*, 1286–1293. [CrossRef]
2. Dunmire, S.K.; Verghese, P.S.; Balfour, H.H. Primary Epstein-Barr virus infection. *J. Clin. Virol.* **2018**, *102*, 84–92. [CrossRef]
3. Sample, J.; Young, L.; Martin, B.; Chatman, T.; Kieff, E.; Rickinson, A.; Kieff, E. Epstein-Barr virus types 1 and 2 differ in their EBNA-3A, EBNA-3B, and EBNA-3C genes. *J. Virol.* **1990**, *64*, 4084–4092.
4. Choi, S.; Jung, S.; Huh, S.; Cho, H.; Kang, H. Phylogenetic comparison of Epstein-Barr virus genomes. *J. Microbiol.* **2018**, *56*, 525–533. [CrossRef]
5. Purtilo, D.T. Epstein-Barr Virus: The Spectrum of Its Manifestations in Human Beings. *South. Med. J.* **1987**, *80*, 943–947. [CrossRef]
6. Epstein, M.A.; Achong, B.G.; Barr, Y.M. Virus Particles in Cultured Lymphoblasts from Burkitt's Lymphoma. *Lancet* **1964**, *1*, 702–703. [CrossRef]
7. Hjalgrim, H.; Askling, J.; Rostgaard, K.; Hamilton-Dutoit, S.; Frisch, M.; Zhang, J.S.; Madsen, M.; Rosdahl, N.; Konradsen, H.B.; Storm, H.H.; et al. Characteristics of Hodgkin's lymphoma after infectious mononucleosis. *N. Engl. J. Med.* **2003**, *349*, 1324–1332. [CrossRef]
8. Zur Hausen, H.; Schulte-Holthausen, H.; Klein, G.; Henle, W.; Henle, G.; Clifford, P.; Santesson, L. EBV DNA in biopsies of Burkitt tumours and anaplastic carcinomas of the nasopharynx. *Nature* **1970**, *228*, 1056–1058. [CrossRef]
9. Lin, J.C.; Wang, W.Y.; Chen, K.Y.; Wei, Y.H.; Liang, W.M.; Jan, J.S.; Jiang, R.S. Quantification of plasma Epstein-Barr virus DNA in patients with advanced nasopharyngeal carcinoma. *N. Engl. J. Med.* **2004**, *350*, 2461–2470. [CrossRef]
10. Murphy, G.; Pfeiffer, R.; Camargo, M.C.; Rabkin, C.S. Meta-analysis shows that prevalence of Epstein-Barr virus-positive gastric cancer differs based on sex and anatomic location. *Gastroenterology* **2009**, *137*, 824–833. [CrossRef]
11. Belbasis, L.; Bellou, V.; Evangelou, E.; Ioannidis, J.P.; Tzoulaki, I. Environmental risk factors and multiple sclerosis: An umbrella review of systematic reviews and meta-analyses. *Lancet Neurol.* **2015**, *14*, 263–273. [CrossRef]
12. Li, Z.X.; Zeng, S.; Wu, H.X.; Zhou, Y. The risk of systemic lupus erythematosus associated with Epstein-Barr virus infection: A systematic review and meta-analysis. *Clin. Exp. Med.* **2019**, *19*, 23–36. [CrossRef]
13. Draborg, A.H.; Duus, K.; Houen, G. Epstein-Barr Virus in Systemic Autoimmune Diseases. *Clin. Dev. Immunol.* **2013**. [CrossRef]
14. Brooks, L.; Yao, Q.Y.; Rickinson, A.B.; Young, L.S. Epstein-Barr virus latent gene transcription in nasopharyngeal carcinoma cells: Coexpression of EBNA1, LMP1, and LMP2 transcripts. *J. Virol.* **1992**, *66*, 2689–2697.
15. Ma, S.; Tsai, M.H.; Romero-Masters, J.C.; Ranheim, E.A.; Huebner, S.M.; Bristol, J.A.; Delecluse, H.J.; Kenney, S.C. Latent Membrane Protein 1 (LMP1) and LMP2A Collaborate To Promote Epstein-Barr Virus-Induced B Cell Lymphomas in a Cord Blood-Humanized Mouse Model but Are Not Essential. *J. Virol.* **2017**, *91*. [CrossRef]
16. Wang, L.W.; Jiang, S.; Gewurz, B.E. Epstein-Barr Virus LMP1-Mediated Oncogenicity. *J. Virol.* **2017**, *91*. [CrossRef]
17. Vrzalikova, K.; Sunmonu, T.; Reynolds, G.; Murray, P. Contribution of Epstein-Barr Virus Latent Proteins to the Pathogenesis of Classical Hodgkin Lymphoma. *Pathogens* **2018**, *7*, 59. [CrossRef]
18. Longnecker, R.; Kieff, E. A second Epstein-Barr virus membrane protein (LMP2) is expressed in latent infection and colocalizes with LMP1. *J. Virol.* **1990**, *64*, 2319–2326.
19. El-Sharkawy, A.; Al Zaidan, L.; Malki, A. Epstein–Barr Virus-Associated Malignancies: Roles of Viral Oncoproteins in Carcinogenesis. *Front. Oncol.* **2018**, *8*, 265. [CrossRef]
20. Young, L.S.; Yap, L.F.; Murray, P.G. Epstein-Barr virus: more than 50 years old and still providing surprises. *Nat. Rev. Cancer* **2016**, *16*, 789–802. [CrossRef]

21. Minamitani, T.; Yasui, T.; Ma, Y.; Zhou, H.; Okuzaki, D.; Tsai, C.Y.; Sakakibara, S.; Gewurz, B.E.; Kieff, E.; Kikutani, H. Evasion of affinity-based selection in germinal centers by Epstein–Barr virus LMP2A. *Proc. Nat.l. Acad. Sci. USA* **2015**, *112*, 11612–11617. [CrossRef]
22. Sokal, E.M.; Hoppenbrouwers, K.; Vandermeulen, C.; Moutschen, M.; Léonard, P.; Moreels, A.; Haumont, M.; Bollen, A.; Smets, F.; Denis, M. Recombinant gp350 vaccine for infectious mononucleosis: A phase 2, randomized, double-blind, placebo-controlled trial to evaluate the safety, immunogenicity, and efficacy of an Epstein-Barr virus vaccine in healthy young adults. *J. Infect. Dis.* **2017**, *196*, 1749–1753. [CrossRef]
23. Van Zyl, D.G.; Mautner, J.; Delecluse, H. Progress in EBV Vaccines. *Front. Oncol.* **2019**, *9*, 104. [CrossRef]
24. Huang, J.; Fogg, M.; Wirth, L.J.; Daley, H.; Ritz, J.; Posner, M.R.; Wang, F.C.; Lorch, J.H. Epstein-Barr virus-specific adoptive immunotherapy for recurrent, metastatic nasopharyngeal carcinoma. *Cancer* **2017**, *123*, 2642–2650. [CrossRef]
25. Chia, W.K.; Teo, M.; Wang, W.W.; Lee, B.; Ang, S.F.; Tai, W.M.; Chee, C.L.; Ng, J.; Kan, R.; Lim, W.T.; et al. Adoptive T-cell transfer and chemotherapy in the first-line treatment of metastatic and/or locally recurrent nasopharyngeal carcinoma. *Mol. Ther.* **2014**, *22*, 132–139. [CrossRef]
26. Trimble, C.L.; Morrow, M.P.; Kraynyak, K.A.; Shen, X.; Dallas, M.; Yan, J.; Edwards, L.; Parker, R.L.; Denny, L.; Giffear, M.; et al. Safety, efficacy, and immunogenicity of VGX-3100, a therapeutic synthetic DNA vaccine targeting human papillomavirus 16 and 18 E6 and E7 proteins for cervical intraepithelial neoplasia 2/3: A randomised, double-blind, placebo-controlled phase 2b trial. *Lancet* **2015**, *386*, 2078–2088. [CrossRef]
27. Aggarwal, C.; Cohen, R.B.; Morrow, M.P.; Kraynyak, K.A.; Sylvester, A.J.; Knoblock, D.M.; Bauml, J.M.; Weinstein, G.S.; Lin, A.; Boyer, J.; et al. Immunotherapy Targeting HPV16/18 Generates Potent Immune Responses in HPV-Associated Head and Neck Cancer. *Clin. Cancer Res.* **2019**, *25*, 110–124. [CrossRef]
28. Lin, M.C.; Lin, Y.C.; Chen, S.T.; Young, T.H.; Lou, P.J. Therapeutic vaccine targeting Epstein-Barr virus latent protein, LMP1, suppresses LMP1-expressing tumor growth and metastasis in vivo. *BMC Cancer* **2017**, *17*, 1. [CrossRef]
29. Lei, L.; Li, J.; Liu, M.; Hu, X.; Zhou, Y.; Yang, S. CD40L-adjuvanted DNA vaccine carrying EBV-LMP2 antigen enhances anti-tumor effect in NPC transplantation tumor animal. *Cent. Eur. J. Immunol.* **2018**, *43*, 117–122. [CrossRef]
30. Levitskaya, J.; Coram, M.; Levitsky, V.; Imreh, S.; Steigerwald-Mullen, P.M.; Klein, G.; Kurilla, M.G.; Masucci, M.G. Inhibition of antigen processing by the internal repeat region of the Epstein-Barr virus nuclear antigen-1. *Nature* **1995**, *375*, 685–688. [CrossRef]
31. Yin, Y.; Manoury, B.; Fåhraeus, R. Self-inhibition of synthesis and antigen presentation by Epstein-Barr virus-encoded EBNA1. *Science* **2003**, *301*, 1371–1374. [CrossRef]
32. Apcher, S.; Komarova, A.; Daskalogianni, C.; Yin, Y.; Malbert-Colas, L.; Fåhraeus, R. mRNA translation regulation by the Gly-Ala repeat of Epstein-Barr virus nuclear antigen 1. *J. Virol.* **2009**, *83*, 1289–1298. [CrossRef]
33. Saridakis, V.; Sheng, Y.; Sarkari, F.; Holowaty, M.N.; Shire, K.; Nguyen, T.; Zhang, R.G.; Liao, J.; Lee, W.; Edwards, A.M.; et al. Structure of the p53 binding domain of HAUSP/USP7 bound to Epstein-Barr nuclear antigen 1 implications for EBV-mediated immortalization. *Mol. Cell* **2005**, *18*, 25–36. [CrossRef]
34. Rothenberger, S.; Burns, K.; Rousseaux, M.; Tschopp, J.; Bron, C. Ubiquitination of the Epstein-Barr virus-encoded latent membrane protein 1 depends on the integrity of the TRAF binding site. *Oncogene* **2003**, *22*, 5614–5618. [CrossRef]
35. Floettmann, J.E.; Rowe, M. Epstein-Barr virus latent membrane protein-1 (LMP1) C-terminus activation region 2 (CTAR2) maps to the far C-terminus and requires oligomerisation for NF-kappaB activation. *Oncogene* **1997**, *15*, 1851–1858. [CrossRef]
36. Winberg, G.; Matskova, L.; Chen, F.; Plant, P.; Rotin, D.; Gish, G.; Ingham, R.; Ernberg, I.; Pawson, T. Latent membrane protein 2A of Epstein-Barr virus binds WW domain E3 protein-ubiquitin ligases that ubiquitinate B-cell tyrosine kinases. *Mol. Cell. Biol.* **2000**, *20*, 8526–8535. [CrossRef]
37. Ikeda, M.; Ikeda, A.; Longan, L.C.; Longnecker, R. The Epstein-Barr virus latent membrane protein 2A PY motif recruits WW domain-containing ubiquitin-protein ligases. *Virology* **2000**, *268*, 178–191. [CrossRef]
38. Fruehling, S.; Swart, R.; Dolwick, K.M.; Kremmer, E.; Longnecker, R. Tyrosine 112 of latent membrane protein 2A is essential for protein tyrosine kinase loading and regulation of Epstein-Barr virus latency. *J. Virol.* **1998**, *72*, 7796–7806.

39. Fotheringham, J.A.; Coalson, N.E.; Raab-Traub, N. Epstein-Barr virus latent membrane protein-2A induces ITAM/Syk- and Akt-dependent epithelial migration through αv-integrin membrane translocation. *J. Virol.* **2012**, *86*, 10308–10320. [CrossRef]
40. Muthumani, K.; Falzarano, D.; Reuschel, E.L.; Tingey, C.; Flingai, S.; Villarreal, D.O.; Wise, M.; Patel, A.; Izmirly, A.; Aljuaid, A.; et al. A synthetic consensus anti–spike protein DNA vaccine induces protective immunity against Middle East respiratory syndrome coronavirus in nonhuman primates. *Sci. Transl. Med.* **2015**, *7*. [CrossRef]
41. Tesone, A.J.; Rutkowski, M.R.; Brencicova, E.; Svoronos, N.; Perales-Puchalt, A.; Stephen, T.L.; Allegrezza, M.J.; Payne, K.K.; Nguyen, J.M.; Wickramasinghe, J.; et al. Satb1 Overexpression Drives Tumor-Promoting Activities in Cancer-Associated Dendritic Cells. *Cell Rep.* **2016**, *14*, 1774–1786. [CrossRef]
42. Perales-Puchalt, A.; Wojtak, K.; Duperret, E.K.; Yang, X.; Slager, A.M.; Yan, J.; Muthumani, K.; Montaner, L.J.; Weiner, D.B. Engineered DNA Vaccination against Follicle-Stimulating Hormone Receptor Delays Ovarian Cancer Progression in Animal Models. *Mol. Ther.* **2019**, *27*, 314–325. [CrossRef]
43. Duperret, E.K.; Perales-Puchalt, A.; Stoltz, R.; Hiranjith, G.H.; Mandloi, N.; Barlow, J.; Chaudhuri, A.; Sardesai, N.Y.; Weiner, D.B. A Synthetic DNA, Multi-Neoantigen Vaccine Drives Predominately MHC Class I $CD8^+$ T-cell Responses, Impacting Tumor Challenge. *Cancer Immunol. Res.* **2019**, *7*, 174–182. [CrossRef]
44. Duperret, E.K.; Liu, S.; Paik, M.; Trautz, A.; Stoltz, R.; Liu, X.; Ze, K.; Perales-Puchalt, A.; Reed, C.; Yan, J.; et al. A Designer Cross-reactive DNA Immunotherapeutic Vaccine that Targets Multiple MAGE-A Family Members Simultaneously for Cancer Therapy. *Clin. Cancer Res.* **2018**, *24*, 6015–6027. [CrossRef]
45. Perales-Puchalt, A.; Svoronos, N.; Villarreal, D.O.; Zankharia, U.; Reuschel, E.; Wojtak, K.; Payne, K.K.; Duperret, E.K.; Muthumani, K.; Conejo-Garcia, J.R.; et al. IL-33 delays metastatic peritoneal cancer progression inducing an allergic microenvironment. *Oncoimmunology* **2019**, *8*, e1515058. [CrossRef]
46. Choi, H.; Kudchodkar, S.B.; Reuschel, E.L.; Asija, K.; Borole, P.; Ho, M.; Wojtak, K.; Reed, C.; Ramos, S.; Bopp, N.E.; et al. Protective immunity by an engineered DNA vaccine for Mayaro virus. *PLoS Negl. Trop. Dis.* **2019**, *13*, e0007042. [CrossRef]
47. Khoshnejad, M.; Patel, A.; Wojtak, K.; Kudchodkar, S.B.; Humeau, L.; Lyssenko, N.N.; Rader, D.J.; Muthumani, K.; Weiner, D.B. Development of Novel DNA-Encoded PCSK9 Monoclonal Antibodies as Lipid-Lowering Therapeutics. *Mol. Ther.* **2019**, *27*, 188–199. [CrossRef]
48. Wan, Y.; Kang, G.; Sreenivasan, C.; Daharsh, L.; Zhang, J.; Fan, W.; Wang, D.; Moriyama, H.; Li, F.; Li, Q. A DNA Vaccine Expressing Consensus Hemagglutinin-Esterase Fusion Protein Protected Guinea Pigs from Infection by Two Lineages of Influenza D Virus. *J. Viro.* **2018**, *92*. [CrossRef]
49. Santra, S.; Korber, B.T.; Muldoon, M.; Barouch, D.H.; Nabel, G.J.; Gao, F.; Hahn, B.H.; Haynes, B.F.; Letvin, N.L. A Centralized Gene-Based HIV-1 Vaccine Elicits Broad Cross-Clade Cellular Immune Responses in Rhesus Monkeys. *Proc. Natl. Acad. Sci. USA* **2008**, *105*, 10489–10494. [CrossRef]
50. Shedlock, D.J.; Aviles, J.; Talbott, K.T.; Wong, G.; Wu, S.J.; Villarreal, D.O.; Myles, D.J.; Croyle, M.A.; Yan, J.; Kobinger, G.P.; et al. Induction of Broad Cytotoxic T Cells by Protective DNA Vaccination Against Marburg and Ebola. *Mol. Ther.* **2013**, *21*, 1432–1444. [CrossRef]
51. Zhou, L.; Chen, J.N.; Qiu, X.M.; Pan, Y.H.; Zhang, Z.G.; Shao, C.K. Comparative analysis of 22 Epstein–Barr virus genomes from diseased and healthy individuals. *J. Gen. Virol.* **2017**, *98*, 96–107. [CrossRef]
52. Tebas, P.; Kraynyak, K.A.; Patel, A.; Maslow, J.N.; Morrow, M.P.; Sylvester, A.J.; Knoblock, D.; Gillespie, E.; Amante, D.; Racine, T.; et al. Intradermal SynCon® Ebola GP DNA Vaccine is Temperature Stable and Safely Demonstrates Cellular and Humoral Immunogenicity Advantages in Healthy Volunteers. *J. Infect. Dis.* **2019**. [CrossRef]
53. Tebas, P.; Roberts, C.C.; Muthumani, K.; Reuschel, E.L.; Kudchodkar, S.B.; Zaidi, F.I.; White, S.; Khan, A.S.; Racine, T.; Choi, H.; et al. Safety and Immunogenicity of an Anti-Zika Virus DNA Vaccine—Preliminary Report. *N. Engl. J. Med.* **2017**. [CrossRef]
54. Heussinger, N.; Büttner, M.; Ott, G.; Brachtel, E.; Pilch, B.Z.; Kremmer, E.; Niedobitek, G. Expression of the Epstein-Barr virus (EBV)-encoded latent membrane protein 2A (LMP2A) in EBV-associated nasopharyngeal carcinoma. *J. Pathol.* **2004**, *203*, 696–699. [CrossRef]
55. Dasari, V.; Bhatt, K.H.; Smith, C.; Khanna, R. Designing an effective vaccine to prevent Epstein-Barr virus-associated diseases: Challenges and opportunities. *Expert Rev. Vaccines* **2017**, *16*, 377–390. [CrossRef]
56. Khan, G.; Hashim, M.J. Global burden of deaths from Epstein-Barr virus attributable malignancies 1990–2010. *Infect. Agent Cancer* **2014**, *9*, 38. [CrossRef]

57. Comoli, P.; Pedrazzoli, P.; Maccario, R.; Basso, S.; Carminati, O.; Labirio, M.; Schiavo, R.; Secondino, S.; Frasson, C.; Perotti, C.; et al. Cell Therapy of Stage IV Nasopharyngeal Carcinoma With Autologous Epstein-Barr Virus–Targeted Cytotoxic T Lymphocytes. *J. Clin. Oncol.* **2005**, *23*, 8942–8949. [CrossRef]
58. Smith, C.; Tsang, J.; Beagley, L.; Chua, D.; Lee, V.; Li, V.; Moss, D.J.; Coman, W.; Chan, K.H.; Nicholls, J.; et al. Effective treatment of metastatic forms of Epstein-Barr virus-associated nasopharyngeal carcinoma with a novel adenovirus-based adoptive immunotherapy. *Cancer Res.* **2012**, *72*, 1116–1125. [CrossRef]
59. Icheva, V.; Kayser, S.; Wolff, D.; Tuve, S.; Kyzirakos, C.; Bethge, W.; Greil, J.; Albert, M.H.; Schwinger, W.; Nathrath, M.; et al. Adoptive Transfer of Epstein-Barr Virus (EBV) Nuclear Antigen 1–Specific T Cells As Treatment for EBV Reactivation and Lymphoproliferative Disorders After Allogeneic Stem-Cell Transplantation. *J. Clin. Oncol.* **2013**, *31*, 39–48. [CrossRef]
60. Bollard, C.M.; Gottschalk, S.; Torrano, V.; Diouf, O.; Ku, S.; Hazrat, Y.; Carrum, G.; Ramos, C.; Fayad, L.; Shpall, E.J.; et al. Sustained Complete Responses in Patients With Lymphoma Receiving Autologous Cytotoxic T Lymphocytes Targeting Epstein-Barr Virus Latent Membrane Proteins. *J. Clin. Oncol.* **2014**, *32*, 798–808. [CrossRef]
61. Pender, M.P.; Csurhes, P.A.; Smith, C.; Douglas, N.L.; Neller, M.A.; Matthews, K.K.; Beagley, L.; Rehan, S.; Crooks, P.; Hopkins, T.J.; et al. Epstein-Barr virus-specific T cell therapy for progressive multiple sclerosis. *JCI Insight* **2018**, *3*. [CrossRef] [PubMed]
62. Yu, M.C.; Yuan, J. Epidemiology of nasopharyngeal carcinoma. *Semin.n Cancer Biol.* **2002**, *12*, 421–429. [CrossRef]
63. Rühl, J.; Citterio, C.; Engelmann, C.; Haigh, T.A.; Dzionek, A.; Dreyer, J.H.; Khanna, R.; Taylor, G.S.; Wilson, J.B.; Leung, C.S.; et al. Heterologous prime-boost vaccination protects against EBV antigen-expressing lymphomas. *J. Clin. Invest.* **2019**, *129*, 2071–2087. [CrossRef] [PubMed]
64. Perales-Puchalt, A.; Duperret, E.K.; Muthumani, K.; Weiner, D.B. Simplifying checkpoint inhibitor delivery through in vivo generation of synthetic DNA-encoded monoclonal antibodies (DMAbs). *Oncotarget* **2019**, *10*, 13–16. [CrossRef]

vaccines

MDPI

Article

In silico Designed Ebola Virus T-Cell Multi-Epitope DNA Vaccine Constructions Are Immunogenic in Mice

Sergei I. Bazhan *, Denis V. Antonets, Larisa I. Karpenko, Svetlana F. Oreshkova, Olga N. Kaplina, Ekaterina V. Starostina, Sergei G. Dudko, Sofia A. Fedotova and Alexander A. Ilyichev

State Research Center of Virology and Biotechnology "Vector", Koltsovo, 630559 Novosibirsk Region, Russia; antonec@nprog.ru (D.V.A.); karpenko@vector.nsc.ru (L.I.K.); sv_oresh@mail.ru (S.F.O.); okaplina@vector.nsc.ru (O.N.K.); starostina_ev@vector.nsc.ru (E.V.S.); s.g.dudko@gmail.com (S.G.D.); hz.smoke.on.the.water@gmail.com (S.A.F.); ilyichev@vector.nsc.ru (A.A.I.)

* Correspondence: bazhan@vector.nsc.ru; Tel.: +7-383-363-47-00 (ext. 2001)

Received: 5 March 2019; Accepted: 27 March 2019; Published: 29 March 2019

Abstract: *Background*: The lack of effective vaccines against Ebola virus initiates a search for new approaches to overcoming this problem. The aim of the study was to design artificial polyepitope T-cell immunogens—candidate DNA vaccines against Ebola virus and to evaluate their capacity to induce a specific immune response in a laboratory animal model. *Method*: Design of two artificial polyepitope T-cell immunogens, one of which (EV.CTL) includes cytotoxic and the other (EV.Th)—T-helper epitopes of Ebola virus proteins was carried out using original TEpredict/PolyCTLDesigner software. Synthesized genes were cloned in pcDNA3.1 plasmid vector. Target gene expression was estimated by synthesis of specific mRNAs and proteins in cells transfected with recombinant plasmids. Immunogenicity of obtained DNA vaccine constructs was evaluated according to their capacity to induce T-cell response in BALB/c mice using IFNγ ELISpot and ICS. *Results*: We show that recombinant plasmids pEV.CTL and pEV.Th encoding artificial antigens provide synthesis of corresponding mRNAs and proteins in transfected cells, as well as induce specific responses both to CD4+ and CD8+ T-lymphocytes in immunized animals. *Conclusions*: The obtained recombinant plasmids can be regarded as promising DNA vaccine candidates in future studies of their capacity to induce cytotoxic and protective responses against Ebola virus.

Keywords: ebola virus disease; artificial T-cell antigens; DNA vaccine constructs; computer design; gene expression; immunogenicity

1. Introduction

Ebola fever or Ebola virus disease (EVD) is an acute disease resulting in high rates of mortality. It is caused by RNA-containing viruses of *Filoviridae* family, genus *Ebolavirus*. Viruses of genus *Ebolavirus* belong to five species with different fatality rates and serologic properties: Zaire ebolavirus, Sudan ebolavirus, Bundibugyo ebolavirus, Tai Forrest ebolavirus, and Reston ebolavirus. The first outbreaks of EVD were registered in 1976 initially in Zaire (currently the Democratic Republic of the Congo) in the Ebola river area (Zaire species, genus Ebola) and almost concurrently in Sudan (Sudan species, genus Ebola). After that, sporadic outbreaks were registered over a period of 40 years in Central Africa countries, affecting from one to several dozens or even hundreds of people. All those outbreaks were successfully and timely controlled. The Ebola fever outbreak in Western Africa in 2014–2015 was found to be significantly extensive. To eliminate it, efforts of several countries across the world were required [1].

The main problems the doctors met with controlling Ebola fever included the absence of a vaccine and prophylactic drugs against this disease. Despite the high fatality rate, an epidemic danger of this agent was always believed to be insignificant. Expensive development of vaccines and therapeutic drugs against rare although lethal disease in each case seemed to be unprofitable and attracted interest only due to a potential bioterrorism threat. The 2014–2015 Ebola fever outbreak claimed more than 11 thousand lives, which enforced studies on countermeasures against this infection. Currently, active studies on development of control measures against the virus are being carried out including small interfering RNA, low-molecular compounds, and antibodies [2,3], drugs based on monoclonal antibodies [3], and, certainly, vaccines. There are a number of approaches to designing vaccines against Ebola virus including DNA vaccines, subunit vaccines, as well as vaccines based on virus-like particles and viral vectors such as adenoviruses HAdV-5, HAdV-26, ChAdV-3, vesicular stomatitis virus (VSV), human cytomegalovirus, and modified vaccinia virus Ankara (MVA) [4–6]. Their protective efficacy was evaluated in non-human primate models. Furthermore, to date, several vaccines to control the virus in humans were described, i.e., rVSV-ZEBOV [7], Ad5-ZEBOV [8], GamEvac-Combi [9], and others.

The majority of developed experimental vaccines were constructed based on genetically modified viruses encoding full-length viral antigens that induce responses of both antibodies and cytotoxic T-lymphocytes (CTL) [10]. However, it should be noted that data on the protective effect of neutralizing antibodies against filoviruses obtained in studies on NHP are contradictory. It was shown that some antibodies protect animals against further infection but fail to neutralize the virus, while others neutralize the virus but fail to protect animals [11]. Consequently, the relative significance of neutralizing antibodies compared with those that can provide protection using other mechanisms (e.g., antibody-dependent cell cytotoxicity or Fc-dependent mechanisms) is still unclear. Besides this, the question deserves to be asked about the role of non-neutralizing antibodies during protection against Ebola virus, considering the well-known effect of antibody-dependent enhancement of infection [12].

A number of Ebola virus vaccine candidates develop base on glycoprotein (GP). However, antibodies induced by such GP vaccines are typically autologous and limited to the other members of the same species. In contrast, T-cell vaccines designed on the basis of conservative regions of the filovirus proteins can protect against different members of the filovirus family. It was shown that simian adenovirus- and poxvirus MVA-vectored vaccines encoding cross-filovirus immunogen provided broad immunogenicity and a solid protection of the BALB/c and C57BL/6J mice against high, lethal challenges with Ebola and Marburg viruses, two distant members of the family [5].

Another promising trend in virus T-cell vaccine design is DNA vaccine. Compared with virus-vectored vaccines, DNA vaccines demonstrate a number of advantages [13]. They are inexpensive, non-infective, and simply produced in large quantities; they can be reused since previously existing immunity is of no importance for DNA-vectors compared to viral vectors. In addition, DNA-vaccination provides the most natural way of antigen presentation by both MHC class I and class II molecules, focusing the immune response only on antigen of interest, providing long-term persistence of immunogenicity, polarizing T-helper cells toward type 1 or type 2, and inducing protective humoral and cellular immune responses. The other important feature of DNA vaccines is the ability to put several antigens or several epitopes from different antigens in the plasmid, resulting in immunization against all of the agents; and a mixture of DNA plasmids can be used to form a broad spectrum of vaccines. At last, in vivo expression of gene of interest ensures the protein resembles the normal eukaryotic structure more closely, with accompanying post-translational modifications. The only disadvantage of DNA vaccine is their relatively low immunogenicity; thus, they require administration of several doses to achieve the desirable immunity [14]. However, this disadvantage can be evaded at present due to the strategy of intramuscular electroporation making it possible to significantly enhance DNA-vaccination efficiency [15–17]. In addition, to increase the immunogenicity of DNA vaccines it is possible to use other methods for delivery, for example, using VLPs [18] that include DNA plasmid, as well as by translating DNA vaccines into RNA vaccine format [19].

One of the promising trends in virus vaccine design is DNA vaccine encoding artificial polyepitope immunogens. These vaccines comprise a combination of conservative cytotoxic T-lymphocytes (CTL)-

and T-helper (Th)-epitopes selected from different viral proteins and combined in one molecule [20–22]. Progress in identifying T-cell epitopes, as well as understanding the mechanisms of processing and presentation of antigens by Major Histocompatibility Complex (MHC) class I and II pathways are instrumental for rational designing of artificial polyepitope vaccines inducing responses of cytotoxic (CD8+) and helper (CD4+) T-lymphocytes [20,22,23].

This study aims to design artificial polyepitope T-cell immunogens—candidate DNA vaccines against Ebola virus using computer-aided molecular design, and to study their capacity to induce a specific immune response in a laboratory animals model.

2. Materials and Methods

2.1. Software

Selection of known T-cell epitopes of Ebola viruses was carried out based on the IEDB—Immune Epitope Database (http://iedb.org) [24]. Prediction of T-cell epitopes was conducted using TEpredict software [25]. Design of polyepitope antigens was performed with PolyCTLDesigner [26]. Genes encoding target immunogens were developed using GeneDesigner software [27]; a compound of codons was optimized to achieve high expression of genes in human cells. Analysis of amino acid sequences of peptides, evaluating their conservatism, statistical analysis of obtained findings, and graph plotting were executed in statistical analysis environment R (version 3.2; https://www.R-project.org/, Vienna, Austria) [28].

2.2. Gene Synthesis and Cloning

Designed genes were synthesized (CJSC Eurogen, Moscow, Russia) and then cloned into pcDNA3.1 eukaryotic plasmid vector and sequenced. The obtained recombinant plasmids pEV.CTL and pEV.Th—candidate DNA vaccines against Ebola virus were used to prove the expression of designed target genes in eukaryotic cells and to assess their immunogenicity in mice of the BALB/c line.

2.3. Evaluation of Target Gene Transcription

Specific mRNA synthesis of target genes was evaluated in eukaryotic cells 293T transfected with pEV.CTL and pEV.Th using MATra-A reagent according to the manufacturer's instruction (PromoKine, Heidelberg, Germany). Cells were cultured in Dulbecco's Modified Eagle's Medium (DMEM) with 10% FBS. 48 h after transfection mRNAs were isolated from cells with a kit for RNA isolation (Promega, Madison, WI, USA). Before reverse transcription all RNA samples were treated with RNase-free DNase. cDNAs were obtained by reverse transcription using RevertAid H Minus First Strand cDNA Synthesis Kit (Thermo Scientific, Berlin, Germany). Further, the obtained cDNA carried out PCR with the use of specific primers to gene *EV.CTL* (f^{CTL}—AACTCAGGCACTCTTCCTGC, r^{CTL}—TCGTACCGGAATCTCAGGGT) and gene *EV.Th* (f^{Th}—ACGTTGACAAGCTGAGGAGG, r^{Th}—GAGAGTCCTCAGCCCAGAGA). The amplification product was analyzed by electrophoresis in 1% agarose gel.

2.4. Immunochemical Staining of Products of Transfected Cells

The presence of target proteins in eukaryotic cells 293T transfected with pEV.CTL and pEV.Th was detected through immunostaining. Cell transfection was carried out using MATra-A reagent according to the manufacturer's instruction (PromoKine, Germany). Cells were cultured in DMEM medium with 10% FBS. 32 h after transfection cells were washed in phosphate buffer solution (PBS), fixed in a mix of ice methanol/acetone (1:1) at 40 °C for 30 min, and then washed in PBS again. The expression products of *EV.CTL* and *EV.Th* gene were detected in immunochemical staining. Staining was carried out using antibodies MAT 29F2/30A6 (JSC Vector-Best, Novosibirsk, Russia) to marker epitope EPFRDYVDRFYKTL being a part of all constructs, and using conjugate of rabbit antibodies to mice IgG with horseradish peroxidase. When staining, 3.3′-Diaminobenzidine was used as substrate.

2.5. Ethics Statement

All experimental procedures in mice were made to minimize animal suffering and carried out in line with the principles of humanity described in the relevant Guidelines of the European Community and Helsinki Declaration. The protocols were approved by the Institutional Animal Care and Use Committee (IACUC) affiliated with State Research Center of Virology and Biotechnology "Vector" (Permit Number: SRC VB "Vector"/10-05.2016).

2.6. Immunization of Experimental Animals Ethics Statement

When immunizing, we used 5–6-week-old BALB/c mice (female) of weight 16–18 g from the State Research Center of Virology and Biotechnology Vector vivarium. Animals were divided into four groups with 5–10 mice in each group including (1) pE-CTL+pE-Th—mice immunized with a mix of DNA-vaccine pEV.CTL and pEV.Th encoding CTL- and Th-epitopes of Ebola virus, respectively; (2) pE-CTL—mice immunized with DNA plasmid pEV.CTL encoding CTL-epitopes of Ebola virus; (3) pDNA3.1—mice immunized with vector plasmid pDNA3.1 (negative control); and (4)—intact non-immunized animals to whom phosphate buffered saline was inoculated (PBS) (pH 7.6) (negative control). Mice were immunized three times intramuscularly with 100 μg DNA vaccine pEV.CTL or pEV.CTL + pEV.Th at 2-week intervals. An equivalent dose of pcDNA3.1 vector plasmid was used for mice from the control group. Two weeks after the last immunization, spleens were removed in animals and splenocytes were isolated to analyze T-cell immune response.

2.7. Detection of T-Cell Immune Response Using IFNγ ELISpot and Intracellular Cytokine Staining (ICS) Assay

Enzyme-Linked ImmunoSpot (ELISpot) and intracellular cytokine staining (ICS) assays were used to characterize the immune response of mice after immunization with DNA vaccines. Stimulation of splenocytes was carried out using a mix of synthetic peptides (KFINKLDALH, NYNGLLSSI, PGPAKFSLL, YFTFDLTALK, EYLFEVDNL, LFLRATTEL, and LYDRLASTV) from the compound of the designed antigens. Peptides were synthesized by Synpeptide Co., Ltd. (Shanghai, China) with >80% purity. Analysis of IFNγ ELISpot was performed with Mouse IFN-γ ELISPOT Set (BD, cat 551083, San Diego, CA, USA) according to the manufacturer's instruction and as previously described [29]. To stimulate splenocytes, we used a mix of peptides at concentration 20 μg/mL of each peptide to 1×10^6 cells followed by co-cultivation for 24 h. IFNγ-producing cells were calculated using an ELISpot-analyzer (Zeiss, Germany). ICS was performed according to the standard protocol of BD Biosciences as previously described [30]. To stimulate splenocytes, we used a mix of peptides at concentration 20 μg/mL of each peptide to 1×10^6 cells and incubated for 20 h at 37 °C and 5% CO_2 and additionally for 5 h with Brefeldin A. Cells were washed with PBS and permeabilized with Cytofix/Cytoperm™ Plus Fixation/Permeabilization Kit (BD Biosciences, San Diego, CA, USA). When staining, the following monoclonal antibodies were used: PerCP Rat Anti-Mouse CD4, FITC Rat Anti-Mouse CD8a, PE Hamster Anti-Mouse CD3ε, and APC Rat Anti-Mouse IFN-γ (BD Pharmingen, San Diego, CA, USA). The samples were analyzed using flow cytometer FACSCalibur (Becton Dickinson, San Jose, CA, USA) and Cell Quest software.

2.8. Statistical Analysis

Statistical analysis of the obtained results was carried out with the R software environment for statistical analysis (version 3.2; https://www.R-project.org/). To evaluate the significance of the differences among the groups, the Kruskal–Wallis test was applied. Pair-wise distribution comparison of the analyzed indices in the experimental and control groups was conducted using one-sided Mann–Whitney test. When multiple testing, FDR procedure was performed to correct p-values.

3. Results and Discussion

3.1. Strategies to Design Polyepitope T-Cell Antigens

To stimulate response of CD8+ T-lymphocytes, viral antigens must be presented to CTL precursors not as full-length molecules, but as short peptides (8–12 amino acid residues) in complex with MHC class I molecules. These epitopes are formed from endogenously synthesized viral antigens in the result of proteasome-mediated processing and then are transferred to ER lumina by means of a transporter associated with antigen processing (TAP) proteins where it binds to emerged MHC class I molecules (see for review [31,32]). Since proteasome-mediated processing functions for antigens synthesized intracellularly, a vaccine inducing T-cell response may be designed as DNA vaccine because in this case the CTL vaccine epitopes are presented in the most natural way—through MHC class I-dependent antigen presentation pathway [33].

Unlike stimulation of CTLs, while stimulating CD4+ T-lymphocytes-helpers response, antigen should be presented to those cells in complex with MHC class II molecules. Usually, antigen processing and presentation occurs for extracellular antigens which are delivered in cells via endocytosis and phagocytosis. In this case, antigen processing takes place in the lysosome.

Thus, when designing artificial polyepitope T-cell immunogens capable of inducing responses of CD4+ and CD8+ T-lymphocytes to all epitopes it comprises, it is necessary to provide efficient proteasome- and/or lysosome-mediated processing of the expression product of the target gene by MHC class I and II pathway.

Different strategies can help achieve this goal:

(1) To combine epitopes in the compound of poly-CTL-epitope construct one may use spacer sequences comprising sites of proteasomal cleavage [34–36] and/or motifs for binding to TAP [37,38].
(2) To combine epitopes in the compound of poly-Th-epitope construct one may use motif [KR][KR] which is a cleavage site for a number of lysosomal cathepsins involved in antigen processing [39,40].
(3) To direct polyepitope immunogen to proteasome and to present CTL-epitopes to CD8+ T-lymphocytes by MHC class I pathway, genetic binding of ubiquitin sequence to its N- or C-terminus is typically used [41].
(4) To degrade polyepitope immunogen and present released Th-epitopes to CD4+ T-lymphocytes by MHC class II pathway, genetic binding of sequence of LAMP-1 (Lysosomal-associated membrane protein 1) tyrosine motif to its C-terminus is typically used to direct polyepitope immunogen from the secretory pathway to the lysosome [42–45].

In our study, two artificial polyepitope T-cell immunogens were designed, one of which comprises cytotoxic (CTL) and the other—T-helper (Th) epitopes identified in Ebola virus proteins GP, VP24, VP30, VP35, L, VP40, and NP (Figure 1). Previously we showed that adding ubiquitin to N-terminus of polyepitope antigen induces CD8+ T-cell response more efficiently as compared to adding the signal peptide and the LAMP-1 C-terminal fragment [30]. Therefore, we added N-terminal ubiquitin to the final poly-CTL-epitope construct, and poly-Th-epitope immunogen was designed using N-terminal signal peptide and LAMP-1 C-terminal fragment. N-terminal signal peptide should direct the polyepitope to the endoplasmic reticulum (ER), and C-terminal fragment of LAMP-1 should redirect the polyepitope from the secretory pathway to the lysosome.

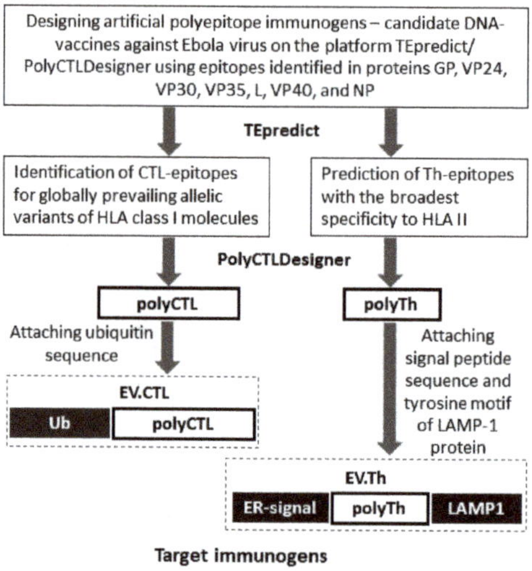

Figure 1. Designing artificial polyepitope antigens of Ebola virus.

3.2. *Design of Artificial Poly-CTL-Epitope Antigen of Ebola Virus*

For the purposes of designing poly-CTL-epitope antigen (EV.CTL), we used Immune Epitope Database (http://iedb.org) [24] to select known T-cell epitopes and peptide fragments of antigens of different Ebola virus strains with an experimentally verified capacity to bind to different allomorphs of MHC molecules. In total, at the time of antigen designing (2016) the database contained information on 1134 unique peptides from 65 antigens of 16 Ebola virus strains verified for their capacity to bind to 60 allomorphs of MHC class I molecules (56 Human Leukocyte Antigen (HLA) allelic variants). To analyze conservation of peptides, we used 14,556 amino acid sequences from NCBI ProteinBank (ncbi.nlm.nih.gov/protein) belonging to different Ebola viruses (Zaire ebolavirus, Sudan ebolavirus, Bundibugyo ebolavirus, Tai Forrest ebolavirus, and Reston ebolavirus). We considered peptides with experimentally verified cytotoxic activity. Furthermore, when designing target immunogens, we selected those with sufficiently high binding affinity to different HLA class I molecule variants (pIC50 > 6.3).

After that, we selected peptides identified at least in 1000 known viral sequences and interacting with at least two allelic HLA molecule variants. In total, we selected 44 peptides which cumulatively were restricted by 34 allelic HLA class I molecule variants including the most globally widespread ones (Table 1). It is known that optimally selected epitopes restricted by ten different HLA class I alleles cover virtually the entire population of any geographic region [46,47].

Based on the selected T-cell epitopes, we designed EV.CTL poly-CTL-epitope antigen using TEpredict/PolyCTLDesigner software we developed earlier [25,26] that we regard as a universal platform for rational design of polyepitope immunogens—candidate DNA vaccines to induce T-cell immunity to infectious as well as oncological diseases. PolyCTLDesigner enables us to select a minimal set of epitopes with known or predicted specificity to different allelic variants of MHC class I molecules covering a selected repertoire of HLA alleles with a preset degree of redundancy. After that, PolyCTLDesigner predicts binding affinity to TAP for the selected set of known or predicted epitopes using a model developed by Peters et al. [48] and when required adds TAP-specific amino acid residues (no more than three) to epitope N-terminus to optimize binding.

Table 1. Predicted CD8+ cytotoxic T-lymphocytes (CTL)-epitopes in the sequences of Ebola virus proteins (antigens).

No.	Epitope	Antigen	Epitope Frequency	HLA Class I Alleles
1	ARLSSPIVL	L	1741	B*27:05; B*39:01; C*07:02
2	EYAPFARLL	NP	1764	A*24:03; A*24:02
3	FAEGVVAFL	GP	3881	B*39:01; A*02:01
4	FIYFGKKQY	L	1737	B*15:01; A*01:01; B*15:17
5	FLLQLNETI	GP	3862	A*02:01; A*24:02
6	FLSFASLFL	NP	1755	A*02:01; A*24:02; C*03:03
7	FPRCRYVHK	GP	3956	B*07:02; B*08:01
8	FRLMRTNFL	NP	1767	B*39:01; B*08:01; C*06:02
9	FRYEFTAPF	L	1744	B*39:01; C*14:02
10	FTPQFLLQL	GP	3868	A*02:01; A*24:02
11	FVHSGFIYF	L	1739	A*24:03;A*23:01;B*35:01;A*26:02;B*15:01; A*02:06; C*03:03
12	GHMMVIFRL	NP	1768	B*39:01; A*02:01; A*24:02
13	GQFLSFASL	NP	1753	B*15:01; B*27:05
14	GYLEGTRTL	L	1748	A*24:03; A*23:01
15	HMMVIFRLM	NP	1768	A*02:01; A*24:02
16	HPLARTAKV	NP	1766	B*07:02; B*51:01
17	IISDLSIFI	L	1713	A*02:01; A*69:01
18	ILMNFHQKK	NP	1711	A*03:01; A*11:01
19	IMYDHLPGF	VP35	1737	B*58:01; C*12:03
20	KQIPIWLPL	VP40	1766	B*40:01; B*27:05
21	KVYWAGIEF	VP24	1702	B*15:01; B*35:01; C*14:02
22	LANETTQAL	GP	1242	B*07:02; B*35:01; C*03:03
23	LANPTADDF	VP30	1686	B*35:01; B*58:01
24	LPQYFTFDL	VP40	1763	B*07:02; B*35:01
25	LSDLCNFLV	VP24	1725	A*01:01; C*05:01
26	MMVIFRLMR	NP	1768	A*03:01; A*11:01
27	NFFHASLAY	L	1750	B*15:01; B*35:01
28	QFLSFASLF	NP	1755	A*24:03; A*24:02
29	RLASTVIYR	GP	3947	A*03:01; A*31:01
30	RLMRTNFLI	NP	1766	A*02:01; A*24:02
31	RTFSILNRK	GP	1207	A*03:01; A*11:01; A*31:01
32	RTSFFLWVI	GP	3802	A*02:01; A*24:02
33	RVPTVFHKK	VP30	1684	A*03:01; A*31:01
34	SFASLFLPK	NP	1756	A*03:01; A*11:01
35	TLASIGTAF	L	1743	B*15:01; B*35:01
36	TPVMSRFAA	L	1738	B*07:02; B*35:01
37	TRSFTTHFL	L	1747	B*39:01; C*06:02
38	TTIGEWAFW	GP	3824	A*24:02; B*58:01; A*68:23; A*32:15; A*32:07
39	TVAPPAPVY	NP	1684	A*11:01; B*35:01
40	VLYHRYNLV	L	1746	A*02:01; A*03:19
41	VQLPQYFTF	VP40	1763	B*15:01; A*24:03
42	YLEGHGFRF	NP	1739	A*02:01; A*24:02
43	YQGDYKLFL	NP	1705	A*02:01; A*24:02
44	YSGNIVHRY	L	1750	A*01:01; B*58:01

At the next step, PolyCTLDesigner analyzes all possible matchings of the selected peptides and detects the optimal spacer sequence for each pair providing an appropriate cleavage of epitopes with a release of proximal peptide C-terminus. To predict proteasomal and/or immunoproteasomal cleavage, PolyCTLDesigner uses models developed by Toes, et al. [49].

When analyzing matchings of epitopes, PolyCTLDesigner forms a direct graph where nodes denote epitopes and ribs correspond to acceptable matchings. Each rib has a relevant weight vector characterized by effective proteasomal cleavage, spacer length, and a number of predicted non-target epitopes at the joint. At the final stage, the software designs the optimal resultant of polyepitope immunogen sequence determined as a full simple way in the formed graph with the least length (weight).

In this study, we used PolyCTLDesigner to predict binding affinity of the selected peptides (Table 1) to TAP; when required software added alanine residue to peptides N-terminus to enhance interaction efficiency. Poly-CTL-epitope fragment of EV.CTL was designed using a degenerated spacer motif [ARSP][DLIT][LGA][VKA] with optimization of proteasomal cleavage and 10% exactness of proteasomal filter.

To test the immunogenicity of the designed vaccine construct in mice using ELISpot and ICS, we selected seven additional peptides with proven ability to induce cytotoxic response of T-lymphocytes in BALB/c mice: *KFINKLDALH, NYNGLLSSI, PGPAKFSLL, YFTFDLTALK, EYLFEVDNL, LFLRATTEL, and LYDRLASTV*. Based on the selected peptides, mouse polyepitope fragment included at C-terminus of the polyepitope construct was designed with PolyCTLDesigner. To verify synthesis of the designed antigen in transfected cells, we included C-terminal marker epitope EPFRDYVDRFYKTLR of p24 HIV-1 protein recognized by monoclonal antibodies 29F2 in the final construct.

Designed amino acid sequence appears as follows (mouse epitopes are italicized):

MMVIFRLMR—**ADLS**—GHMMVIFRL—**KK**—VQLPQYFTF—**ADLS**—KQIPIWLPL—**RK**—EYAPFA
RLL—RVPTVFHKK—FIYFGKKQY—**R**—VLYHRYNLV—**ADL**—YQGDYKLFL—AFPRCRYVHK—ATP
VMSRFAA—AFAEGVVAFL—KVYWAGIEF—**R**—TVAPPAPVY—TLASIGTAF—**R**—TTIGEWAFW—
RK—LANETTQAL—FLLQLNETI—**R**—FVHSGFIYF—**K**—IISDLSIFI—**R**—NFFHASLAY—**RR**—LAN
PTADDF—**K**—ILMNFHQKK—**ADLS**—FTPQFLLQL—YSGNIVHRY—**ADLA**—RTSFFLWVI—RTF
SILNRK—**RK**—LSDLCNFLV—**ADLV**—HMMVIFRLM—**ADLK**—IMYDHLPGF—ALPQYFTFDL—YL
EGHGFRF—**R**—FLSFASLFL—**R**—TRSFTTHFL—RLMRTNFLI—**ADG**—FRLMRTNFL—**R**—GQFLSFA
SL—**R**—SFASLFLPK—RLASTVIYR—ARLSSPIVL—AHPLARTAKV—QFLSFASLF—**R**—GYLEGTRTL
—**R**—FRYEFTAPF—**KK**—*YFTFDLTALK*—*EYLFEVDNL*—**R**—*PGPAKFSLL*—**RK**—*LFLRATTEL*—**RK**—
NYNGLLSSI—**R**—*LYDRLASTV*—**R**—*KFINKLDALH*—SGSG—**EPFRDYVDRFYKTLR**

The length of the designed polyepitope EV.CTL is 547 amino acids; a share of spacer sequences is 12.76%. To target polyepitope immunogen into proteasome, we added ubiquitin sequence to N-terminus of the final poly-CTL-epitope construct.

3.3. Design of Poly-Th-Epitope Ebola Virus

To achieve the most efficient induction of T-cell immune response, one should induce not only responses of CD8+ but also CD4+ T-lymphocytes; therefore, in the following steps, we constructed poly-Th-epitope fragment (EV.Th). We used Th-epitopes predicted for humans and showing the broadest specificity regarding HLA class II molecules. For the purpose, TEpredict [25] predicted Th-epitopes in Ebola virus proteins. PolyCTLDesigner [26] was used to select eight fragments of the length of 35–40 amino acid residues comprising the most of the Th-epitopes with the broadest specificity regarding different HLA class II allomorphs. N-terminus of the selected peptides was extended up to 5 amino acid residues as compared to the beginning of the first epitope, and C-terminus—up to 5 amino acid residues as compared to the end of the last epitope (Table 2).

Additionally included at C-terminus of the construct: universal Th-epitope PADRE (PAn DR Epitope)—AKFVAAWTLKAAA; marker epitope EPFRDYVDRFYKTLR of p24 HIV-1 protein recognized by monoclonal antibodies 29F2, and a C-terminal fragment of LAMP-1 protein—RKRSHAGYQTI. According to the literature, adding the signal peptide concurrently with LAMP-1 C-terminus fragment to the target antigen raises the level of CD4+ T-lymphocyte response significantly [50–53]. As a signal peptide, we selected the sequence of an N-terminal fragment of Ebola virus surface glycoprotein comprising MGVTGILQLPRDR leader peptide. Using the SignalP server [54] we predicted that the leader peptide in the designed artificial polypeptide is functional and should efficiently split out. Poly-Th-epitope antigen EV.Th was designed using K/R-K/R spacer sequences that form cleavage sites by lysosomal cathepsins [39,40]:

MGVTGILQLPRDR—FKRTSFFLWVIILFQRTFSIPLGVIHNSTLQVSDVDKL—**RR**—TNTNHFN
MRTQRVKEQLSLKMLSLIRSNILKFINKLDA—**RR**—LTLDNFLYYLTTQIHNLPHRSLRILKPTFK

HASVMSRL—**RR**—TQTYHFIRTAKGRITKLVNDYLKFFLIVQALKHNGTWQAE—**RR**—WDRQ SLIMFITAFLNIALQLPCESSAVVVSGLRTLVPQSD—**RR**—SSAFILEAMVNVISGPKVLMKQIPIW LPLGVADQKTYSF—**RR**—QYPTAWQSVGHMMVIFRLMRTNFLIKFLLIHQGMHMVAGH—**RR**—ES ADSFLLMLCLHHAYQGDYKLFLESGAVKYLE—**RR**—**AKFVAAWTLKAAA**—SGSG—**EPFRDY VDRFYKTLR**—SGSG—**RKRSHAGYQTI**

MGVTGILQLPRDR—signal peptide; AKFVAAWTLKAAA—PADRE epitope; EPFRDYVDRF YKTLR—marker epitope; RKRSHAGYQTI—C-terminal fragment of LAMP-1 protein.

Table 2. Predicted CD4+ T-helper (Th)-epitopes in the sequences of Ebola virus proteins (antigens) *.

Peptide	Protein	Fragment	Number of HLA-DR Allomorphs	Number of Epitopes
FKRTSFFLWVIILFQRTFSIPLGVIHNSTLQVSDVDKL	GP	14–51	48	11
TNTNHFNMRTQRVKEQLSLKMLSLIRSNILKFINKLDA	VP24	129–166	49	8
LTLDNFLYYLTTQIHNLPHRSLRILKPTFKHASVMSRL	L	1486–1523	50	5
TQTYHFIRTAKGRITKLVNDYLKFFLIVQALKHNGTWQAE	L	2111–2150	48	10
WDRQSLIMFITAFLNIALQLPCESSAVVVSGLRTLVPQSD	VP30	230–269	47	8
SSAFILEAMVNVISGPKVLMKQIPIWLPLGVADQKTYSF	VP40	70–108	42	8
QYPTAWQSVGHMMVIFRLMRTNFLIKFLLIHQGMHMVAGH	NP	186–225	50	13
ESADSFLLMLCLHHAYQGDYKLFLESGAVKYLE	NP	68–100	47	5

*—Table demonstrates peptide sequence, antigen name, the beginning and the end of the selected peptide, the number of HLA class II allomorphs interacting with a fragment, the number of Th epitopes predicted in a fragment.

3.4. Designing Artificial Genes and Producing Recombinant Plasmids—Candidate DNA Vaccines Against Ebola Virus Encoding Polyepitope Immunogens of Ebola Virus

Artificial genes encoding EV.CTL and EV.Th-immunogens of Ebola virus were designed using GeneDesigner software [27]. Reverse translation of amino acid sequences was conducted considering the frequency of codons in humans [55]. Kozak sequence (CCGCCACC) is located ahead of ATG initiating codon. At the end of the encoding sequence, three stop-codons (TAGTGATGA) were added. Designed genes—*EV.CTL* and *EV.Th* were synthesized and cloned in pcDNA 3.1 vector plasmid. As the result, we constructed two recombinant plasmids pEV.CTL and pEV.Th—candidate DNA vaccines against Ebola virus.

3.5. Analysis of Target Gene Expression

The genes expression of DNA vaccines was evaluated with two methods: specific mRNA synthesis assay and immunostaining of the transfected cells. To evaluate synthesis of specific mRNA, we isolated total RNA from 293T cells transfected with plasmids pEV.CTL and pEV.Th and obtained cDNA in RT. The obtained cDNA was used to carry out PCR using pairs of primers (f^{CTL}, r^{CTL}) and (f^{Th}, r^{Th}) to genes *EV.CTL* and *EV.Th*, respectively.

The results in Figure 2 demonstrate that the sizes of the amplified fragments correspond to the theoretically calculated sizes of amplification products, i.e., 891 bps for *EV.CTL* gene and 495 bps for *EV.Th* gene. Similar PCR fragments were obtained when using initial target plasmids pEV.CTL and pEV.Th (positive control) as a matrix. The findings indicate presence of specific mRNA in the total cell RNA fraction.

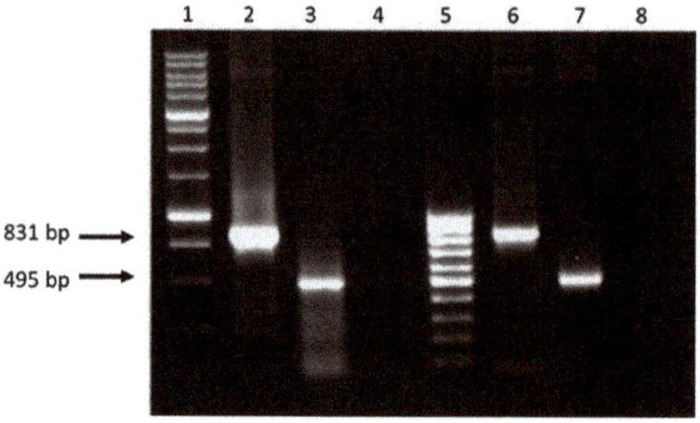

Figure 2. Electrophoregram on 1% agarose gel of PCR products: 1 - Molecular weight marker (M12, SibEnzyme); 2 and 3—PCR fragments of 831 and 495 bps obtained using cDNA as a matrix with primers (fCTL, rCTL) and (fTh, rTh), respectively; 4 and 8—The results of PCR with primers (fCTL, rCTL) and (fTh, rTh) and total RNA isolated from 293T cells transfected with plasmids pEV.CTL and pEV.Th, respectively (without reverse transcription; control for the absence of target plasmids in isolated samples of total RNA); 5—Molecular weight marker (M15, SibEnzyme); 6 and 7—PCR fragments obtained using plasmids pEV.CTL and pEV.Th as a matrix, respectively (positive control).

Immunohistochemical staining of cells transfected with pEV.CTL and pEV.Th plasmids was evaluated using MAT 29F2/30A6 antibodies to EPFRDYVDRFYKTL marker epitope, included in all constructs. The results depicted in Figure 3 demonstrate the presence of specific proteins. The findings confirm the expression of the target genes both at the level of transcription and translation.

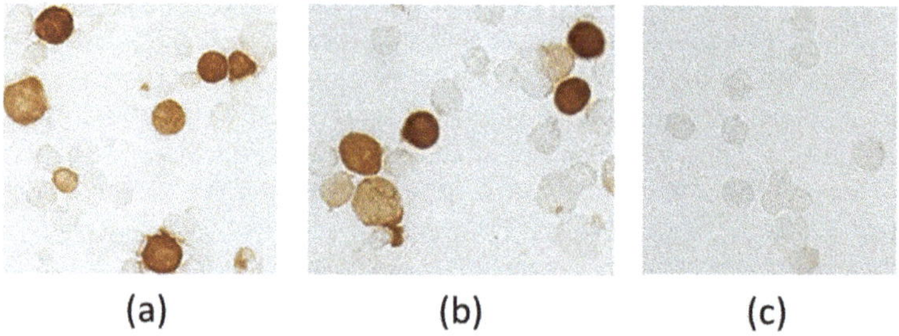

Figure 3. Evidence of genes expression in cells transfected with plasmids pEV.CTL and pEV.Th by immunohistochemical staining. (**a**) 293T-cells transfected with p*EV.CTL* plasmid. (**b**) 293T-cells transfected with p*EV.Th* plasmid. (**c**) 293T-cells transfected with pcDNA3.1 vector plasmid.

3.6. Immunogenicity Study of DNA-Vaccine Constructs Encoding Multiple T-Cell Epitopes of Ebola Virus

Immunogenicity of the target DNA vaccine constructs was evaluated regarding their capacity to induce a T-cell response in BALB/c mice 14 days after the third immunization. The level of T-cell immune response was detected using IFNγ-ELISpot and ICS.

ELISpot results (Figure 4) demonstrate that the induction of specific response was registered in both experimental groups [pE-CTL+pE-Th] and [pE-CTL], especially in the animal group immunized with a mix of target DNA vaccine constructs [pE-CTL+pE-Th]. Significant differences from both negative controls were observed only in [pE-CTL+pE-Th] group (Table 3).

The capacity of vaccine constructs to induce IFNγ-producing CD4+ and CD8+ T-cells was tested by ICS after stimulating splenocytes with specific peptides. The results of ICS (Figure 5) revealed that statistically significant difference from control (Table 4) was demonstrated by IFNγ-producing CD8+ T-lymphocytes in animal groups immunized both with pEV.CTL and a mix (pEV.CTL + pEV.Th) DNA vaccines as well as by IFNγ-producing CD4+ T-helpers in the group immunized with only a mix of vaccine constructs (pEV.CTL + pEV.Th). The maximal responses of IFNγ-producing CD8+ T-lymphocytes ($p = 0.024$) and CD4 + T-cells ($p = 0.012$) were registered in the animal group immunized with a mix of vaccine constructs. This is believed to be caused by the synergistic effect of CD8+ and CD4+ T-lymphocytes.

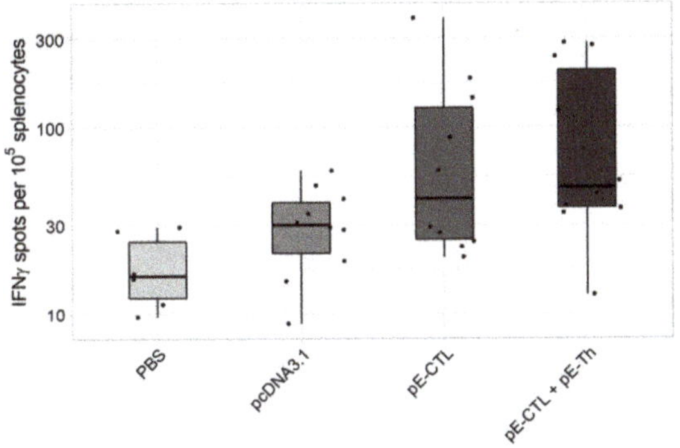

Figure 4. The results of IFNγ-producing T-cell count in IFNγ-ELISpot assay in BALB/c mice immunized with DNA-vaccine constructs encoding target immunogens (n = 6 for phosphate buffer solution (PBS) control group and n = 10 for the other groups). The figure represents spot count (i.e., IFNγ-producing T-cells) in different experimental and control animal groups.

Table 3. Results of statistical data analysis in ELISpot.

Animal Groups	Phosphate Buffer Solution (PBS)	pcDNA3.1	pE-CTL
pcDNA3.1	0.070	–	–
pE-CTL	0.029	0.148	–
pE-CTL + pE-Th	0.009	0.0296	0.264

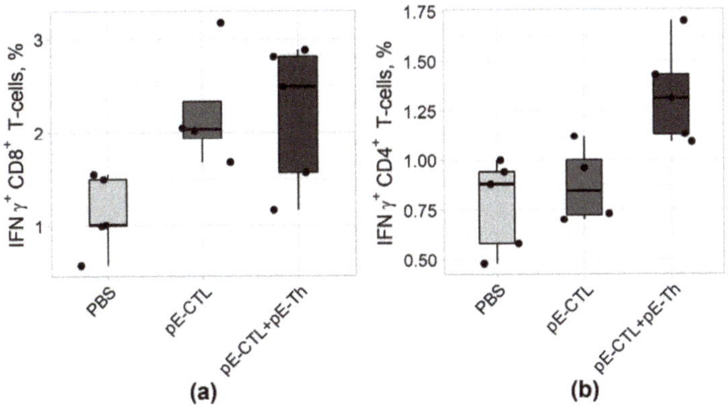

Figure 5. The results of IFNγ-producing CD4+ (A) and CD8+ (B) T-cell count using intracellular cytokine staining (ICS) approach in BALB/c mice immunized with DNA vaccine constructs encoding target immunogens (n = 5).

To design the target antigens, we used PolyCTLDesigner software that we had developed for rational design of artificial polyepitope vaccine constructs [26]. It enables us to calculate amino acid sequence of polyepitope antigen by detecting the best spacer sequences for each pair of epitopes and optimal relative positions of epitopes in the construct considering state-of-the-art knowledge about the specificity of proteasomal processing of antigens and interaction between peptides and TAP.

The findings revealed that the designed artificial DNA vaccine constructs encoding CTL and Th-epitopes of Ebola virus antigens provide expression of the target genes, as well as induce virus-specific responses of CD4+ and CD8+ T-lymphocytes in immunized mice.

Table 4. Statistical analysis results obtained using intracellular cytokine staining (ICS).

Animal Groups	CD8+IFNγ+		CD4+IFNγ+	
	PBS	**pE-CTL**	**PBS**	**pE-CTL**
pE-CTL	0.024	–	0.278	–
pE-CTL+pE-Th	0.024	0.635	0.012	0.024

4. Conclusions

Our original developed TEpredict/PolyCTLDesigner software was used in the study to predict cytotoxic and T-helper epitopes in a compound of seven Ebola virus proteins (GP, VP24, VP30, VP35, L, VP40, and NP) and to design two polyepitope immunogens EV.CTL and EV.Th on the base of those epitopes. Recombinant plasmids, candidate DNA vaccines against Ebola virus encoding the designed antigens, were obtained. We show that the designed DNA vaccine constructs provide a synthesis of corresponding mRNA and proteins in a eukaryotic cell culture, as well as induce statistically significant responses both of CD4+ and CD8+ T-lymphocytes in immunized animals, and consequently are promising candidates for further studies of their capacity to induce cytotoxic and protective responses.

Author Contributions: Conceptualization, S.I.B., A.A.I. and D.V.A.; Methodology, S.I.B., L.I.K. and D.V.A.; software, D.V.A.; validation, S.I.B., L.I.K., O.N.K. and D.V.A.; Formal analysis, D.V.A.; Investigation, S.F.O., O.N.K., E.V.S., S.G.D. and S.A.F.; data curation, S.I.B. and D.V.A.; Writing—Original Draft preparation, S.I.B. and D.V.A.; Writing—Review and Editing all authors; visualization, S.I.B., L.I.K. and D.V.A.; supervision, A.A.I. and S.I.B.

Funding: The study was funded by GZ-25/16 state assignment.

Conflicts of Interest: The authors declare no conflict of interest, financial or otherwise.

References

1. WHO Ebola Response Team; Agua-Agum, J.; Ariyarajah, A.; Aylward, B.; Blake, I.M.; Brennan, R.; Cori, A.; Donnelly, C.A.; Dorigatti, I.; Dye, C.; et al. West African Ebola epidemic after one year—Slowing but not yet under control. *N. Engl. J. Med.* **2015**, *372*, 584–587. [CrossRef] [PubMed]
2. Wong, G.; Qiu, X.; Olinger, G.G.; Kobinger, G.P. Post-exposure therapy of filovirus infections. *Trends Microbiol.* **2014**, *22*, 456–463. [CrossRef] [PubMed]
3. Saphire, E.O. An update on the use of antibodies against the filoviruses. *Immunotherapy* **2013**, *5*, 1221–1233. [CrossRef] [PubMed]
4. Lázaro-Frías, A.; Gómez-Medina, S.; Sánchez-Sampedro, L.; Ljungberg, K.; Ustav, M.; Liljeström, P.; Muñoz-Fontela, C.; Esteban, M.; García-Arriaza, J. Distinct Immunogenicity and Efficacy of Poxvirus-Based Vaccine Candidates against Ebola Virus Expressing GP and VP40 Proteins. *J. Virol.* **2018**, *92*. [CrossRef] [PubMed]
5. Rahim, M.N.; Wee, E.G.; He, S.; Audet, J.; Tierney, K.; Moyo, N.; Hannoun, Z.; Crook, A.; Baines, A.; Korber, B.; et al. Complete protection of the BALB/c and C57BL/6J mice against Ebola and Marburg virus lethal challenges by pan-filovirus T-cell epigraph vaccine. *PLoS Pathog.* **2019**, *15*, e1007564. [CrossRef]
6. Marzi, A.; Feldmann, H. Ebola virus vaccines: An overview of current approaches. *Expert Rev Vaccines* **2014**, *13*, 521–531. [CrossRef] [PubMed]
7. Henao-Restrepo, A.M.; Camacho, A.; Longini, I.M.; Watson, C.H.; Edmunds, W.J.; Egger, M.; Carroll, M.W.; Dean, N.E.; Diatta, I.; Doumbia, M.; et al. Efficacy and effectiveness of an rVSV-vectored vaccine in preventing Ebola virus disease: Final results from the Guinea ring vaccination, open-label, cluster-randomised trial (Ebola Ça Suffit!). *Lancet* **2017**, *389*, 505–518. [CrossRef]
8. Wu, L.; Zhang, Z.; Gao, H.; Li, Y.; Hou, L.; Yao, H.; Wu, S.; Liu, J.; Wang, L.; Zhai, Y.; et al. Open-label phase I clinical trial of Ad5-EBOV in Africans in China. *Hum. Vaccin. Immunother.* **2017**, *13*, 2078–2085. [CrossRef]

9. Dolzhikova, I.V.; Zubkova, O.V.; Tukhvatulin, A.I.; Dzharullaeva, A.S.; Tukhvatulina, N.M.; Shcheblyakov, D.V.; Shmarov, M.M.; Tokarskaya, E.A.; Simakova, Y.V.; Egorova, D.A.; et al. Safety and immunogenicity of GamEvac-Combi, a heterologous VSV- and Ad5-vectored Ebola vaccine: An open phase I/II trial in healthy adults in Russia. *Hum. Vaccin. Immunother.* **2017**, *13*, 613–620. [CrossRef] [PubMed]
10. Shedlock, D.J.; Aviles, J.; Talbott, K.T.; Wong, G.; Wu, S.J.; Villarreal, D.O.; Myles, D.J.; Croyle, M.A.; Yan, J.; Kobinger, G.P.; et al. Induction of broad cytotoxic T cells by protective DNA vaccination against Marburg and Ebola. *Mol. Ther.* **2013**, *21*, 1432–1444. [CrossRef]
11. Krause, P.R.; Bryant, P.R.; Clark, T.; Dempsey, W.; Henchal, E.; Michael, N.L.; Regules, J.A.; Gruber, M.F. Immunology of protection from Ebola virus infection. *Sci. Transl. Med.* **2015**, *7*. [CrossRef]
12. Takada, A.; Ebihara, H.; Feldmann, H.; Geisbert, T.W.; Kawaoka, Y. Epitopes required for antibody-dependent enhancement of Ebola virus infection. *J. Infect. Dis.* **2007**, *196* (Suppl. 2), S347–S356. [CrossRef]
13. Khan, K.H. DNA vaccines: Roles against diseases. *Germs* **2013**, *3*, 26–35. [CrossRef] [PubMed]
14. Lu, S.; Wang, S.; Grimes-Serrano, J.M. Current progress of DNA vaccine studies in humans. *Expert Rev. Vaccines* **2008**, *7*, 175–191. [CrossRef] [PubMed]
15. Grant-Klein, R.J.; Van Deusen, N.M.; Badger, C.V.; Hannaman, D.; Dupuy, L.C.; Schmaljohn, C.S. A multiagent filovirus DNA vaccine delivered by intramuscular electroporation completely protects mice from ebola and Marburg virus challenge. *Hum. Vaccin. Immunother.* **2012**, *8*, 1703–1706. [CrossRef] [PubMed]
16. Petkov, S.; Starodubova, E.; Latanova, A.; Kilpeläinen, A.; Latyshev, O.; Svirskis, S.; Wahren, B.; Chiodi, F.; Gordeychuk, I.; Isaguliants, M. DNA immunization site determines the level of gene expression and the magnitude, but not the type of the induced immune response. *PLoS ONE* **2018**, *13*, e0197902. [CrossRef]
17. Lambricht, L.; Lopes, A.; Kos, S.; Sersa, G.; Préat, V.; Vandermeulen, G. Clinical potential of electroporation for gene therapy and DNA vaccine delivery. *Expert Opin. Drug Deliv.* **2016**, *13*, 295–310. [CrossRef]
18. Karpenko, L.I.; Bazhan, S.I.; Eroshkin, A.M.; Antonets, D.V.; Chikaev, A.N.; Ilyichev, A.A. Artificial Epitope-Based Immunogens in HIV-Vaccine Design. Available online: https://www.intechopen.com/books/advances-in-hiv-and-aids-control/artificial-epitope-based-immunogens-in-hiv-vaccine-design (accessed on 5 November 2018).
19. Öhlund, P.; García-Arriaza, J.; Zusinaite, E.; Szurgot, I.; Männik, A.; Kraus, A.; Ustav, M.; Merits, A.; Esteban, M.; Liljeström, P.; et al. DNA-launched RNA replicon vaccines induce potent anti-Ebolavirus immune responses that can be further improved by a recombinant MVA boost. *Sci. Rep.* **2018**, *8*, 12459. [CrossRef]
20. Bazhan, S.I.; Karpenko, L.I.; Ilyicheva, T.N.; Belavin, P.A.; Seregin, S.V.; Danilyuk, N.K.; Antonets, D.V.; Ilyichev, A.A. Rational design based synthetic polyepitope DNA vaccine for eliciting HIV-specific CD8+ T cell responses. *Mol. Immunol.* **2010**, *47*, 1507–1515. [CrossRef]
21. Hanke, T.; McMichael, A.J. Design and construction of an experimental HIV-1 vaccine for a year-2000 clinical trial in Kenya. *Nat. Med.* **2000**, *6*, 951–955. [CrossRef]
22. Karpenko, L.I.; Bazhan, S.I.; Antonets, D.V.; Belyakov, I.M. Novel approaches in polyepitope T-cell vaccine development against HIV-1. *Expert Rev. Vaccines* **2014**, *13*, 155–173. [CrossRef] [PubMed]
23. Khan, M.A.; Hossain, M.U.; Rakib-Uz-Zaman, S.M.; Morshed, M.N. Epitope-based peptide vaccine design and target site depiction against Ebola viruses: an immunoinformatics study. *Scand. J. Immunol.* **2015**, *82*, 25–34. [CrossRef] [PubMed]
24. Vita, R.; Overton, J.A.; Greenbaum, J.A.; Ponomarenko, J.; Clark, J.D.; Cantrell, J.R.; Wheeler, D.K.; Gabbard, J.L.; Hix, D.; Sette, A.; et al. The immune epitope database (IEDB) 3.0. *Nucleic Acids Res.* **2015**, *43*, D405–D412. [CrossRef] [PubMed]
25. Antonets, D.V.; Maksiutov, A.Z. TEpredict: software for T-cell epitope prediction. *Mol. Biol. (Mosk.)* **2010**, *44*, 130–139. [CrossRef] [PubMed]
26. Antonets, D.V.; Bazhan, S.I. PolyCTLDesigner: A computational tool for constructing polyepitope T-cell antigens. *BMC Res. Notes* **2013**, *6*, 407. [CrossRef] [PubMed]
27. Villalobos, A.; Welch, M.; Minshull, J. In silico design of functional DNA constructs. *Methods Mol. Biol.* **2012**, *852*, 197–213. [PubMed]
28. R Development Core Team. R: A Language and Environment for Statistical Computing. Vienna, Austria: The R Foundation for Statistical Computing. Available online: https://www.r-project.org/ (accessed on 22 March 2019).

29. Karpenko, L.I.; Ilyichev, A.A.; Eroshkin, A.M.; Lebedev, L.R.; Uzhachenko, R.V.; Nekrasova, N.A.; Plyasunova, O.A.; Belavin, P.A.; Seregin, S.V.; Danilyuk, N.K.; et al. Combined virus-like particle-based polyepitope DNA/protein HIV-1 vaccine design, immunogenicity and toxicity studies. *Vaccine* **2007**, *25*, 4312–4323. [CrossRef] [PubMed]
30. Reguzova, A.; Antonets, D.; Karpenko, L.; Ilyichev, A.; Maksyutov, R.; Bazhan, S. Design and evaluation of optimized artificial HIV-1 poly-T cell-epitope immunogens. *PLoS ONE* **2015**, *10*, e0116412. [CrossRef] [PubMed]
31. Van de Weijer, M.L.; Luteijn, R.D.; Wiertz, E.J.H.J. Viral immune evasion: Lessons in MHC class I antigen presentation. *Semin. Immunol.* **2015**, *27*, 125–137. [CrossRef]
32. Yewdell, J.W. DRiPs solidify: Progress in understanding endogenous MHC class I antigen processing. *Trends Immunol.* **2011**, *32*, 548–558. [CrossRef]
33. Kutzler, M.A.; Weiner, D.B. DNA vaccines: Ready for prime time? *Nat. Rev. Genet.* **2008**, *9*, 776–788. [CrossRef] [PubMed]
34. Livingston, B.D.; Newman, M.; Crimi, C.; McKinney, D.; Chesnut, R.; Sette, A. Optimization of epitope processing enhances immunogenicity of multiepitope DNA vaccines. *Vaccine* **2001**, *19*, 4652–4660. [CrossRef]
35. Depla, E.; Van der Aa, A.; Livingston, B.D.; Crimi, C.; Allosery, K.; De Brabandere, V.; Krakover, J.; Murthy, S.; Huang, M.; Power, S.; et al. Rational design of a multiepitope vaccine encoding T-lymphocyte epitopes for treatment of chronic hepatitis B virus infections. *J. Virol.* **2008**, *82*, 435–450. [CrossRef] [PubMed]
36. Schubert, B.; Kohlbacher, O. Designing string-of-beads vaccines with optimal spacers. *Genome Med.* **2016**, *8*, 9. [CrossRef] [PubMed]
37. Uebel, S.; Wiesmüller, K.H.; Jung, G.; Tampé, R. Peptide libraries in cellular immune recognition. *Curr. Top. Microbiol. Immunol.* **1999**, *243*, 1–21.
38. Cardinaud, S.; Bouziat, R.; Rohrlich, P.-S.; Tourdot, S.; Weiss, L.; Langlade-Demoyen, P.; Burgevin, A.; Fiorentino, S.; van Endert, P.; Lemonnier, F.A. Design of a HIV-1-derived HLA-B07.02-restricted polyepitope construct. *AIDS* **2009**, *23*, 1945–1954. [CrossRef]
39. Schneider, S.C.; Ohmen, J.; Fosdick, L.; Gladstone, B.; Guo, J.; Ametani, A.; Sercarz, E.E.; Deng, H. Cutting edge: Introduction of an endopeptidase cleavage motif into a determinant flanking region of hen egg lysozyme results in enhanced T cell determinant display. *J. Immunol.* **2000**, *165*, 20–23. [CrossRef]
40. Zhu, H.; Liu, K.; Cerny, J.; Imoto, T.; Moudgil, K.D. Insertion of the dibasic motif in the flanking region of a cryptic self-determinant leads to activation of the epitope-specific T cells. *J. Immunol.* **2005**, *175*, 2252–2260. [CrossRef]
41. Varshavsky, A.; Turner, G.; Du, F.; Xie, Y. Felix Hoppe-Seyler Lecture 2000. The ubiquitin system and the N-end rule pathway. *Biol. Chem.* **2000**, *381*, 779–789. [CrossRef]
42. Rowell, J.F.; Ruff, A.L.; Guarnieri, F.G.; Staveley-O'Carroll, K.; Lin, X.; Tang, J.; August, J.T.; Siliciano, R.F. Lysosome-associated membrane protein-1-mediated targeting of the HIV-1 envelope protein to an endosomal/lysosomal compartment enhances its presentation to MHC class II-restricted T cells. *J. Immunol.* **1995**, *155*, 1818–1828.
43. Ruff, A.L.; Guarnieri, F.G.; Staveley-O'Carroll, K.; Siliciano, R.F.; August, J.T. The enhanced immune response to the HIV gp160/LAMP chimeric gene product targeted to the lysosome membrane protein trafficking pathway. *J. Biol. Chem.* **1997**, *272*, 8671–8678. [CrossRef] [PubMed]
44. Wu, T.C.; Guarnieri, F.G.; Staveley-O'Carroll, K.F.; Viscidi, R.P.; Levitsky, H.I.; Hedrick, L.; Cho, K.R.; August, J.T.; Pardoll, D.M. Engineering an intracellular pathway for major histocompatibility complex class II presentation of antigens. *Proc. Natl. Acad. Sci. USA* **1995**, *92*, 11671–11675. [CrossRef]
45. Guarnieri, F.G.; Arterburn, L.M.; Penno, M.B.; Cha, Y.; August, J.T. The motif Tyr-X-X-hydrophobic residue mediates lysosomal membrane targeting of lysosome-associated membrane protein 1. *J. Biol. Chem.* **1993**, *268*, 1941–1946. [PubMed]
46. Sette, A.; Sidney, J. HLA supertypes and supermotifs: a functional perspective on HLA polymorphism. *Curr. Opin. Immunol.* **1998**, *10*, 478–482. [CrossRef]
47. Sidney, J.; Grey, H.M.; Kubo, R.T.; Sette, A. Practical, biochemical and evolutionary implications of the discovery of HLA class I supermotifs. *Immunol. Today* **1996**, *17*, 261–266. [CrossRef]
48. Peters, B.; Bulik, S.; Tampe, R.; Van Endert, P.M.; Holzhütter, H.-G. Identifying MHC class I epitopes by predicting the TAP transport efficiency of epitope precursors. *J. Immunol.* **2003**, *171*, 1741–1749. [CrossRef] [PubMed]

49. Toes, R.E.; Nussbaum, A.K.; Degermann, S.; Schirle, M.; Emmerich, N.P.; Kraft, M.; Laplace, C.; Zwinderman, A.; Dick, T.P.; Müller, J.; et al. Discrete cleavage motifs of constitutive and immunoproteasomes revealed by quantitative analysis of cleavage products. *J. Exp. Med.* **2001**, *194*, 1–12. [CrossRef] [PubMed]
50. Bonehill, A.; Heirman, C.; Tuyaerts, S.; Michiels, A.; Breckpot, K.; Brasseur, F.; Zhang, Y.; Van Der Bruggen, P.; Thielemans, K. Messenger RNA-electroporated dendritic cells presenting MAGE-A3 simultaneously in HLA class I and class II molecules. *J. Immunol.* **2004**, *172*, 6649–6657. [CrossRef]
51. Bonini, C.; Lee, S.P.; Riddell, S.R.; Greenberg, P.D. Targeting antigen in mature dendritic cells for simultaneous stimulation of CD4+ and CD8+ T cells. *J. Immunol.* **2001**, *166*, 5250–5257. [CrossRef]
52. Kim, T.W.; Hung, C.-F.; Boyd, D.; Juang, J.; He, L.; Kim, J.W.; Hardwick, J.M.; Wu, T.-C. Enhancing DNA vaccine potency by combining a strategy to prolong dendritic cell life with intracellular targeting strategies. *J. Immunol.* **2003**, *171*, 2970–2976. [CrossRef]
53. Fassnacht, M.; Lee, J.; Milazzo, C.; Boczkowski, D.; Su, Z.; Nair, S.; Gilboa, E. Induction of CD4(+) and CD8(+) T-cell responses to the human stromal antigen, fibroblast activation protein: implication for cancer immunotherapy. *Clin. Cancer Res.* **2005**, *11*, 5566–5571. [CrossRef]
54. Petersen, T.N.; Brunak, S.; von Heijne, G.; Nielsen, H. SignalP 4.0: Discriminating signal peptides from transmembrane regions. *Nat. Methods* **2011**, *8*, 785–786. [CrossRef]
55. Deml, L.; Bojak, A.; Steck, S.; Graf, M.; Wild, J.; Schirmbeck, R.; Wolf, H.; Wagner, R. Multiple effects of codon usage optimization on expression and immunogenicity of DNA candidate vaccines encoding the human immunodeficiency virus type 1 Gag protein. *J. Virol.* **2001**, *75*, 10991–11001. [CrossRef]

vaccines MDPI

Article

The Increase of the Magnitude of Spontaneous Viral Blips in Some Participants of Phase II Clinical Trial of Therapeutic Optimized HIV DNA Vaccine Candidate

Ekaterina Akulova [1], Boris Murashev [2], Sergey Verevochkin [1], Alexey Masharsky [1], Ruslan Al-Shekhadat [1], Valeriy Poddubnyy [3], Olga Zozulya [3], Natalia Vostokova [3] and Andrei P. Kozlov [1,2,*]

[1] Laboratory of Molecular Biology of HIV, Research Institute of Ultra Pure Biologicals, St. Petersburg 197110, Russia
[2] The Biomedical Center, St. Petersburg 194044, Russia
[3] Innovative Pharma, Mosco 143026, Russia
* Correspondence: contact@biomed.spb.ru

Received: 29 March 2019; Accepted: 14 August 2019; Published: 20 August 2019

Abstract: We developed a candidate DNA vaccine called "DNA-4"consisting of 4 plasmid DNAs encoding Nef, Gag, Pol(rt), and gp140 HIV-1 proteins. The vaccine was found to be safe and immunogenic in a phase I clinical trial. Here we present the results of a phase II clinical trial of "DNA-4". This was a multicenter, double-blind, placebo-controlled clinical trial of safety, and dose selection of "DNA-4" in HIV-1 infected people receiving antiretroviral therapy (ART). Fifty-four patients were randomized into 3 groups (17 patients—group DNA-4 0.25 mg, 17 patients—group DNA-4 0.5 mg, 20 patients—the placebo group). All patients were immunized 4 times on days 0, 7, 11, and 15 followed by a 24-week follow-up period. "DNA-4" was found to be safe and well-tolerated at doses of 0.25 mg and 0.5 mg. We found that the amplitudes of the spontaneous viral load increases in three patients immunized with the candidate DNA vaccine were much higher than that in placebo group—2800, 180,000 and 709 copies/mL, suggesting a possible influence of therapeutic DNA vaccination on viral reservoirs in some patients on ART. We hypothesize that this influence was associated with the reactivation of proviral genomes.

Keywords: HIV; AIDS; DNA vaccine; clinical trial; therapeutic vaccine

---

1. Introduction

Since AIDS was first described in 1981 about 60 million people have been infected with HIV, and about 30 million have died of AIDS. In Russia more than 1.2 million infected individuals (59 per 100,000 of citizens) have been detected [1]. Despite significant progress having been made in the field of antiretroviral therapy (ART), the pandemic of HIV infection is yet to be contained. The development of vaccines against HIV/AIDS, both preventive and therapeutic, is the necessary step to stop further spread of the epidemic.

Our group has developed a candidate DNA vaccine called "DNA-4" which consists of 4 plasmid DNAs encoding Nef, Gag, Pol(rt), and gp140 HIV-1 proteins of the Eastern European subtype A. The candidate vaccine has passed preclinical studies in laboratory animals [2] and phase I clinical trials in healthy volunteers [3]. The vaccine was found to be safe and well-tolerated. Intramuscular immunization with "DNA-4" induced the development of HIV-specific mostly cellular immune responses in all trial participants. Some of the induced immune reactions, e.g., TNFα, were similar to the reactions discovered in exposed seronegative individuals, who remain HIV uninfected despite repeated unprotected exposure to the virus [3,4].

Here we present the results of a phase II clinical trial of the candidate vaccine "DNA-4" in HIV-1 infected people receiving ART. The objectives of the clinical trial were to assess safety and to determine an optimal dose of the vaccine for HIV-positive patients. We also were looking for the possible influence of vaccination on spontaneous increase of the viral load.

2. Materials and Methods

2.1. Study Vaccine

A candidate DNA-vaccine "DNA-4" has been developed at The Biomedical Center (St. Petersburg, Russia) in collaboration with the Research Institute of Ultra Pure Biologicals (St. Petersburg, Russia). The vaccine contains four plasmid DNA encoding consensus sequences of *nef*, *gag*, *rt*, or *gp140* HIV-1 FSU subtype A genes [2]. Amino acid sequences of viral proteins were modified to increase their expression level and optimize their immunological properties. Nucleotide sequences were designed to replace most wild-type codons with codons from highly expressed human genes. In reverse transcriptase (RT), N-terminal methionine and hystidines were introduced to replace catalytic aspartic acids residues 110, 185, and 186 within the active site of RT. In Nef, glycine residues 2 and 3 were deleted to remove the myristylation site. In gp140, the signal peptide was replaced with the signal sequence of human tissue plasminogen activator to increase its transport and secretion; the transmembrane and cytoplasmic regions of gp160 (amino acids 676–860) were removed to obtain a soluble form of the HIV-1 envelope glycoprotein, region 500–534 containing the cleavage site and fusion peptide domain was removed to prevent the proteolytic processing of the envelope, to stabilize the protein by linking it covalently to the gp41 extracellular domain, and to reduce toxicity; and region 589–618 containing the sequence between the heptad repeats was removed to stabilize the formation of trimers and eliminate formation of the hairpin intermediate [2].

Each gene was inserted into the vector pBMC that had been created at The Biomedical center. Inserted genes were expressed in eukaryotic cells under the control of the cytomegalovirus promoter and the bovine growth hormone polyadenylation signal [2].

DNA-4 was manufactured by the production facility of the Research Institute of Ultra Pure Biologicals (St. Petersburg, Russia) in accordance with the existing Russian federal regulations. The plasmids were equally formulated in 0.5 mL of sterile saline solution with overall plasmid concentration of 0.25 mg/mL. No adjuvants were added to the vaccine. Placebo vials contained 0.5 mL of saline solution without plasmids.

2.2. Phase II Clinical Trial Design

Phase II clinical trial was a multicenter, double-blind, placebo-controlled study. It was conducted to assess the safety of two "DNA-4" doses (0.5 mg and 0.25 mg) in patients with HIV-1 receiving ART by the analysis of frequency and severity of adverse events.

The study was conducted in 7 Centers for the Prevention and Control of AIDS and Infectious Diseases situated in different Russian cities: Moscow region, Kazan, Tolyatti, Volgograd, Lipetsk, Kaluga, Izhevsk.

During screening (visit 1) the following data were obtained: medical history, assessment of weight and height, electrocardiography, chest X-ray (both direct and lateral projection), laboratory tests of blood and urine were performed, viral load, levels of CD4 and CD8 T cells. For women pregnancy tests were performed. Patients eligible for inclusion were included in the study. The inclusion and exclusion criteria used in the study are listed in Appendix A. All trial participants were randomized into three equal groups and vaccinated four times with corresponding dose (0.5 mg or 0.25 mg or placebo) on days 1, 7, 11, and 15 with a 22-week follow-up period. Vaccine doses were selected based on the results of the phase I clinical trials of DNA-4 vaccine [3]. The highest dose of 1.0 mg/mL was excluded from this study since it did not show the enhancement of the immunogenicity.

Randomization was performed centrally by an unblinded study monitor according to the randomization list and stratum. At screening, each subject was allocated an individual registration. Investigator completed the Inclusion form including following information: screening date, site number, subject number, subject initials, date of birth, and basic ART. At Randomization visit the eligible patients were randomized to one of three treatment groups with the ratio 1:1:1. Trial participants were stratified by basic ART. Investigator indicated basic ART for each subject during randomization: 2NRTI + NNRTI or 2NRTI + PI. Patients with different basic ART were allocated equally to one of three treatment groups.

A dose of the studied vaccine was blinded by using two types of packages for each patient (box A and box B). Each package contained 4 ampoules with the DNA-4 vaccine with a dosage of 0.25 mg or with placebo.

Patients from 0.25 mg DNA-4 group were immunized with one ampoule from box A with DNA-4 vaccine of 0.25 mg intramuscularly strictly to the deltoid muscle of the right shoulder and one ampoule from box B with placebo intramuscularly to the deltoid muscle of the left shoulder.

Patients from 0.5 mg DNA-4 group were immunized with one ampoule from box A with DNA-4 vaccine of 0.25 mg intramuscularly strictly to the deltoid muscle of the right shoulder and one ampoule from box B with DNA-4 vaccine of 0.25 mg intramuscularly to the deltoid muscle of the left shoulder.

Patients from the placebo group were immunized with one ampoule from box A with placebo intramuscularly strictly to the deltoid muscle of the right shoulder and one ampoule from box B with placebo intramuscularly to the deltoid muscle of the left shoulder.

The candidate vaccine was administered intramuscularly in 1 mL of sterile saline solution in the deltoid muscle of each shoulder. Figure 1 shows the clinical trial design.

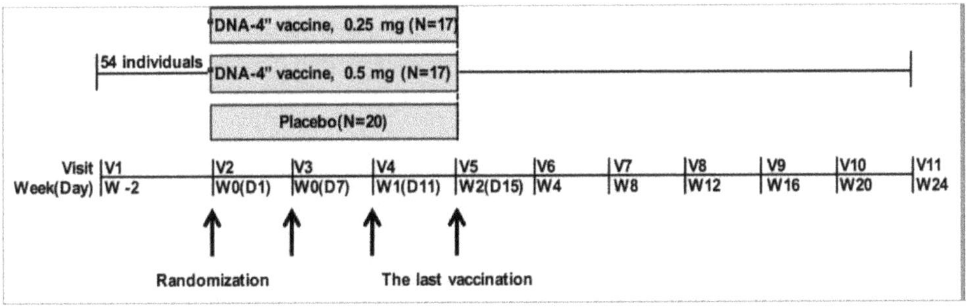

Figure 1. Trial scheme. Arrows show days of immunization.

Safety and tolerability were evaluated by the frequency and severity of adverse events (AE) according to subjective complaints from the patient's diary, vital signs, physical examination, laboratory tests and development of local reactions. The severity of AE was assigned in accordance with the DAIDS scale, Version 1.0, December 2004. Each adverse event was graded using a 4-grade scale: 1—mild, 2—moderate, 3—severe, 4—potentially life threatening.

Association of AE with vaccine administration was determined as associated, possibly associated, unlikely associated, or not associated. AE associated with the vaccine injection should meet the following criteria: occurs in a short time after injection, accompanies a known response to the use of the vaccine, terminates after cessation of the vaccination, re-occurs after the resumption of the vaccination.

The viral load was assessed at screening and at visits 2 and 6–11 by real-time PCR analysis. "AmpliSense HIV-Monitor-M-FL" kit (Russia) were used to detect transient viral increases above 50 copies/mL (the sensitivity of the kit was 20 copies/mL). The magnitude of viral blips, the number of viral increases as well as the number of patients with viral increases were compared between vaccinated groups and placebo group.

The quantity and ratio of CD4 and CD8 T cells were measured by flow cytometry analysis.

The viral load and CD4 and CD8 T cell levels at visit 2 were the baselines for assessing the dynamics of the viral load.

2.3. Ethical Compliance

The study was reviewed and approved by the Ethical Committee of the Ministry of Health of the Russian Federation (clinical trial approval number 222 of 22 April 2014). The volunteers provided written informed consent following protocol review, as well as discussion and counseling with the clinical study team.

3. Results

3.1. Adherence and Tolerability

54 HIV-1 infected individuals receiving ART participated in the study. All participants were randomized into three equivalent groups: 0.5 mg of vaccine—17 individuals, 0.25 mg—17 individuals, and placebo—20 individuals. Demographic characteristics of trial participants are presented in Table 1.

Table 1. Demographic characteristics of trial participants.

Group	Placebo	0.25 mg	0.5 mg	Total
Number of participants randomized	20	17	17	54
Number of men	9	5	9	23
Number of women	11	12	8	31
Average age	33.6 ± 6.2	36.9 ± 9.4	37.1 ± 8.5	35.7 ± 8.0

Vaccination was fully completed in 53 trial participants. One individual from group vaccinated with 0.25 mg of the vaccine was prematurely withdrawn from the study after first vaccine application due to a cold caused by a respiratory virus. There was no temporal association with vaccine administration, so this AE was determined as unlikely to be associated with the vaccination. However, data on safety and tolerability were analyzed in this participant.

The diagram describing the course of the study is presented at Figure 2.

Adverse events were registered in 17 out of 54 trial participants (31.8%). In the vaccinated groups (0.25 mg and 0.5 mg combined) 35 AE in 12 patients were detected (35.3%), in the placebo group—13 AE in 5 patients (25.0%). In the group receiving 0.25 mg of the vaccine AE were found twice as often as in the group receiving the 0.5 mg dose (47.1% and 23.5% respectively). The total data on the adverse events registered in trial participants are presented in Table 2. Statistically significant differences between the frequencies of adverse events in vaccinated and placebo groups were not found (Fisher's exact test).

Pain in the left arm and hyperemia at the injection site were associated with immunization with the studied candidate vaccine. Fourteen cases of AE were determined to be possibly associated with vaccination including leukopenia, neutropenia, fever, itching at the injection site, hypersecretion from the genital tract, and menstrual disorders.

No deaths were detected. Most adverse events had mild or moderate severity. In the vaccinated groups, 4 cases of 3rd grade AE (3 cases in the 0.25 mg group and 1 case in the 0.5 mg group) and 1 case of 4th grade AE (in the 0.25 mg group) were registered, all of them neutropenias. This did not lead to an interruption of the vaccination. In all cases neutropenias were completely resolved.

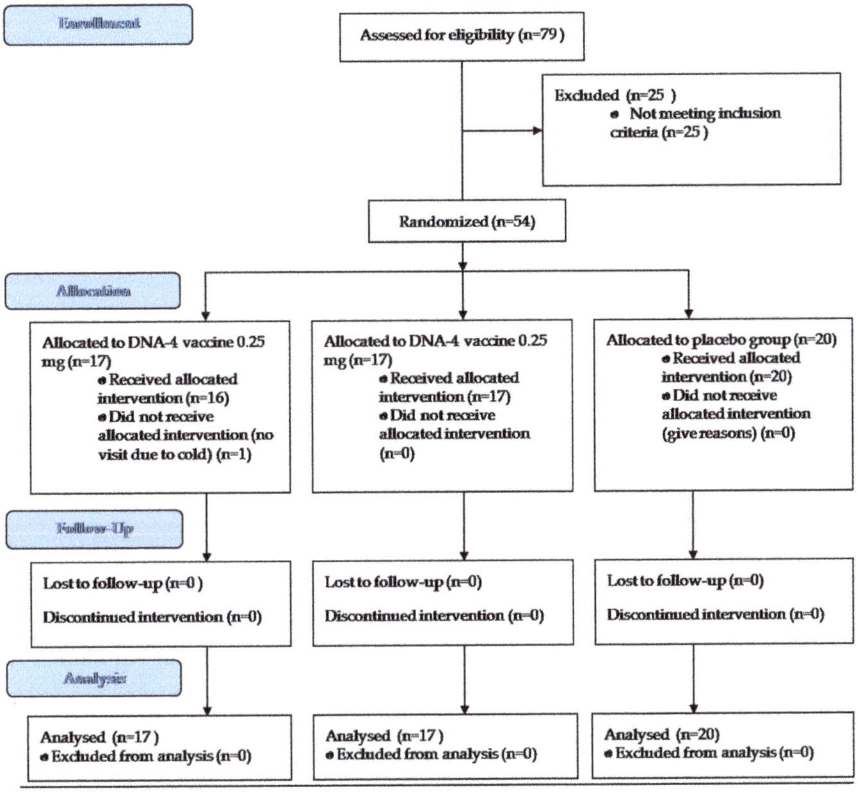

Figure 2. Consort diagram of the study.

Table 2. Adverse events registered in trial participants.

Adverse Event	DNA-4 0.25 mg		DNA-4 0.5 mg		Placebo	
Number	17		17		20	
	N	%	N	%	N	%
Fever	1	5.9	0	0.0	2	10.0
Feeling of acid in the mouth	0	0.0	0	0.0	1	5.0
Toothache	0	0.0	0	0.0	1	5.0
Weakness	0	0.0	0	0.0	1	5.0
Left arm pain	0	0.0	0	0.0	1	5.0
Itching at the injection site	1	5.9	0	0.0	1	5.0
Hyperemia at the injection site	1	5.9	0	0.0	0	0.0
Menstrual disorders	2	18.2	0	0.0	0	0.0
Hypersecretion from the genital tract (subjective analysis)	1	5.9	0	0.0	0	0.0
Cold	3	17.6	3	17.6	0	0.0
Gastrointestinal infection	1	5.9	0	0.0	0	0.0
High blood pressure	1	5.9	0	0.0	0	0.0
Neutropenia	3	17.6	1	5.9	1	5.0
Increased bilirubin	1	5.9	0	0.0	1	5.0
Leukopenia	2	11.8	2	11.8	1	5.0

Table 2. *Cont.*

Adverse Event	DNA-4 0.25 mg		DNA-4 0.5 mg		Placebo	
Number	17		17		20	
	N	%	N	%	N	%
Anemia	1	5.9	0	0.0	1	5.0
Increase in alanine aminotransferase	1	5.9	0	0.0	0	0.0
Increase in gamma-glutamyl transferase	1	5.9	0	0.0	0	0.0
Erythropenia	0	0.0	1	5.9	0	0.0
Proteinuria	0	0.0	1	5.9	0	0.0
Irritability	0	0.0	1	5.9	0	0.0

$p > 0.05$.

3.2. *Viral Load Dynamics*

A viral load was measured at screening and at visits 2 and 6–11 by real-time PCR analysis. Transient viral increases above 50 copies/mL (viral blips) were analyzed. Table 3 presents the data on viral load analysis.

Table 3. Data on viral load increases registered in trial participants.

Group	0.25 mg		0.5 mg		Placebo	
The number of viral blips (>50 copies/mL)	8/88	9.1%	6/89	6.7%	7/95	7.4%
The number of participants with viral blips	4/17	23.5%	6/17	35.3%	6/20	30.0%

$p > 0.1$.

The relative frequency of the viral blips as well as the number of patients with viral blips in the placebo group and the vaccinated groups did not differ (Table 3). But the magnitude of some transient viral increases was much higher in groups receiving the candidate DNA vaccine. The biggest blips were detected in the group receiving 0.25 mg of the vaccine (patients # 21 and 37) and made up 2800 and 18,000 copies/mL, respectively. There were gradual increases and then decreases of the viral load in participant #21. The third largest blip, 709 copies/mL, was found in 0.5 mg group in patient #43 (Appendix B Table A1).

3.3. *CD4 and CD8 T Cells Measurement*

The number of CD4 and CD8 T cells were measured by flow cytometry at visits 2, 6, 7, 9, and 11. At visit 2 blood donation was performed before the first vaccination. Results at visit 2 present the data on the CD4 and CD8 level at the time of study entry. The results are shown in Tables 4 and 5.

There was a weak trend to increase in the absolute number of CD4 T cells in the group receiving 0.25 mg of the studied vaccine, but the differences with the placebo group were not statistically significant.

Table 4. Data on CD4 T cells number in trial participants at different visits (cells × 10^9/L).

Group		Visit						
		Screening	**2**	**6**	**7**	**9**	**11**	***t* test**
0.25 mg	N	17	16	17	15	15	13	0.132
	Mean	0.669	0.593	0.619	0.722	0.703	0.756	
	SD	0.224	0.223	0.241	0.152	0.223	0.187	
	Min	0.289	0.246	0.288	0.506	0.354	0.348	
	Max	1.086	1.114	1.290	1.176	1.121	1.056	
0.5 mg	N	17	17	17	14	14	11	0.104
	Mean	0.707	0.769	0.714	0.710	0.671	0.797	
	SD	0.259	0.282	0.278	0.278	0.255	0.323	
	Min	0.289	0.307	0.333	0.346	0.232	0.361	
	Max	1.157	1.281	1.267	1.275	1.093	1.196	
Placebo	N	20	20	20	17	16	12	-
	Mean	0.567	0.558	0.620	0.603	0.555	0.650	
	SD	0.197	0.202	0.183	0.213	0.127	0.211	
	Min	0.336	0.189	0.353	0.278	0.239	0.367	
	Max	1.159	1.063	1.018	1.009	0.749	1.009	

Table 5. Data on CD8 T cells number in trial participants at different visits (cells × 10^9/L).

Group		Visit						
		Screening	**2**	**6**	**7**	**9**	**11**	***t* test**
0.25 mg	N	17	16	17	15	15	13	0.306
	Mean	0.926	0.939	0.937	1.059	1.014	0.937	
	SD	0.413	0.540	0.450	0.533	0.534	0.293	
	Min	0.347	0.312	0.316	0.301	0.390	0.352	
	Max	1.776	2.376	1.926	2.199	2.230	1.406	
0.5 mg	N	17	17	17	14	14	11	0.969
	Mean	1.023	1.037	0.992	0.902	0.847	1.033	
	SD	0.477	0.479	0.380	0.276	0.390	0.451	
	Min	0.358	0.422	0.322	0.507	0.262	0.469	
	Max	1.871	2.020	1.870	1.287	1.635	2.033	
Placebo	N	20	20	20	17	16	12	-
	Mean	0.975	0.976	0.976	0.940	0.923	1.086	
	SD	0.436	0.549	0.484	0.408	0.349	0.500	
	Min	0.299	0.285	0.332	0.364	0.437	0.476	
	Max	2.169	2.506	2.059	1.711	1.604	2.365	

4. Discussion

Different therapeutic vaccine strategies including tools based on DNA, viral vectors such as modified vaccinia Ankara (MVA) and vesicular stomatitis virus (VSV), RNA, peptide, or protein, Lentiviral vector and dendritic cell have been used in numerous clinical trials. Despite the major advances in our immunological understanding of HIV-1 specific T cell responses and HIV-1 reservoir, we have not been able to achieve a cure and none of these vaccines have proven to be effective [5]. Combination strategies are now being considered as the most promising approach for therapeutic HIV vaccine development. Interleukins, immune checkpoint inhibitors and Treg modulation were suggested as candidates for effective vaccine, but failed to yield any significant clinical benefit [5]. At the CROI 2017 conference data on clinical trial BCN02 were presented. It was the combined use of therapeutic vaccination with a vaccine based on the MVA vector (MVA.HIVconsv vaccine) and Romidepsin, specific drugs that can reactivate latent virus from the reservoir (Kick and kill strategies) followed by ART treatment interruption. At the time of the report 11 patients had interrupted treatment, 7 of them had to resume ART within the first 4 weeks while 4 participants (36%) remained off ART after 7, 12, 14, and 22 weeks, respectively. The authors suggested that therapeutic vaccination targeting conserved regions of HIV-1 combined with HIV latency reactivation strategies may facilitate clearance of the viral reservoir in early-treated individuals [6]. The DNA vaccine, since it induces HIV specific cytotoxic T cells, in case of latent viral reservoirs destruction may be an ideal strategy for HIV eradication.

In our previous studies we have developed a candidate DNA vaccine against HIV-1 consisting of four plasmids encoding four HIV-1 subtype A genes: *gag*, *env*, *rt*, and *nef* [2]. The preclinical studies and phase I clinical trial of the vaccine were conducted [2,3]. The phase I trial was conducted to access safety, tolerability and immunogenicity of the DNA-4 HIV vaccine in healthy HIV-1-negative adult volunteers. We found that our DNA vaccine was safe and well-tolerated at three used doses (0.25 mg, 0.5 mg, and 1.0 mg). Altogether, T-cell immune responses were elicited in all participants. We observed the increase in lymphocyte proliferation after fourth immunization that can show the advantage of fourfold against triple immunization. The frequency of detection positive cytokine responses decreases with increasing the vaccine dose. The humoral responses were induced in 5 people (24%). We did not observe any correlation between the antibody production and the DNA-4 vaccine doses. We also found the important correlation with our results obtained for the HIV specific immune responses in exposed seronegative individuals, i.e., TNFa production in immunized group [3].

This study was conducted as a multicenter, double-blind, placebo-controlled study of safety and dose selection of a candidate HIV vaccine for HIV-infected people receiving ART. It can be concluded that the DNA-4 candidate vaccine at doses of 0.25 mg and 0.5 mg was safe and well-tolerated by HIV-infected individuals receiving ART. In vaccinated groups, three spontaneous increases of viral load with largest amplitude were detected.

The proportion of trial participants who demonstrated adverse events associated or possibly associated with the vaccine administration was 7.4% higher in the vaccinated group than in the placebo group. The frequency of local reactions in group immunized with 0.25 mg of the vaccine and the placebo group was similar, and in the group immunized with 0.5 mg no local reactions were revealed. This is in contrast with other AE, which were highest in the group receiving 0.25 mg of the vaccine.

Immunogenicity of the DNA-4 vaccine was performed in Phase I clinical trial using IFNγ-ELISpot, intracellular cytokine staining (ICS) of IFNγ, TNFα and IL-2, lymphocyte proliferation assay (LPA) and ELISA [3]. For specific T cell stimulation, a panel of 451 overlapping peptides spanning HIV-1 subtype A-Eastern European (EE) Env, Gag, RT, and Nef proteins was used. Peptides were synthesized at the Research Institute of Ultra Pure Biologicals (St. Petersburg, Russia). HIV-specific cellular immune responses were detected in 21/21 (100%) trial participants: 9 patients were IFNγ-ELISpot reactive, 18 patients expressed cytokines to specific antigen stimulation, and 12 patients had positive lymphocyte proliferation. Using ICS we detected the increased TNFα expression by CD4 T cells in response to the specific peptide stimulation in 3/21 trial participants [3]. The humoral response was induced in 5 people (24%). The titer of HIV-specific antibodies did not exceed 1/100.

For complete eradication of the HIV infection the destruction of latent viral reservoirs is necessary, and this cannot be achieved by modern ART. The only example of HIV cure is the so-called "Berlin patient" who underwent allogeneic hematopoietic stem-cell transplantation (HSCT) from a donor carrying homozygous mutation in the HIV coreceptor CCR5 [7,8]. Recently information about HIV-1 remission maintained over a further 18 months after a similar procedure has been published [9]. However, this procedure is very expensive, high-risk and cannot be widely used.

One of the approaches used for eliminating viral reservoirs is reactivation of latent proviral genomes during ART treatment by histone deacetylase inhibitors and some cytokines [10,11].

Another way is enhancement of cellular immunity in HIV-infected individuals using therapeutic vaccines capable of inducing functional $CD8^+$ T cells specific for HIV-1 epitopes [12–16]. The next generation of therapeutic vaccines will also be combined with reservoir activating agents [17]. DNA vaccines, in case of provirus activation, may be an ideal drug for viral reservoirs eradication.

Proviral genome reactivation may be caused by TNFα expression. TNFα activates transcription factor NFkB and HIV transcription [12,18]. DNA-4 vaccination induced increased TNFα expression in some individuals, as shown in a phase I clinical trial by intracellular cytokine staining followed by flow cytometry [3]. The expression of TNFα was also demonstrated by us in a cohort of exposed, seronegative individuals [4]. That is why we hypothesized that therapeutic "DNA-4" vaccine immunization may activate latent provirus and destroy at least some virus reservoirs. In order to measure that, we assessed the frequency and magnitude of transient viral load increases above 50 copies/mL (blips). Such spontaneous viral load increases occurring during ART treatment may be associated with latent viral reservoirs activation.

To investigate the possible effects of DNA vaccination on viral reservoirs we analyzed the magnitude and frequency of the blips in the placebo and immunized groups (Table 3). Neither relative frequency of the blips nor relative numbers of patients with blips differ between groups. But the amplitudes of blips in patients 21 and 37 immunized with 0.25 mg of the candidate DNA vaccine were much higher than that in placebo group—2800 and 18,000 copies/mL, respectively. In participant #21 an increase of the viral load was detected from the 6th to the 10th visit with the dynamics of increasing, peak and decreasing of the viral load, while most of the other blips were detected only during a single visit. The third largest blip, 709 copies/mL, was found in trial participant 43 vaccinated with 0.5 mg of DNA vaccine.

The number of patients is small. However, the largest increases were registered in double-blinded vaccinated groups. The results suggest that the lower DNA concentration (0.25 mg) is more active than 0.5 mg. This is in correspondence with more AE in the group vaccinated with 0.25 mg.

These results may have several explanations. The participation of therapeutic DNA-4 vaccination during ART in destruction of latent viral reservoirs in some patients due to the reactivation of a latent provirus by TNFα is possible but is not proved. The destruction of latent cells containing viral RNA can be the source of the viral blips."Repliclones", populations of replicating cells with HIV's genome nested inside them can also produce new virions [19].

The studied vaccine contains Nef protein which has been shown to have an ability to induce viral reactivation. It was demonstrated that exogenous Nef activated virus production in latent cell lines and in peripheral blood mononuclear cells isolated from asymptomatic HIV-infected individuals [20]. Early production of Nef during viral reactivation might enhance latent T cell activation.

Nef increases the production of exosomes containing activated ADAM17 (a disintegrin and metalloprotease domain 17), an enzyme that converts pro-TNF-α into its active form. The uptake of ADAM17-containing exosomes by target cells can induce the release of TNF-α, which subsequently binds to TNF receptor type 1 and activates NF-κB and c-Jun N-terminal kinase (JNK) pathways [20].

On the other hand, Nef is able to selectively downregulate surface CD4 and HLA-I molecules that may lead to evade immune surveillance by reactivated cells. Moreover, Nef can counteract multiple apoptotic pathways and promote cell survival could further hinder the clearance of reactivating reservoirs [20]. So, Nef protein can has dual effect on latent viral reservoirs reactivation.

5. Conclusions

The further studies of these effects are necessary. As far as we know, no systematic studies of blips in vaccinated patients have been performed before. The measurement of the magnitude of spontaneous increases of viral load could become the part of monitoring the results of immunotherapy of HIV-infected patients in the future.

In conclusion, we demonstrated safety of the candidate DNA vaccine in HIV-infected patients receiving ART, and detected unusual blips effects in vaccinated individuals, which may be of interest for the future studies.

Author Contributions: Conceptualization, A.P.K. and B.M.; methodology, E.A., R.A.-S., V.P., O.Z., and N.V.; validation, E.A., V.P., O.Z., and N.V.; formal analysis, E.A., V.P., and O.Z.; investigation, E.A., V.P., and O.Z.; resources, S.V. and A.M.; data curation, V.P., O.Z., and N.V.; writing—original draft preparation, E.A.; writing—review and editing, A.P.K.; visualization, E.A.; supervision, A.P.K.; project administration, A.P.K.; funding acquisition, A.P.K.

Funding: This research was funded by The Ministry of Industry and Trade Russia, government contract number 13411.1008799.13.160.

Acknowledgments: We wish to thank all trial participants for their devotion to the project.

Conflicts of Interest: The authors declare no conflict of interest.

Appendix A

The inclusion and exclusion criteria used in the study:

1. Inclusion criteria:

- Informed consent to participate in the study;
- HIV positive men and women over 18 years old receiving stable first-line ART for at least 6 months and not more than 2 years;
- Stable clinical course of HIV infection (clinical stage 1 or 2 according to WHO classification);
- HIV viral load less than 50 copies/mL at screening;
- Number of CD4 T cells more than 250 cells/mm^3 at screening;
- blood parameters: leukocytes—$\geq$2900/mm^3 (2.9×10^9 cells/L), absolute neutrophil count—$\geq$1500/mm^3 (1.5×10^9 cells/L), platelets—$\geq$100,000/mm^3 (100×10^9 cells/L), hemoglobin—$\geq$9.0 g/dL, bilirubin—$\leq 1.5 \times$ upper limit of normal, ALT and AST—$\leq 2.5 \times$ upper limit of normal;
- Glomerular filtration rate (GFR)—>60 mL/min.
- Consent to use adequate contraceptive methods throughout the study (condom with spermicide).

2. Exclusion criteria:

- Acute hepatitis or cirrhosis of any etiology; anti-HCV or HBsAg, at screening;
- Opportunistic infections that meet the Category C classification of the Centers for Disease Control and Prevention (CDC) of 2008, with the exception of Kaposi's sarcoma that does not require systemic therapy;
- Tuberculosis;
- Malignant neoplasms;
- Participation in other clinical studies within 3 months before screening;
- Reception of immunomodulators (interferons, interleukins), immunosuppressive (cyclosporine), glucocorticosteroids within 3 months before screening;
- Any vaccination within 6 months before screening;
- Significant alcohol or drug addiction;
- Hypersensitivity to any component of the study vaccine;
- Severe concomitant diseases, such as disorders of the nervous, respiratory, cardiovascular, renal, hepatic, endocrine system and the gastrointestinal tract;
- Systemic autoimmune diseases or connective tissue diseases requiring treatment with systemic glucocorticosteroids, cytostatics or penicillamine;
- Pregnancy or breastfeeding. Women planning a pregnancy during a clinical trial; women who do not use adequate methods of contraception;
- The inability to read or write, failure to understand and follow research protocol procedures.

Appendix B

Table A1. Data on viral load measured in trial participants.

Group	Participant Number	Visit							
		Screening	2	6	7	8	9	10	11
Placebo	01	20	440	20	39	20	20	80	20
	02	20	20	565	20	71	39	20	20
	03	20	200	39	20	20	39	43	20
	04	20	55	20	47	52	20	20	20
	05	40	57	20	20	20	20	39	20
	06	20	20	20	20	20	20	20	20
	07	20	39	20	39	n/a	n/a	n/a	n/a
	08	42	232	95	20	n/a	n/a	n/a	n/a
	09	20	20	39	20	n/a	n/a	n/a	n/a
	10	20	39	20	20	20	20	20	20
	11	20	20	20	20	80	20	n/a	n/a
	12	40	39	20	20	20	20	n/a	n/a
	13	40	20	39	20	20	n/a	n/a	n/a
	14	40	20	20	20	n/a	20	20	n/a
	15	20	20	20	20	20	20	20	20
	16	40	39	39	20	20	39	39	42
	17	20	39	20	41	20	20	20	20
	18	40	39	39	39	50	20	20	20
	19	20	20	20	20	20	20	52	n/a
	20	20	20	20	n/a	n/a	20	n/a	20
	N	20	20	20	19	15	16	13	12
	Median	20	39	20	20	20	20	20	20
	SD	9.9	104.8	121.2	9.6	20.9	7.7	18.4	6.4
	Min	20	20	20	20	20	20	20	20
	Max	42	440	565	47	80	39	80	42
	>50	0	5	2	0	3	0	2	0
0.25 mg	21	20	39	101	59	129	2800	39	20
	22	20	20	20	20	39	20	20	20
	23	20	20	20	20	20	50	20	20
	24	20	20	20	20	20	20	20	20
	25	20	46	20	20	20	20	20	20
	26	20	20	20	39	n/a	59	80	39
	27	20	20	39	20	20	20	57	n/a
	28	20	39	39	39	20	n/a	n/a	n/a
	29	20	20	20	20	20	20	20	20
	30	20	49	39	20	20	20	20	20
	31	20	20	n/a	20	20	20	20	20
	32	20	20	20	20	20	n/a	n/a	n/a
	33	20	20	20	20	20	20	20	20
	34	20	20	20	n/a	20	40	20	20
	35	20	20	20	20	39	39	20	20
	36	40	39	39	20	20	20	20	20
	37	20	20	20	18,000	n/a	n/a	n/a	n/a
	N	17	17	16	16	15	14	14	13
	Median	20	20	20	20	20	20	20	20
	SD	4.9	10.8	20.8	4493.7	28.2	740.9	18.3	5.3
	Min	20	20	20	20	20	20	20	20
	Max	40	49	101	18000	129	2800	80	39
	>50	0	0	1	2	1	2	2	0

Table A1. *Cont.*

Group	Participant Number	Visit							
		Screening	2	6	7	8	9	10	11
0.5 mg	38	20	39	62	20	20	20	20	20
	39	20	20	39	20	20	20	20	20
	40	20	42	44	49	61	20	20	20
	41	20	39	20	20	20	20	20	20
	42	40	20	20	20	71	20	20	20
	43	20	20	20	20	709	20	20	n/a
	44	20	20	20	20	20	20	20	n/a
	45	40	20	39	20	20	20	n/a	n/a
	46	20	20	39	20	n/a	n/a	n/a	n/a
	47	20	20	20	20	20	20	20	20
	48	40	39	58	20	20	20	39	20
	49	20	20	20	39	n/a	n/a	n/a	n/a
	50	40	39	40	39	20	20	39	20
	51	40	20	20	20	20	20	20	20
	52	40	39	39	57	39	39	20	n/a
	53	40	39	20	46	20	20	20	39
	54	20	20	20	20	20	20	20	20
	N	17	17	17	17	15	15	14	11
	Median	20	20	20	20	20	20	20	20
	SD	10.1	9.9	14.3	12.8	176.6	4.9	6.9	5.7
	Min	20	20	20	20	20	20	20	20
	Max	40	42	62	57	709	39	39	39
	>50	0	0	2	1	3	0	0	0

SD—standard deviation; Min—minimum value; max—maximum value; 20 copies/mL—a method sensitivity limit, means undetectable viral load.

References

1. Federal Service for Surveillance on Consumer Rights Protection and Human Wellbeing. Available online: https://www.rospotrebnadzor.ru/en/ (accessed on 29 March 2019).
2. Murashev, B.; Kazennova, E.; Kozlov, A.; Murasheva, I.; Dukhovlinova, E.; Galachyants, Y.; Dorofeeva, E.; Dukhovlinov, I.; Smirnova, G.; Masharsky, A.; et al. Immunogenicity of candidate DNA vaccine based on subtype A of human immunodeficiency virus type 1 predominant in Russia. *Biotechnol. J.* **2007**, *2*, 871–888. [CrossRef]
3. Akulova, E.; Murashev, B.; Nazarenko, O.; Verevochkin, S.; Masharsky, A.; Krasnoselskih, T.; Lioznov, D.; Sokolovsky, E.; Kozlov, A.P. Immune Responses Induced by Candidate Optimized HIV DNA Vaccine in Phase I Clinical Trial. *Madridge J. Vaccines* **2017**, *1*, 34–43. [CrossRef]
4. Murashev, B.V.; Nazarenko, O.V.; Akulova, E.B.; Artemyeva, A.K.; Verevochkin, S.V.; Shaboltas, A.V.; Skochilov, R.V.; Toussova, O.V.; Kozlov, A.P. The high frequency of HIV type 1-specific cellular immune responses in seronegative individuals with parenteral and/or heterosexual HIV type 1 exposure. *AIDS Res. Hum. Retroviruses* **2012**, *28*, 1598–1605. [CrossRef] [PubMed]
5. Seddiki, N.; Levy, Y. Therapeutic HIV-1 vaccine: Time for immunomodulation and combinatorial strategies. *Curr. Opin. HIV AIDS* **2018**, *13*, 119–127. [CrossRef] [PubMed]
6. Mothe, B. Viral control induced by HIVconsv vaccines & romidepsin in early treated individuals. In Proceedings of the CROI 2017, Seattle, WA, USA, 13–16 February 2017.
7. Hutter, G.; Nowak, D.; Mossner, M.; Ganepola, S.; Müssig, A.; Allers, K.; Schneider, T.; Hofmann, J.; Kücherer, C.; Blau, O.; et al. Long-Term Control of HIV by CCR5 Delta32/Delta32 Stem-Cell Transplantation. *N. Engl. J. Med.* **2009**, *360*, 692–698. [CrossRef]
8. Allers, K.; Hütter, G.; Hofmann, J.; Loddenkemper, C.; Rieger, K.; Thiel, E.; Schneider, T. Evidence for the cure of HIV infection by CCR5Δ32/Δ32 stem cell transplantation. *Blood* **2011**, *117*, 2791–2799. [CrossRef]

9. Gupta, R.K.; Abdul-Jawad, S.; McCoy, L.E.; Mok, H.P.; Peppa, D.; Salgado, M.; Martinez-Picado, J.; Nijhuis, M.; Wensing, A.M.J.; Lee, H.; et al. HIV-1 remission following CCR5Δ32/Δ32 haematopoietic stem-cell transplantation. *Nature* **2019**, *568*, 244–248. [CrossRef]
10. Vandergeeten, C.; Fromentin, R.; Chomont, N. The role of cytokines in the establishment, persistence and eradication of the HIV reservoir. *Cytokine Growth Factor Rev.* **2012**, *23*, 143–149. [CrossRef] [PubMed]
11. Folks, T.M.; Clouse, K.A.; Justement, J.; Rabson, A.; Duh, E.; Kehrl, J.H.; Fauci, A.S. Tumor necrosis factor alpha induces expression of human immunodeficiency virus in a chronically infected T-cell clone. *Proc. Natl. Acad. Sci. USA* **1989**, *86*, 2365–2368. [CrossRef] [PubMed]
12. Katlama, C.; Deeks, S.G.; Autran, B.; Martinez-Picado, J.; van Lunzen, J.; Rouzioux, C.; Miller, M.; Vella, S.; Schmitz, J.E.; Ahlers, J.; et al. Barriers to a cure for HIV: New ways to target and eradicate HIV-1 reservoirs. *Lancet* **2013**, *381*, 2109–2117. [CrossRef]
13. Li, J.Z.; Brumme, C.J.; Lederman, M.M.; Brumme, Z.L.; Wang, H.; Spritzler, J.; Carrington, M.; Medvik, K.; Walker, B.D.; Schooley, R.T.; et al. Characteristics and outcomes of initial virologic suppressors during analytic treatment interruption in a therapeutic HIV-1 gag vaccine trial. *PLoS ONE* **2012**, *7*, e34134. [CrossRef] [PubMed]
14. Lisziewicz, J.; Bakare, N.; Calarota, S.A.; Bánhegyi, D.; Szlávik, J.; Ujhelyi, E.; Tőke, E.R.; Molnár, L.; Lisziewicz, Z.; Autran, B.; et al. Single DermaVirimmunization: Dose-dependent expansion of precursor/memory T cells against all HIV antigens in HIV-1 infected individuals. *PLoS ONE* **2012**, *7*, e35416. [CrossRef] [PubMed]
15. García, F.; Climent, N.; Assoumou, L.; Gil, C.; González, N.; Alcamí, J.; León, A.; Romeu, J.; Dalmau, J.; Martínez-Picado, J.; et al. A therapeutic dendritic cell-based vaccine for HIV-1 infection. *J. Infect. Dis.* **2011**, *203*, 473–478. [CrossRef] [PubMed]
16. Achenbach, C.J.; Assoumou, L.; Deeks, S.G.; Wilkin, T.J.; Berzins, B.; Casazza, J.P.; Lambert-Niclot, S.; Koup, R.A.; Costagliola, D.; Calvez, V.; et al. Effect of therapeutic intensification followed by HIV DNA prime and rAd5 boost vaccination on HIV-specific immunity and HIV reservoir (EraMune02): A multicentre randomised clinical trial. *Lancet HIV* **2015**, *2*, e82–e91. [CrossRef]
17. Barouch, D.H.; Deeks, S.G. Immunologic strategies for HIV-1 remission and eradication. *Science* **2014**, *345*, 169–174. [CrossRef]
18. Van Lint, C.; Bouchat, S.; Marcello, A. HIV-1 transcription and latency: An update. *Retrovirology* **2013**, *10*, 67. [CrossRef]
19. Cohen, J. Tests identify HIV's final redoubt. *Science* **2019**, *363*, 1260–1261. [CrossRef]
20. Kuang, X.T.; Brockman, M.A. Implications of HIV-1 Nef for "Shock and Kill" Strategies to Eliminate Latent Viral Reservoirs. *Viruses* **2018**, *10*, 677. [CrossRef]

vaccines

Review

Plasmid DNA-Based Alphavirus Vaccines

Kenneth Lundstrom

PanTherapeutics, 1095 Lutry, Switzerland; lundstromkenneth@gmail.com; Tel.: +41-79-776-6351

Received: 14 February 2019; Accepted: 4 March 2019; Published: 8 March 2019

Abstract: Alphaviruses have been engineered as vectors for high-level transgene expression. Originally, alphavirus-based vectors were applied as recombinant replication-deficient particles, subjected to expression studies in mammalian and non-mammalian cell lines, primary cell cultures, and in vivo. However, vector engineering has expanded the application range to plasmid DNA-based delivery and expression. Immunization studies with DNA-based alphavirus vectors have demonstrated tumor regression and protection against challenges with infectious agents and tumor cells in animal tumor models. The presence of the RNA replicon genes responsible for extensive RNA replication in the RNA/DNA layered alphavirus vectors provides superior transgene expression in comparison to conventional plasmid DNA-based expression. Immunization with alphavirus DNA vectors revealed that 1000-fold less DNA was required to elicit similar immune responses compared to conventional plasmid DNA. In addition to DNA-based delivery, immunization with recombinant alphavirus particles and RNA replicons has demonstrated efficacy in providing protection against lethal challenges by infectious agents and tumor cells.

Keywords: alphaviruses; layered RNA/DNA vectors; DNA vaccines; RNA replicons; recombinant particles; tumor regression; protection against tumor challenges and infectious agents

---

1. Introduction

The classic approach for the development of vaccines for infectious diseases has comprised of immunization with live attenuated or inactivated agents [1]. The introduction of genetic engineering expanded the approaches of vaccine development to the application of recombinantly expressed antigens and immunogens as immunization agents [2]. Both viral and non-viral vectors expressing surface proteins and antigens have been used for immunization, first in animal models followed by human clinical trials [3]. Taking this approach has elicited strong humoral and cellular immune responses and has provided protection against challenges with lethal doses of infectious agents [4]. Similarly, recombinantly expressed tumor antigens and tumor cell proteins have elicited immune responses in vaccinated animals and provided protection against challenges with tumor cells [5].

The standard procedure for non-viral vector-based immunization involves the application of conventional DNA plasmids for the expression of the antigen in question [6]. Various approaches to improve the efficacy of delivery and the expression of antigens include polymer and liposome-based coating of plasmid vectors [7,8]. DNA delivery based on both microparticles and nanoparticles has provided promising strategies for vaccine development. Microparticle systems promote the passive targeting of antigen presenting cells (APCs) through size exclusion and supports sustained DNA presentation to cells through the degradation and release of encapsulated vaccines [7]. On the other hand, nanoparticle encapsulation provides increased internalization, enhanced transfection efficiency, and improved uptake across mucosal surfaces. Appropriate biomaterial selection can enhance immune stimulation and activation through triggering innate immune response receptors [7]. Moreover, nanoparticle-based delivery can target DNA to professional APCs. Encapsulation also adds flexibility to administration routes generating systemic and mucosal immunity resulting in more effective humoral and cellular protective immune responses.

One alternative has been to apply alphavirus-based vectors, which due to the presence of the alphavirus replicon provides a self-amplifying mechanism generating substantial gene amplification and thereby enhanced expression of the gene of interest. The increased expression levels relate to improved immune responses, but also allows the potential use of reduced quantities of plasmid DNA for vaccinations. Although the focus in this review concerns DNA-based genetic antigen preparations, a short presentation of application of alphavirus RNA replicons and alphavirus replicon particles is included. The basics of the self-amplifying replicon function is briefly described below.

2. Alphavirus Vectors

Alphaviruses are single stranded RNA viruses possessing a positive strand polarity [9]. The genome is encapsulated in a capsid protein structure covered by a membrane protein envelope structure. After the release of the alphavirus RNA genome in infected cells, the non-structural alphavirus proteins (nsP1-4) forms the RNA replicase complex responsible for extensive RNA replication. In expression vectors, which were first engineered for RNA replicon and replicon particle delivery, the alphavirus structural genes were replaced by the foreign gene of interest [10]. This approach required the in vitro transcription of RNA from a plasmid DNA construct, which then was directly transfected into host cells for immediate transgene expression. Alternatively, co-transfection of in vitro transcribed RNA from an alphavirus vector carrying the alphavirus structural genes allowed packaging of replication-deficient recombinant alphavirus particles. These so-called "suicide particles" are capable of one round of infection of a broad range of host cells generating high levels of transgene expression.

To be able to use alphavirus-based plasmid DNA vectors for direct immunization, a mammalian host cell compatible eukaryotic RNA polymerase II type promoter such as CMV was engineered upstream of the replicon genes [11]. DNA-based alphavirus vectors provide high biosafety levels with no risk of production of new viral progeny, but still generating high levels of transgene expression due to the presence of the alphavirus replicon. However, the host cell range is dependent on the efficacy of available transfection methods. Another issue related to plasmid DNA delivery concerns the improvement of transfer to the nucleus by the introduction of nuclear localization signals (NLS) in the vector [12].

3. Immunization with Alphavirus Vectors

As described above, alphavirus vectors have been utilized for vaccine development as recombinant viral particles, RNA replicons and plasmid DNA [10,11]. As the main focus here is on DNA-based vaccines, immunization studies based of recombinant alphavirus particles and alphavirus RNA replicons are only described briefly.

3.1. DNA-Based Immunization

Alphavirus-based DNA plasmids have been frequently used for immunization studies in animal models targeting infectious agents and different types of cancers (Table 1). For instance, a Sindbis virus (SIN) DNA vector expressing the herpes simplex virus type 1 glycoprotein B (HSV-1-gB) elicited a broad spectrum of immune responses including virus-specific antibodies and cytotoxic T cells in mice [13]. Furthermore, a single intramuscular immunization with SIN-HSV-1-gB protected mice from lethal challenges with HSV-1. In another study, a Semliki Forest virus (SFV) DNA vector expressing the bovine viral diarrhea virus (BVDV) p80 (NS3) was evaluated in BALB/c mice [14]. The administration of SFV-BVDV p80 DNA into the quadricep muscles of mice generated statistically significant cytotoxic T-lymphocyte (CTL) activity and cell mediated immune (CMI) responses against cytopathic and noncytopathic BVDV. Related to measles virus (MV), SIN DNA vectors expressing the MV hemagglutinin (pMSIN-H) and fusion protein (pMSINH-FdU) were administered either alone or boosted with a live measles virus vaccine in cotton rats [15]. The study demonstrated that neutralizing antibodies, mucosal and systemic antibody-secreting cells, memory B cells, and interferon-γ (IFN-γ)-secreting T cells were obtained after priming, further enhanced after boosting.

Table 1. Immunization with DNA-based alphavirus vectors in animal models.

Disease	DNA Vector	Amount (μg)	Target	Model/Delivery	Response	Ref
Infections						
HSV	SIN	0.01–3	HSV-1-gB	mouse/i.m.	Protection against HSV-1 challenges	[13]
BVDV	SFV	100	BVDV p80	mouse/i.m.	CTL and CMI immune responses	[14]
MV	SIN	100	MV-H, MV-HFdU	rat/i.m.	Protection against MV challenges	[15]
CSFV	SFV	100	CSFV E2 + rAdV	pig/i.m.	No viremia in immunized pigs	[16]
HIV	SFV	0.2	Env, Gag-Pol-Nef	mouse/i.m.	Efficient low dose priming	[17]
HCV	SFV	0.5–50	Core-E1-E2 + MVA	mouse/i.m.	Humoral immune response	[18]
EBOV	SFV	5	EBOV GP, VP40	mouse/i.d.	Binding & neutralizing antibodies	[19]
EBOV	SFV	10	EBOV GP + VP40	mouse/i.m.	Humoral & cellular immune responses	[20]
TB	SIN	0.5–50	Ag85A	mouse/s.c.	Protection against *M. tuberculosis*	[21]
TB	VEE	20	Acr-Ag85B fusion	mouse/i.m.	Protection against *M. tuberculosis*	[22]
TP	SFV	100	TgNTPAse-II	mouse/i.m.	Protection against *T. gondii*	[23]
Toxins						
BoNT/A	SFV	100	BoNT/A + GM-CSF	mouse/i.m.	Prolonged survival after BoNT/A challenge	[24]
Cancer						
Metastasis	SFV	2	HPV E7/Hsp70	mouse/gg	Potency against metastatic tumors	[25]
Cervix CA	SFV	0.05	HPV E6-E7	mouse/i.d.	Protection against HPV	[26]
Breast CA	SIN	100	neu	mouse/i.m.	Reduced tumor incidence and tumor mass	[27]
Breast CA	SIN	100	neu + Dox & Pac	mouse/i.m.	Tumor reduction	[28]
Breast CA	SIN	100	neu + Ad-neu	mouse/i.m.	Prolonged survival in mice	[29]
Tumors	SIN	3	TRP1	mouse/gg	Activation of innate immune pathways	[30]
Melanoma	SIN	50	MUC18	mouse/i.m.	Protection against tumor challenges	[31]
Melanoma	SFV	50	VEGFR2-IL-12 + Survivin-βhCG Ag	mouse/i.m.	Prolonged survival in mice	[32]
Brain CA	SIN	100	gp100, IL-18	mouse	Anti-tumor and protective effects	[33]

Acr, α-crystallin; Ad, adenovirus; Ag, antigen; BoNT/A, Botulinum neurotoxin serotype A; BVDV, bovine viral diarrhea virus; CA, cancer; CMI, cell mediated immune; CTL, cytotoxic T-lymphocyte; Dox, doxorubcin; CSFV, classical swine fever virus; EBOV, Ebola virus; gB, glycoprotein B; gg, gene gun; GM-CSF, granulocyte-macrophage colony-stimulating factor; GP, glycoprotein; H, hemagglutinin; HCV, hepatitis C virus; HPV E7, human papilloma virus E7 protein; Hsp70, heat shock protein 70 from Mycobacterium tuberculosis; HSV, herpes simplex virus; i.d., intradermal; IL-18, intereukin-18; i.m., intramuscular; MV, measles virus; MVA, modified vaccinia virus Ankara; MV-HFdU, measles virus hemagglutinin fusion protein; MUC18, melanoma cell adhesion molecule; neu, neu oncogene; Pac, paclitaxel; s.c., subcutaneous; SFV, Semliki Forest virus; SIN, Sindbis virus; TB, tuberculsois; TgNTPase-II, Toxoplasma gondii nucleoside triphosphate hydrolase-II; TP, toxoplasmosis; TRP1, tyrosine related protein-1; VEE, Venezuelan equine encephalitis virus; VEGFR2, vascular epithelial growth factor receptor-2; VP40, matrix viral protein.

Protection against pulmonary measles was achieved after immunization with pMSIN-H, whereas pMSINH-FdU provided protection only after boosting with a live measles virus vaccine. In another approach, an SFV DNA vector was compared to a recombinant adenovirus expressing the classical swine fever virus (CSFV) E2 glycoprotein in pigs [16]. Significantly higher titers of CSFV-specific neutralizing antibodies were obtained after a pSFV1CS-E2/rAdV-E2 heterologous prime-boost immunization strategy compared to double immunizations with rAdV-E2 alone. Moreover, the heterologous prime-boost immunization regimen prevented viremia and clinical symptoms in pigs. In contrast, these symptoms were seen in one of five pigs vaccinated with rAdV-E2 alone. Related to HIV vaccines, an SFV DNA plasmid and a poxvirus Ankara (MVA) vector expressing an HIV Env and a Gag-Pol-Nef fusion protein were subjected to a prime-boost study [17]. It was revealed that efficient priming of HIV-specific T cell and IgG responses was achieved with a low dose of 0.2 μg SFV DNA and the priming effect seemed to relate to the number of prime administrations rather than dose. In another prime-boost study, four novel alphavirus DNA replicon vectors were engineered to express structural Core-E1-E2 or nonstructural p7-NS2-NS3 hepatitis C virus (HCV) [18]. Prime immunization with alphavirus DNA-HCV vectors followed by a heterologous boost with a vaccinia virus expressing the nearly full-length HCV genome (MVA-HCV) elicited long-lasting HCV-specific $CD4^+$ and $CD8^+$ T cell responses in mice presenting a promising approach for prophylactic and therapeutic HCV vaccine development. Moreover, alphavirus DNA vectors were subjected to the expression of the Ebola virus (EBOV) glycoprotein (GP) gene alone or together with the EBOV VP40 gene of Sudan or Zaire EBOV strains [19]. Both binding and neutralizing antibodies were detected in immunized mice. The alphavirus-based DNA vaccine showed superior immunogenicity in comparison to recombinant MVA vaccines. In another study, the co-expression of EBOV GP and VP40 elicited significantly higher antibody levels than for immunization with GP or VP40 alone [20]. SFV-DNA EBOV GP and VP40 co-vaccination induced EBOV-specific humoral and cellular immune responses in mice [20].

In the context of *Mycobacterium tuberculosis*, a SIN DNA vector expressing the p85 antigen (Ag85) was highly immunogenic in mice and provided enhanced long-term protection against challenges with *M. tuberculosis* [21]. In another study, the alphavirus-based Venezuelan equine encephalitis virus (VEE) DNA vector expressing a fusion of the *M. tuberculosis* antigens α-crystallin (Acr) and Ag85B named Vrep-Acr/Ag85B was evaluated in a mouse model of pulmonary tuberculosis [22]. Immunization studies elicited antigen-specific $CD4^+$ and $CD8^+$ T cell responses, which persisted for at least ten weeks and also induced T cell responses in lung tissues. Moreover, bacterial growth was inhibited in lungs and spleen after aerosol challenges with *M. tuberculosis*. Related to toxoplasmosis, the *Toxoplasma gondii* nucleoside triphosphate hydrolase-II (TgNTPase-II) gene expressed from an SFV DNA vector was intramuscularly delivered to mice [23]. Specific humoral responses were obtained as well as cellular immune responses associated with high levels of IFN-γ, IL-2, and IL-10 cytokines and low levels of IL-4. Partial protection against acute infection with the virulent RH strain and chronic infection with the PRU cyst strain of *T. gondii* was obtained in immunized mice.

Related to toxins, alphavirus DNA vectors expressing the Hc gene of botulinum neurotoxin serotype A (BoNT/A) demonstrated specific antibody and lymphoproliferative responses in immunized BALB/c mice [24]. Co-delivery or co-expression of granulocyte-macrophage colony-stimulating factor (GM-CSF) enhanced the immunogenicity and survival rates in immunized mice were significantly prolonged after challenges with BoNT/A. Furthermore, co-immunization with aluminum phosphate adjuvant improved the survival.

In the context of cancer, an SFV DNA vector expressing the human papilloma virus type 16 (HPV-16) E7 protein as a fusion protein with the *M. tuberculosis* heat shock protein 70 (Hsp70) elicited significantly higher E7-specific T cell-mediated immune responses in comparison to E7 expressed alone in mice [25]. Moreover, the E7/Hsp70 fusion construct showed superior potency against established E7-expressing metastatic tumors. In another study on HPV, the SFV based DNA encoding the HPV E6 and E7 antigens was subjected to intradermal administration followed by electroporation, which provided effective and therapeutic anti-tumor activity resulting in approximately 85% tumor-free mice [26]. Related to breast cancer, the HER2/neu gene was targeted due to its role in increased metastasis and poor prognosis [27]. Intramuscular administration of SIN-neu DNA elicited strong antibody responses against the A2L2 mouse breast cancer cell line expressing neu. Moreover, challenges with A2L2 cells reduced tumor incidence and tumor mass in immunized mice. Intradermal vaccination required 80% less SIN-neu DNA to reach the same efficacy compared to intramuscular administration. Furthermore, the vaccination protected against development of spontaneous breast tumors and reduction in metastasis from HER2/neu expressing tumors. In another study, mice injected in the mammary fat pad with A2L2 tumor cells were evaluated for the combination treatment of SIN-neu DNA and chemotherapy [28]. Neither immunization with SIN-neu DNA nor chemotherapy with doxorubicin or paclitaxel alone reduced tumor growth. In contrast, chemotherapy followed by vaccination with SIN-neu DNA reduced tumor growth significantly. In another study, the effect of SIN-DNA immunizations was evaluated in a solid mammary tumor model and a lung metastasis model [29]. When mice were immunized with SIN-neu DNA or an Adenovirus (Ad-neu) vector prior to challenges with A2L2 tumor cells, tumor growth was significantly inhibited. In contrast, vaccination two days after tumor cell challenges was ineffective. However, in a regimen with SIN-neu DNA priming and Ad-neu boosting, significantly prolonged survival of mice was observed.

In an immunotherapy approach SIN-DNA expressing the self/tumor antigen tyrosine-related protein-1 (TRP1) was demonstrated to activate innate immune pathways providing improved immunization efficacy of naked DNA [30]. Related to melanoma, the melanoma cell adhesion molecule /MCAM/MUC18) was expressed from a SIN DNA plasmid (SIN-MUC18) and mice were vaccinated against B16F10 mouse melanoma cells [31]. The immunization provided protection of mice from lethal challenges with melanoma expressing mouse MUC18 in both primary and metastatic tumor models. In the context of brain tumors, immunization with SIN DNA expressing human gp100 and interleukin-18 (IL-18) enhanced both protective and therapeutic effects on malignant brain tumors [33]. The anti-tumor and protective effects were mediated by both $CD4^+$/$CD8^+$ T cells and IFN-γ and the survival rate was significantly improved in mice with implanted B16 tumors. The synergistic approach of targeting tumor cells and angiogenesis was simultaneously executed by co-immunization studies with an SFV DNA replicon vector carrying 1-4 domains of murine vascular epidermal growth factor receptor-2 (VEGFR2) and IL-12 and another SFV DNA replicon expressing the survivin and β-hCG antigens [32]. The combined vaccines elicited strong humoral and cellular immune responses against survivin, β-hCG and VEGFR2, inhibited tumor growth and prolonged survival in a B16 melanoma mouse model.

3.2. Recombinant Viral Particles

Numerous immunization studies conducted with recombinant alphavirus replicon particles have been described previously [34] and as the focus on this review is on DNA-based alphavirus vectors, only two examples of comparative studies on replicon particles and DNA vectors are presented here. In this context, a study on the immunogenicity and protective efficacy of DNA-based SIN and recombinant SIN particles expressing the medium (M) or small (S) gene segments of the Seoul virus (SEOV) was conducted in Syrian hamsters [35]. Both DNA-SIN and recombinant SIN particles elicited anti-SEOV immune responses and protection against SEOV challenges was observed for all animals vaccinated with SEOV-M, but only for a small number immunized with SEOV-S. Furthermore, the study revealed that hamsters immunized with SIN-DNA developed neutralizing antibodies faster and at higher titers compared to SIN replicon particle-based delivery.

In another study, recombinant SFV particles and RNA replicons were applied for expression of the HIV-1C gag, env, and polRT genes [36]. Immunization of mice elicited significant antigen-specific IFN-γ T cell responses. Moreover, SFV-based Gag and Env expression generated TNF-α secreting $CD4^+$ and $CD8^+$ T-cells and IL-2 secreting T cells, respectively. In this study, superior immunogenicity was obtained for SFV particle administration in comparison to RNA replicon delivery.

3.3. RNA-Based Delivery

Similar to recombinant alphavirus particle delivery, RNA replicon administration has proven efficient in vaccine development [34]. For example, a single intramuscular injection of 0.1 μg SFV-LacZ replicon RNA generated antigen-specific antibody and $CD8^+$ T cell responses in immunized mice [37]. Immunization with SFV-LacZ RNA prior to challenges by colon tumors provided protection in mice. Moreover, the therapeutic vaccination of animals with pre-existing tumors resulted in prolonged survival. Interestingly, the levels of antigen production for RNA replicons in vitro were not significantly higher than those observed for conventional DNA vaccines, but in vivo the enhanced efficacy correlated with a caspase-dependent apoptotic cell death. In another approach, a SIN RNA replicon expressing the rabies virus glycoprotein gene was applied for immunization studies with 10 μg of SIN-Rab-G RNA in comparison to a conventional rabies DNA vaccine and the commercial cell culture vaccine Rabipur [38]. The SIN-Rab-G RNA immunization elicited similar cellular and humoral IgG responses in comparison to the rabies DNA vaccine. Moreover, the alphavirus RNA vaccine provided similar protection to the rabies DNA vaccine against challenges with the lethal rabies virus CVS strain.

In addition to naked RNA delivery, alphavirus vectors have also been subjected to nanoparticle encapsulation procedures [39]. An in vivo expression comparison of 1×10^6 IU recombinant VEE particles, 1 μg of naked replicon RNA, 1 μg of replicon RNA encapsulated in lipid nanoparticles (RNA/LNPs), 10 μg of conventional plasmid DNA, and 10 μg of replicon DNA expressing firefly luciferase was carried out in mice 7 days after bilateral intramuscular administration. The luciferase levels were similar for RNA/LNPs and VEE particles, but significantly higher than for naked replicon RNA, replicon DNA, and plasmid DNA. The immunogenicity of delivery modes was evaluated by heterologous expression of the respiratory syncytial virus fusion protein (RSV-F) after intramuscular administration. The F-specific IgG response to 1 μg RNA/LNPs was equivalent to that of 1×10^6 IU of VEE particles. In contrast, plasmid DNA/LNPs at a dose of 0.1 μg and 20 μg of electroporated plasmid DNA elicited much lower IgG titers. RNA/LNPs, replicon RNA, VEE particles and an RSV-F subunit vaccine were evaluated for protection against viral challenges after intranasal RSV challenges in cotton rats. All replicon RNA vaccines protected animals for RSV challenges reducing the viral load more than 1000-fold in the lungs. The RNA/LNPs (1 μg) elicited similar responses as VEE particles. However, the recombinant F subunit vaccine formulated with alum showed the highest potency. In another study, naked RNA from SFV replicon (rSFV-NP) and poliovirus (rDELTA1-E-NP) vectors expressing the influenza type A virus nucleoprotein (NP) were intramuscularly administered in C57BL/6 mice [40]. Both rSFV-NP and rDELTA1-E-NP elicited antibodies against the influenza virus NP, but CTL responses against the immunodominant H-2D(b) epitope NP366 was only obtained with the SFV replicon RNA. Furthermore, reduced virus load was demonstrated for rSFV-NP after challenges with a mouse-adapted influenza A/PR/8/34 virus in immunized mice. The protective potential for RNA replicon immunization was similar to what has previously been achieved for plasmid DNA immunizations.

4. Comparison to Conventional DNA Immunization

In attempts to evaluate the feasibility of alphavirus DNA replicons as vaccine vectors, a direct comparison to conventional DNA vaccines has been an essential component. In this context, both the conventional DNA plasmid pWRG7077 and the SIN DNA replicon expressing SEOV M and S gene segments showed potential as vaccine vectors as described above [35]. However, there were substantial and to some extent surprising differences. In vitro expression levels were consistently higher from the conventional DNA vector than from the SIN DNA replicon. However, higher titers were obtained in vivo for vaccinations with SIN DNA replicons than for the conventional DNA plasmid. It has been suggested that the enhanced immune response relates to certain alphavirus vector genes promoting cell death and inducing interferon responses [41]. Moreover, as described above, immunization with SIN-TRP1 DNA broke tolerance and provided immunity to melanoma, which was not the case for conventional DNA vaccines [30]. Similarly, the long-term protection against *M. tuberculosis* obtained by immunization with SIN-Ag85 DNA was not achieved by vaccination with a conventional DNA plasmid in mice [21].

Several studies have demonstrated that in general, significantly lower doses of alphavirus DNA replicon are required to achieve the same level of response as seen for conventional DNA vaccines [14,17]. For instance, 100-fold to 1000-fold lower doses of SIN-HSV-1-gB were needed to elicit antibody responses and protection against lethal virus challenges. Moreover, a single dose of 10 ng elicited strong immune responses in mice. In the context of cervical cancer vaccines, while a conventional DNA-based vaccine failed to prevent tumor growth, immunization with a 200-fold lower equimolar dose of 0.05 μg of the SFV DNA replicon resulted in complete tumor regression in 85% of immunized mice [26]. In attempts to enhance the immune responses, the alphavirus DNA replicon vector expressing the multiclade HIV-1 T cell immunogen HIVconsv (DREP.HIVconsv) was subjected to intradermal delivery followed by in vivo electroporation and compared to the conventional DNA plasmid pTH.HIVconsv [42]. HIV-1-specific $CD8^+$ T cell responses were obtained in mice with 1 μg of pTH.HIVconsv compared to only 3.2 ng of DREP.HIVconsv, which represents a 625-fold molar dose reduction. These responses could be further enhanced for both the conventional DNA plasmid and the alphavirus DNA replicon by heterologous vaccine boosts with MVA-HIVconsv and attenuated chimpanzee adenovirus ChAdV63.HIVconsv. Additionally, immunization of rhesus macaques demonstrated that application of alphavirus DNA replicon vectors allowed to reduce the dose by at least 20-fold compared to conventional plasmid DNA vectors. For this reason, the manufacturing of large batches of GMP grade material for clinical trials and marketed products is easier and more feasible. Another feature of importance related to DNA replicon vaccines is that the expression is transient and lytic, eliminating such biosafety risks as chromosomal integration and the induction of immunological tolerance [43].

5. Conclusions

Several studies have confirmed that alphavirus DNA replicon vectors elicit strong immune responses in vaccinated animal models targeting both infectious agents and tumor antigens. Moreover, protection against lethal challenges by viruses, bacteria, and tumor cells have also been established. In many cases, DNA replicon vaccines have proven superior to conventional DNA plasmid vaccines or at least as efficient. However, it has been confirmed that significantly lower doses of DNA replicon vaccines are needed to achieve the same immune responses and protection as for conventional DNA vaccines. In the context of alphaviruses, in addition to DNA replicon vectors, RNA replicons and recombinant alphavirus particles have also been subjected to vaccine studies. So far, there is no clear indication of which delivery format is the best and it seems more like the ranking order varies from one target to another.

Related to the biosafety of DNA vaccines, the probability of stable chromosomal integration of transfected DNA presents some concern. In this context, it was confirmed that an intramuscularly administered DNA vector expressing a luciferase reporter gene could be detected in the skeletal muscle for more than 19 months [44]. However, the DNA was only present as an extrachromosomal plasmid. When intramuscular immunization was followed by electroporation, low-level random chromosomal integration occurred, although the frequency was significantly lower than observed for spontaneous gene mutations [45]. Another study demonstrated that DNA administration into the skeletal muscles resulted in the presence of a majority of the DNA at the injection site with only minor amounts detected in other organs [46]. Moreover, no genomic plasmid DNA integration was discovered. Related to immune responses, no anti-DNA antibodies were observed after repeated intramuscular injections in primates [47]. Another issue relates to the presence of prokaryotic elements such as antibiotic resistance genes in DNA vaccines [48]. However, no transfer of such elements has been documented so far.

Another concern of alphavirus DNA replicon vaccines relates to the difficulties in transferring the strong immune responses detected in rodents to larger animals and most importantly to humans. Disappointingly, this has also been verified in clinical trials which have supported the need of dose optimization [49–51]. Recent studies have indicated that prime-boost strategies combining alphavirus-based vaccines with other viral-based vaccines have enhanced the immunogenicity, which is important, especially in clinical settings. Another approach briefly mentioned in this review relates to the improved delivery and stability of DNA-based vaccines through polymer and lipid encapsulation procedures. Moreover, efforts are being made to target dendritic cells in order to generate better immune responses for future vaccines. Overall, alphavirus-based DNA vaccines have the potential to provide a flexible and inexpensive alternative to current existing approaches.

Funding: This research received no external funding.

Conflicts of Interest: The author declares no conflict of interest.

References

1. Delrue, I.; Verzele, D.; Madder, A.; Nauwynck, H.J. Inactivated virus vaccines: From chemistry to prophylaxis: Merits, risks and challenges. *Expert Rev. Vaccines* **2012**, *11*, 695–719. [CrossRef] [PubMed]
2. Deng, M.P.; Hu, Z.H.; Wang, H.L.; Deng, F. Developments of subunit and VLP vaccines against influenza A virus. *Virol. Sin.* **2012**, *27*, 145–153. [CrossRef] [PubMed]
3. Apostolopoulos, V. Vaccine delivery methods into the future. *Vaccines* **2016**, *4*, 9. [CrossRef] [PubMed]
4. Lundstrom, K. Alphavirus-based vaccines. *Viruses* **2014**, *6*, 2392–2415. [CrossRef] [PubMed]
5. Zajakina, A.; Spunde, K.; Lundstrom, K. Application of Alphaviral Vectors for Immunomodulation in Cancer Therapy. *Curr. Pharmaceut. Design* **2017**, *23*, 1–27.
6. Chiarella, P.; Massi, E.; De Robertis, M.; Fazio, V.M.; Signori, E. Strategies for effective naked-DNA against infectious diseases. *Recent Pat. Antiinfect. Drug Discov.* **2008**, *3*, 93–101. [CrossRef] [PubMed]
7. Farris, E.; Brown, D.M.; Ramer-Tait, A.E.; Pannier, A.K. Micro- and nano-particulates for DNA vaccine delivery. *Exp. Biol. Med.* **2016**, *241*, 919–929. [CrossRef]
8. Tejeda-Mansir, A.; Garcia-Rendon, A.; Guerrero-German, P. Plasmid-DNA lipid and polymer nanovaccines: A new strategic in vaccines development. *Biotechnol. Genet. Eng. Rev.* **2018**, *26*, 1–23. [CrossRef]
9. Strauss, J.H.; Strauss, E.G. The Alphaviruses: Gene Expression, Replication and Evolution. *Micobiol. Rev.* **1994**, *58*, 491–562.
10. Liljestrom, P.; Garoff, H. A new generation of animal cell expression vectors based on the Semliki Forest virus replicon. *Biotechnology* **1991**, *9*, 1356–1361. [CrossRef]
11. DiCiommo, D.P.; Bremner, R. Rapid, high level protein production using DNA-based Semliki Forest virus vectors. *J. Bio. Chem.* **1998**, *273*, 18060–18066. [CrossRef]
12. Lechardeur, D.; Lukacs, G.L. Nucleocytoplasmic transport of plasmid DNA: A perilous journey from the cytoplasm to the nucleus. *Hum. Gene Ther.* **2006**, *17*, 882–889. [CrossRef] [PubMed]
13. Hariharan, M.J.; Driver, D.A.; Townsend, K.; Brumm, D.; Polo, J.M.; Belli, B.A.; Catton, D.J.; Hsu, D.; Mittelstaedt, D.; McCormack, J.E. DNA immunization against herpes simplex virus: Enhanced efficacy using a Sindbis virus-based vector. *J. Virol.* **1998**, *72*, 950–958. [PubMed]
14. Reddy, J.R.; Kwang, J.; Varthakavi, V.; Lechtenberg, K.F.; Minocha, H.C. Semliki Forest virus vector carrying the bovine viral diarrhea virus NS3 (p80) cDNA induced immune responses in mice and expressed BVDV protein in mammalian cells. *Comp. Immunol. Microbiol. Infect. Dis.* **1999**, *22*, 231–246. [CrossRef]
15. Pasetti, M.F.; Ramirez, K.; Resendiz-Albor, A.; Ulmer, J.; Barry, E.M.; Levine, M.M. Sindbis virus-based measles DNA vaccines protect cotton rats against respiratory measles: relevance of antibodies, mucosal and systemic antibody-secreting cells, memory B cells, and Th1-type cytokines as correlates of immunity. *J. Virol.* **2009**, *83*, 2789–2794. [CrossRef] [PubMed]
16. Sun, Y.; Li, N.; Li, H.Y.; Li, M.; Qiu, H.J. Enhanced immunity against classical swine fever in pigs induced by prime-boost immunization using an alphavirus replicon-vectored DNA vaccine and a recombinant adenovirus. *Vet. Immunol. Immunopathol.* **2010**, *137*, 20–27. [CrossRef] [PubMed]
17. Knudsen, M.L.; Ljungberg, K.; Tatoud, R.; Weber, J.; Esteban, M.; Liljeström, P. Alphavirus replicon DNA expressing HIV antigens is an excellent prime for boosting with recombinant Ankara (MVA) or with HIV gp140 protein antigen. *PLoS ONE* **2015**, *10*, e0117042. [CrossRef]

18. Marin, M.Q.; Perez, P.; Ljungberg, K.; Sorzano, C.Ó.S.; Gómez, C.E.; Liljeström, P.; Esteban, M.; García-Arriaza, J. Potent Anti-Hepatitis C (HCV) T Cell Immune Responses Induced in Mice Vaccinated with DNA-launched RNA Replicons and MVA-HCV. *J. Virol.* **2019**. [CrossRef]
19. Öhlund, P.; Garcia-Arriaza, J.; Zusinaite, E.; Szurgot, I.; Männik, A.; Kraus, A.; Ustav, M.; Merits, A.; Esteban, M.; Liljeström, P. DNA-launched RNA replicon vaccines induce potent anti-Ebolavirus immune responses that can be further improved by a recombinant MVA boost. *Sci. Rep.* **2018**, *8*, 12459. [CrossRef]
20. Ren, S.; Wei, Q.; Cai, L.; Yang, X.; Xing, C.; Tan, F.; Leavenworth, J.W.; Liang, S.; Liu, W. Alphavirus Replicon DNA Vectors Expressing Ebola GP and VP40 Antigens Induce Humoral and Cellular Immune Responses in Mice. *Front. Microbiol.* **2018**, *8*, 2662. [CrossRef]
21. Kirman, J.R.; Turon, T.; Su, H.; Li, A.; Kraus, C.; Polo, J.M.; Belisle, J.; Morris, S.; Seder, R.A. Enhanced immunogenicity to Mycobacterium tuberculosis by vaccination with an alphavirus plasmid replicon expressing antigen 85A. *Infect. Immun.* **2003**, *71*, 575–579. [CrossRef]
22. Dalmia, N.; Klimstra, W.B.; Mason, C.; Ramsay, A.J. DNA-Launched Alphavirus Replicons Encoding a Fusion of Mycobacterial Antigens Acr and Ag85B Are Immunogenic and Protective in a Murine Model of TB Infection. *PLoS ONE* **2015**, *10*, e0136635. [CrossRef] [PubMed]
23. Zheng, L.; Hu, Y.; Hua, Q.; Luo, F.; Xie, G.; Li, X.; Lin, J.; Wan, Y.; Ren, S.; Pan, C. Protective immune response in mice induced by a suicidal DNA vaccine encoding NTPase-II gene of Toxoplasma gondii. *Acta Trop.* **2017**, *166*, 336–342. [CrossRef]
24. Li, N.; Yu, Y.Z.; Yu, W.Y.; Sun, Z.W. Enhancement of the immunogenicity of DNA replicon vaccine of Clostridium botulinum neurotoxin serotype A by GM-CSF gene adjuvant. *Immunopharmacol. Immunotoxicol.* **2011**, *33*, 211–219. [CrossRef] [PubMed]
25. Hsu, K.F.; Hung, C.F.; Cheng, W.F.; He, L.; Slater, L.A.; Ling, M.; Wu, T.C. Enhancement of suicidal DNA vaccine potency by linking Mycobacterium tuberculosis heat shock protein 70 to an antigen. *Gene Ther.* **2001**, *8*, 376–383. [CrossRef] [PubMed]
26. Van de Wall, S.; Ljungberg, K.; Ip, P.P.; Boerma, A.; Knudsen, M.L.; Nijman, H.W.; Liljeström, P.; Daemen, T. Potent therapeutic efficacy of an alphavirus replicon DNA vaccine expressing human papilloma virus E6 and E7 antigens. *Oncoimmunology* **2018**, *7*, e1487913. [CrossRef] [PubMed]
27. Lachman, L.B.; Rao, X.M.; Kremer, R.H.; Ozpolat, B.; Kiriakova, G.; Price, J.E. DNA vaccination against neu reduces breast cancer incidence and metastasis in mice. *Cancer Gene Ther.* **2001**, *8*, 259–268. [CrossRef]
28. Eralp, Y.; Wang, X.; Wang, J.P.; Maughan, M.F.; Polo, J.M.; Lachman, L.B. Doxorubicin and paclitaxel enhance the antitumor efficacy of vaccines directed against HER2/neu in a murine mammary carcinoma model. *Breast Cancer Res.* **2004**, *6*, R275–R283. [CrossRef]
29. Wang, X.; Wang, J.P.; Rao, X.M.; Price, J.E.; Zhou, H.S.; Lachman, L.B. Prime-boost vaccination with plasmid and adenovirus gene vaccines control HER2/neu+ metastatic breast cancer in mice. *Breast Cancer Res.* **2005**, *7*, R580–R588. [CrossRef]
30. Leitner, W.W.; Hwang, L.N.; deVeer, M.J.; Zhou, A.; Silverman, R.H.; Williams, B.R.; Dubensky, T.W.; Ying, H.; Restifo, N.P. Alphavirus-based DNA vaccine breaks immunological tolerance by activating innate antiviral pathways. *Nat. Med.* **2003**, *9*, 33–39. [CrossRef]
31. Leslie, M.C.; Zhao, Y.J.; Lachman, L.B.; Hwu, P.; Wu, G.J.; Bar-Eli, M. Immunization against MUC18/MCAM, a novel antigen that drives melanoma invasion and metastasis. *Gene Ther.* **2007**, *14*, 316–323. [CrossRef] [PubMed]
32. Yin, X.; Wang, W.; Zhu, X.; Wang, Y.; Wu, S.; Wang, Z.; Wang, L.; Du, Z.; Gao, J.; Yu, J. Synergistic antitumor efficacy of combined DNA vaccines targeting tumor cells and angiogenesis. *Biochem. Biophys. Res. Commun.* **2015**, *465*, 239–244. [CrossRef] [PubMed]
33. Yamanaka, R.; Xanthopoulos, K.G. Induction of antigen-specific immune responses against malignant barin tumors by intramuscular injection of Sindbis DNA encoding gp100 and IL-18. *DNA Cell Biol.* **2005**, *24*, 317–324. [CrossRef] [PubMed]
34. Lundstrom, K. Self-Replicating RNA Viruses for RNA Therapeutics. *Molecules* **2018**, *23*, 3310. [CrossRef] [PubMed]
35. Kamrud, K.I.; Hooper, J.W.; Elgh, F.; Schmaljohn, C.S. Comparison of the protective efficacy of naked DNA, DNA-based Sindbis replicon, and packaged Sindbis replicon vectors expressing Hantavirus structural genes in hamsters. *Virology* **1999**, *263*, 209–219. [CrossRef]

36. Ajbani, S.P.; Velhal, S.M.; Kadam, R.B.; Patel, V.V.; Lundstrom, K.; Bandivdekar, A.H. Immunogenicity of virus-like Semliki Forest virus replicon particles expressing Indian HIV-1C gag, env and pol RT genes. *Immunol. Lett.* **2017**, *190*, 221–232. [CrossRef] [PubMed]
37. Ying, H.; Zaks, T.Z.; Wang, R.-F.; Irvine, K.R.; Kammula, U.S.; Marincola, F.M.; Leitner, W.W.; Restifo, N.P. Cancer therapy using a self-replicating RNA vaccine. *Nat. Med.* **1999**, *5*, 823–827. [CrossRef]
38. Saxena, S.; Sonwane, A.A.; Dahiya, S.S.; Patel, C.L.; Saini, M.; Rai, A.; Gupta, P.K. Induction of immune responses and protection in mice against rabies using a self-replicating RNA vaccine encoding rabies virus glycoprotein. *Vet. Microbiol.* **2009**, *136*, 36–44. [CrossRef]
39. Geall, A.J.; Verma, A.; Otten, G.R.; Shaw, C.A.; Hekele, A.; Banerjee, K.; Cu, Y.; Beard, C.W.; Brito, L.A.; Krucker, T. Nonviral delivery of self-amplifying RNA vaccines. *Proc. Natl. Acad. Sci. USA* **2012**, *109*, 14604–14609. [CrossRef]
40. Vignuzzi, M.; Gerbaud, S.; van der Werf, S.; Escriou, N. Naked RNA immunization with replicons derived from poliovirus and Semliki Forest virus genomes for the generation of a cytotoxic T cell response against the influenza A virus nucleoprotein. *J. Gen. Virol.* **2001**, *82*, 1737–1747. [CrossRef]
41. Leitner, W.W.; Hwang, L.N.; Bergmann-Leitner, E.S.; Finkelstein, S.E.; Frank, S.; Restifo, N.P. Apoptosis is essential for the increased efficacy of alphaviral replicase-based DNA vaccines. *Vaccine* **2004**, *22*, 1537–1544. [CrossRef] [PubMed]
42. Knudsen, M.L.; Mbewe-Mvula, A.; Rosario, M.; Johansson, D.X.; Kakoulidou, M.; Bridgeman, A.; Reyes-Sandoval, A.; Nicosia, A.; Ljungberg, K.; Hanke, T. Superior induction of T cell responses to conserved HIV-1 regions by electroporated alphavirus replicon DNA compared to that with conventional plasmid DNA vaccine. *J. Virol.* **2012**, *86*, 4082–4090. [CrossRef] [PubMed]
43. Berglund, P.; Smerdou, C.; Fleeton, M.N.; Tubulekas, I.; Liljeström, P. Enhancing immune responses using suicidal DNA vaccines. *Nat. Biotechnol.* **1998**, *16*, 562–565. [CrossRef] [PubMed]
44. Wolff, J.A.; Ludtke, J.J.; Acsadi, G.; Williams, P.; Jani, A. Long-term persistence of plasmid DNA and foreign gene expression in mouse muscle. *Hum. Mol. Genet.* **1992**, *1*, 363–369. [CrossRef]
45. Wang, Z.; Troilo, P.J.; Wang, X.; Griffiths, T.G.; Pacchione, S.J.; Barnum, A.B.; Harper, L.B.; Pauley, C.J.; Niu, Z.; Denisova, L. Detection of integration of plasmid DNA into host genomic DNA following intramuscular injection and electroporation. *Gene Ther.* **2004**, *11*, 711–721. [CrossRef] [PubMed]
46. Manam, S.; Ledwith, B.J.; Barnum, A.B.; Troilo, P.J.; Pauley, C.J.; Harper, L.B.; Griffiths, T.G., 2nd; Niu, Z.; Denisova, L.; Follmer, T.T. Plasmid DNA vaccines: Tissue distribution and effects of DNA sequence, adjuvants and delivery method on integration into host DNA. *Intervirology* **2000**, *43*, 273–281. [CrossRef] [PubMed]
47. Jiao, S.; Williams, P.; Berg, R.K.; Hodgeman, B.A.; Liu, L.; Repetto, G.; Wolff, J.A. Direct gene transfer into nonhuman primate myofibers in vivo. *Hum. Gene Ther.* **1992**, *3*, 21–33. [CrossRef]
48. Mairhofer, J.; Lara, A.R. Advances in host and vector development for the production of plasmid DNA vaccines. *Methods Mol. Biol.* **2014**, *1139*, 505–541.
49. Bernstein, D.I.; Reap, E.A.; Katen, K.; Watson, A.; Smith, K.; Norberg, P.; Olmsted, R.A.; Hoeper, A.; Morris, J.; Negri, S. Randomized, double-blind, Phase I trial of an alphavirus replicon vaccine for cytomegalovirus in CMV seronegative adult volunteers. *Vaccine* **2009**, *28*, 484–493. [CrossRef]
50. Morse, M.A.; Hobelka, A.C.; Osada, T.; Berglund, P.; Hubby, B.; Negri, S.; Niedzwiecki, D.; Devi, G.R.; Burnett, B.K.; Clay, T.M. An alphavirus vector overcomes the presence of neutralizing antibodies and elevated Tregs to induce to induce immune responses in humans with advanced cancers. *J. Clin. Investig.* **2010**, *120*, 3234–3241. [CrossRef]
51. Wecker, M.; Gilbert, P.; Russell, N.; Hural, J.; Allen, M.; Pensiero, M.; Chulay, J.; Chiu, Y.L.; Abdool Karim, S.S.; Burke, D.S. Phase I Safety and Immunogenicity Evaluations on an Alphavirus Replicon HIV-1 Subtype C gag Vaccine in Healthy HIV-1-Uninfected Adults. *Clin. Vaccine Immunol.* **2012**, *19*, 1651–1660. [CrossRef] [PubMed]

vaccines

MDPI

Article

Recombinant BCG Expressing HTI Prime and Recombinant ChAdOx1 Boost Is Safe and Elicits HIV-1-Specific T-Cell Responses in BALB/c Mice

Athina Kilpeläinen [1,2], Narcís Saubi [1,2], Núria Guitart [1], Alex Olvera [3,4], Tomáš Hanke [5,6], Christian Brander [3,4,7,8] and Joan Joseph [1,2,*]

1 Catalan Center for HIV Vaccine Research and Development, AIDS Research Unit, Infectious Diseases Department, Hospital Clínic/IDIBAPS, 08036 Barcelona, Catalonia, Spain
2 Vall d'Hebron Research Institute, Hospital Universitari Vall d'Hebron, 08035 Barcelona, Catalonia, Spain
3 Irsicaixa AIDS Research Institute, 08916 Badalona, Catalonia, Spain
4 Universitat de Vic-Universitat Central de Catalunya (UVic-UCC), 08500 Vic, Barcelona, Spain
5 Nuffield Department of Medicine, The Jenner Institute, University of Oxford, Oxford OX3 7DQ, UK
6 International Research Center of Medical Sciences (IRCMS), Kumamoto University, Kumamoto 860-0811, Japan
7 ICREA, Pg. Lluís Companys 23, 08010 Barcelona, Catalonia, Spain
8 AELIX Therapeutics, 08028 Barcelona, Catalonia, Spain
* Correspondence: jjoseph@vhebron.net

Received: 10 May 2019; Accepted: 24 July 2019; Published: 2 August 2019

Abstract: Despite the availability of anti-retroviral therapy, HIV-1 infection remains a massive burden on healthcare systems. Bacillus Calmette-Guérin (BCG), the only licensed vaccine against tuberculosis, confers protection against meningitis and miliary tuberculosis in infants. Recombinant BCG has been used as a vaccine vehicle to express both HIV-1 and Simian Immunodeficiemcy Virus (SIV) immunogens. In this study, we constructed an integrative *E. coli*-mycobacterial shuttle plasmid, p2auxo.HTI.int, expressing the HIVACAT T-cell immunogen (HTI). The plasmid was transformed into a lysine auxotrophic *Mycobacterium bovis* BCG strain (BCGΔ*Lys*) to generate the vaccine BCG.HTI$^{2auxo.int}$. The DNA sequence coding for the HTI immunogen and HTI protein expression were confirmed, and working vaccine stocks were genetically and phenotypically characterized. We demonstrated that the vaccine was stable in vitro for 35 bacterial generations, and that when delivered in combination with chimpanzee adenovirus (ChAd)Ox1.HTI in adult BALB/c mice, it was well tolerated and induced HIV-1-specific T-cell responses. Specifically, priming with BCG.HTI$^{2auxo.int}$ doubled the magnitude of the T-cell response in comparison with ChAdOx1.HTI alone while maintaining its breadth. The use of integrative expression vectors and novel HIV-1 immunogens can aid in improving mycobacterial vaccine stability as well as specific immunogenicity. This vaccine candidate may be a useful tool in the development of an effective vaccine platform for priming protective responses against HIV-1/TB and other prevalent pediatric pathogens.

Keywords: BCG; HIV; vaccine; rBCG; HTI; T-cell

1. Introduction

According to the latest reports, there are currently 37 million people infected with HIV, the majority of whom live in sub-Saharan Africa [1]. Despite the existence of anti-retroviral therapy, 1.8 million people were newly infected in 2017, and almost one million people died due to HIV-related disease [1]. Developing a safe, efficacious, and accessible HIV vaccine would be the optimal solution for the prevention of HIV-1 infection as well as reduction of HIV-related diseases. Evidence demonstrating the role of T-cell responses directed against HIV-1 in the control of viral replication is growing [2,3].

HIV-1-specific CD8$^+$ T-cells have been detected in exposed seronegative individuals, and CD8$^+$ cytotoxic T-lymphocytes (CTL) responses targeting HIV-1 Gag have been associated with reduced viral loads in infected individuals [4–6].

The "HIVACAT T-cell immunogen" (HTI) was designed to cover T-cell targets, against which T-cell responses are predominantly observed in HIV-1-infected individuals with low HIV-1 viral loads [7]. This immunogen has been manufactured as naked DNA, as well as introduced into viral vaccine vectors and an immunization regimen consisting of three injections of DNA encoding HTI followed by a boost with modified vaccinia Ankara (MVA)-vectored HTI has been shown in C57BL/6 mice to result in the induction of HIV-1 specific T-cell responses to most antigen regions included in its design. High magnitudes of HIV-1 specific T-cells were also induced in macaques following three injections of DNA.HTI and two injections of MVA.HTI [7]. It is well known that delivering a boosting injection of an immunogen using a viral vector such as MVA can boost the response of DNA immunization and increase the magnitude of responses. Such heterologous prime-boost regimens have been used for a number of immunogens in the context of HIV [8].

Upon intramuscular delivery, DNA vaccines are thought to induce cellular immunity through antigen synthesis and presentation to T-cells. The immunity is induced by the direct transfection of antigen-presenting cells (APCs) or through cross-presentation by APCs [9,10]. Similar to DNA, the *Mycobacterium bovis* strain, Bacillus Calmette-Guérin (BCG), when used as a vaccine vector also induces immunity by targeting APCs, although this occurs not through transfection, but rather through infection. Recombinant BCG is a promising live attenuated bacterial vaccine vector for inducing T-cell immunity, as it is a slow-growing organism that provides a persistent low-level antigenic exposure upon the infection of macrophages and APCs, and could drive effector and memory T-cell responses [11]. In the context of anti-tuberculosis (anti-TB) immunity, the pathogen for which BCG currently is licensed as a vaccine, immune responses in humans are predominantly T helper 1 (Th1)-cell mediated. Infected dendritic cells migrate to lymph nodes and activate antigen-specific CD4$^+$ T-cells in the presence of cytokines such as interleukin (IL)-18 and IL-12 [12]. The T-cell repertoire induced by vaccination is broad, targeting multiple mycobacterial antigens [13]. BCG is safe and is currently administered to 80% of infants in countries where it is part of the national childhood immunization program [14]. Aside from the induction of anti-TB immune responses, vaccination has been linked to decreased mortality due to other infections in infants [15,16]. This phenomenon has been related to the enhanced monocyte function observed in humans following vaccination, which is characterized by CD11b, TLR-4 expression, and increased cytokine production [17].

Recombinant BCG (rBCG) has been utilized as a vector to express HIV-1/Simian Immunodeficiency Virus (SIV) antigens and assessed regarding the induction of specific T-cell responses in several animal models [18]. The need for adjuvants is overcome as its cell-wall peptidoglycans and lipoproteins act as an adjuvant on their own [19–22]. BCG also has several advantages as a live vaccine vehicle, it is easy to mass-produce with low cost, and is heat stable [23]. It is also suitable for neonates, as vaccination is not affected by maternal antibodies [24,25]. Finally, it has a proven safety record after having been delivered as a TB vaccine to over three billion individuals [26]. As with DNA vaccination, rBCG-based HIV vaccines on their own may induce low-level specific immune responses, and thus they are often combined with virally vectored immunogens in heterologous prime-boost vaccination regimens where they have been shown to increase HIV-1 specific immune responses [27–30]. However, a rBCG expressing HIV-1 group M consensus Env vaccine on its own was shown to induce comparable immune responses both in the female reproductive tract and lungs when compared with adenovirus prime/recombinant vaccinia virus boost immunization [31]. The applicability of rBCG as a priming agent was demonstrated by Ami *et al.*, where priming with rBCG and boosting with a replication-deficient vaccinia virus strain expressing SIVgag was able to confer protection in Cynomolgus macaques against mucosal challenge with pathogenic SHIV. Interestingly, effective protection was not achieved in animals receiving the opposite combination or the vaccine modalities delivered on their own [32]. These data support the use of rBCG as a priming vector for an HIV-1 vaccine, whereby the use of rBCG could potentially strengthen or qualitatively modify the immune response when combined with DNA and/or a viral vector expressing an HIV-1 immunogen.

Here, we present the construction and characterization of recombinant BCG expressing the HTI immunogen, the BCG.HTI$^{2auxo.int}$ vaccine, harboring the integrated 2auxo expression cassette in their chromosome. The HTI immunogen has previously been assessed in mice and macaques when delivered as a prime-boost regimen vectored by DNA and MVA [7]. We demonstrate that BCG.HTI$^{2auxo.int}$ delivered in combination with ChAdOx1.HTI increases the HIV-1 specific T-cell responses in adult BALB/c mice. Priming with wild type BCG (BCGwt) was also shown to similarly increase the magnitude of the response, but significantly decreased the breadth of the T-cell responses. Furthermore, we demonstrate that priming with rBCG, in some mice, can alter the immunodominance profile of the vaccine-induced T-cell response.

2. Materials and Methods

2.1. Construction of the BCG.HTI$^{2auxo.int}$ Strain Using an Antibiotic-Free Plasmid Selection System

The double auxotrophic *E. coli*–mycobacterial shuttle integrative vector, the p2auxo.int plasmid, was previously constructed in our laboratory [33]. This vector contains the *glyA* and *LysA* genes, which function as an antibiotic-free selection and maintenance system in the auxotrophic strains of *E. coli* M15Δ*glyA* and BCGΔ*Lys*, respectively. It also contains sites (*attP*) for integration into the BCG genome at the *attB* site. The synthetic sequence of HTI [7] was codon-optimized for BCG expression to match the G+C rich mycobacterial codon usage for enhanced expression [34]. The HTI G+C rich DNA sequence was synthesized by Geneart (USA) and ligated to the integrative p2auxo.int plasmid fused to the 19-kDa lipoprotein secretion signal sequence generating p2auxo.HTI^{int}. The ligation products were subsequently transformed into the *E. coli* M15Δ*glyA* strain for growth and selection.

2.2. Bacterial Cultures and Transformation

Cells of the glycine auxotrophic strain of *E. coli*, M15Δ*Gly*, provided by Dr. Pau Ferrer (Universitat Autònoma de Barcelona, Spain), were cultured in LB supplemented with glycine (70 μg/mL). The *E. coli* M15Δ*Gly* cells were transformed with the p2auxo.HTI^{int} plasmid by electroporation. For this, the *E. coli* cultures were grown to an optical density of 0.125 at 600 nm, as well as concentrated and transformed using a Bio-Rad gene pulser electroporator at 2.5 kV, 25 μF, and 200 Ω. The transformed cells were subsequently cultured on M9-D agar plates (minimal M9-derivative medium: Na_2HPO_4, 6.78 g/L; KH_2PO_4, 3 g/L; NaCl, 0.5 g/L; NH_4Cl, 1 g/L, glucose, 10 g/L; $MgSO_4$, 2 mmol/L; $CaCl_2$, 0.1 mmol/L; thiamine, 0.1 g/L; $FeCl_3$, 0.025 g/L; $AlCl_3{\cdot}6H_2O$, 0.13 mg/L; $ZnSO_4{\cdot}7H_2O$, 2.6 mg/L; $CoCl_2{\cdot}6H_2O$, 0.47 mg/L; $CuSO_4{\cdot}H_2O$, 4.6 mg/L; H_3BO_3, 0.03 mg/L; $MnCl_2{\cdot}4H_2O$, 4.2 mg/L; $NiCl_2{\cdot}6H_2O$, 0.02 mg/L; $Na_2MoO_4{\cdot}2H_2O$, 0.06 mg/L, with 1.5% bactoagar added) without glycine supplementation for selection or with glycine supplementation as a control. The QIAprep Spin Miniprep Kit was used according to the manufacturer's instructions (Qiagen, Hilden, Germany) to extract plasmid DNA from *E. coli*. The resulting plasmids were tested for identity and correct insertion by PCR and restriction enzyme profiling. The selected plasmid was transformed into BCGΔ*lys*.

The lysine auxotrophic BCG strain, BCGΔ*lys*, kindly provided by W.R. Jacobs Jr., B.R. Bloom, and T. Hsu (Albert Einstein College of Medicine, New York, NY, USA), was transformed with p2auxo.HTI^{int} plasmid by electroporation. The mycobacteria were cultured in Middlebrook 7H9 broth medium or on Middlebrook agar 7H10 medium supplemented with albumin–dextrose–catalase (ADC; Difco Laboratories, Franklin Lakes, NJ, USA) containing 0.05% Tween 80. L-lysine monohydrochloride (Sigma) was dissolved in distilled water and used as a supplement at a final concentration of 40 μg/mL. For transformation, BCG was cultured to an optical density of 1.5 at 600 nm, washed with 10% glycerol, concentrated, and transformed using a Bio-Rad gene pulser electroporator at 2.5 kV, 25 μF, and 1000 Ω. Then, the transformants were cultured on ADC-supplemented Middlebrook agar 7H10 medium containing 0.05% Tween 80 without lysine supplementation. The resulting colonies were assessed for plasmid insertion, integrity, and HTI expression. From a selected colony, a Master Seed (MS) and a Working Vaccine Stock (WVS) were produced according to the seed lot system. For the BCG substrain identification assay, the commercial BCG Danish 1331 strain (Pfizer, New York, NY, USA) kindly provided by Dr. Neus Altet (Urology Department at Hospital Clínic de Barcelona, Barcelona, Spain), and the commercial BCG Connaught strain (ImmuCyst, Aventis, Paris, France) were used as standards.

2.3. Sodium Dodecyl Sulfate–Polyacrylamide Gel Electrophoresis and Western Blot Analysis

Cell lysates of mid-logarithmic phase BCG transformants were prepared by sonication in a protein extraction buffer (50 mmol/L Tris–HCl pH 7.5, 5 mmol/L Ethylenediaminetetraacetic acid (EDTA), 0.6% sodium dodecyl sulfate) containing protease inhibitor cocktail (Sigma-Aldrich, St Louis, MO, USA). Cell lysates supernatants were subsequently separated by a Novex 4–12% Bis-Tris SDS-PAGE gel (Thermo Fisher Scientific, Waltham, MA, USA), and electroblotted onto a pretreated polyvinylidene difluoride membrane using an iBlot kit (Thermo Fisher Scientific, Waltham, MA, USA). The HTI protein was stained using the primary anti-HTI monoclonal antibodies n63 and n69 at 5 μg/mL overnight kindly provided by Aelix Therapeutics (Barcelona) followed by secondary goat anti-mouse Immunoglobulin G-Horse Radish Peroxidase(IgG–HRP) antibody (Jackson ImmunoResearch, Cambridgeshire, UK) for 1 h diluted at 1:10,000. The membrane was developed using the SuperSignal™ West Femto Maximum Sensitivity Substrate kit (Thermo Fisher Scientific, Waltham, MA, USA).

2.4. In Vitro Stability of the BCG.HTI^{int} Strain

Five subcultures (~35 bacterial generations) from the MS of BCG.HTI$^{2auxo.int}$ harboring the p2auxo.HTI^{int} plasmid DNA (two selected clones) containing the lysine complementing gene were cultured in 7H9 Middlebrook broth with and without L-lysine selection. Subcultures were performed every 7 days by transferring 100 μL of the stationary phase culture to 5 mL of fresh medium. PCR analysis of the HTI DNA coding sequence were performed using insert specific primers designed at both HTI 3′ and 5′ sequences. PCR product size from the p2auxo.HTI.int plasmid and subcultures were compared.

2.5. Mycobacterial Genomic DNA Preparation for the Multiplex PCR Assay and for attR and attL DNA Regions PCR

For isolation of DNA from BCGwt, BCG.HTI$^{2auxo.int}$; 2 mL of mycobacterial culture was centrifuged at 5000 rpm for 10 min at room temperature. The pellet was resuspended in 200 μL of distilled water and heated at 95 °C for 20 min to inactivate and lyse bacterial cells. The sample was next centrifuged at a speed of 13,000× *g*. A total of 5 μL of supernatant was used for the amplification reaction. The commercial BCG strains were treated similarly, except in this case, 400 μL of the reconstituted freeze-dried flasks were used.

2.6. Multiplex PCR Assay for M. bovis BCG Substrain Pasteur Identification

The multiplex PCR assay was performed as described previously by Bedwell *et al.* [35], using 5 μL of mycobacterial DNA isolated from BCG.HTI$^{2auxo.int}$, BCG wt (Pasteur strain, kindly provided by W.R. Jacobs Jr., B.R. Bloom, and T. Hsu (Albert Einstein College of Medicine, New York, NY, USA)), and commercial BCG strains as template in a final reaction volume of 50 μL.

2.7. Immunization of Mice and Isolation of Splenocytes

Groups of eight adult (seven-week-old) female BALB/c mice were immunized intradermally in one footpad, and two groups were left unimmunized. The first group received 10^5 colony-forming units (CFU) of BCG.HTI$^{2auxo.int}$ (Group A), the second group received 10^6 CFU of BCG wt (Group B), both groups in one footpad. Two groups were left unimmunized (Groups C and D). ChAdOx1.HTI was constructed as previously described [36], and groups A–C were boosted intramuscularly with

10^9 viral particles (vp) after five weeks, while group D was left unimmunized. All the mice were sacrificed two weeks after the boost for immunogenicity analyses. Immediately following sacrifice of the animals, splenocytes were harvested and homogenized using 70 μm cell strainers (Falcon; Becton Dickinson, Franklin Lakes, NJ, United States) and 5-ml syringe rubber plungers. Red blood cells were removed with ACK lysing buffer (Lonza, Barcelona, Spain), and the splenocytes were washed and resuspended in complete medium (R10 (RPMI 1640 supplemented with 10% fetal calf serum and penicillin–streptomycin), 20 mmol/L of HEPES, and 15 mmol/L of 2-mercaptoethanol).

2.8. IFN-γ ELISpot Analysis

The Enzyme-linked immune absorbent spot (ELISpot) assay was performed using the commercial murine IFN-γ ELISpot kit (Mabtech, Nacka Strand, Sweden) according to the manufacturer's instructions. The ELISpot plates (MSISP4510, 96-well plates with polyvinylidene difluoride membranes, Millipore, USA) were 70% EtOH treated and coated with purified anti-mouse interferon-γ (IFN-γ) capture monoclonal antibody diluted in phosphate-buffered saline (PBS) to a final concentration of 5 μg/mL at 4 °C overnight. Then, 250,000 fresh splenocytes were added to each well and stimulated with 17 peptide pools containing a total of 147 15 mer overlapping peptides (OLP) spanning the HTI sequence, at a concentration of 10 μg/mL per peptide. Tuberculin purified protein derivative (PPD, AJ vaccines, Copenhagen, Denmark,) at a concentration of 5 μg/mL was used to assess TB-specific responses. All the samples and controls were plated in duplicate wells. ELISpot assays were incubated for 16 h at 37 °C, 5% CO_2. The plates were subsequently washed 5× with PBS, incubated for 2 h with a biotinylated anti-IFN-γ monoclonal antibody (mAb) diluted in PBS 2% Fetal Calf Serum (FCS) to a final concentration of 2 μg/mL, washed 5× in PBS, and incubated with the streptavidin–alkaline phosphatase conjugate in PBS 2% FCS. Then, plates were washed 5× with PBS before incubating with 100 μL of 5-bromo-4-chloro-3-indolyl phosphate (BCIP)/nitro blue tetrazolium (NBT) substrate solution (Sigma-Aldrich, St Louis, MO, USA). After 5–10 min, the plates were washed with tap water, dried, and the resulting spots counted using an ELISPOT reader (Autoimmune Diagnostika GmbH, Strassberg, Germany). For each animal, the mean of background responses was subtracted individually from all the wells to enable a comparison of the IFN-γ spot forming cells (SFC)/10^6 between groups. To define positive responses, a threshold was defined as at least five spots per well, and responses exceeding the mean number of spots in negative control wells plus three standard deviations of the negative control wells.

2.9. Statistical Analysis

Immunogenicity data is represented as group means of the total IFN-γ SFC/10^6 response or as medians for individual antigens/pools. Statistical differences were assessed by ordinary one-way analysis of variance when comparing total ELISpot responses or the Kruskal–Wallis test when comparing responses to individual pools. (* $p < 0.05$; ** $p < 0.01$; *** $p < 0.001$). GraphPad Prism 6.0 (Graphpad, San Diego, CA, USA) software was used. Body mass data are shown as group means with error bars indicating standard deviation as well as means ± 2 standard deviation (SD) from naïve mice. Statistical analyses were performed using the Kruskal–Wallis test.

2.10. Ethics Statement

The animal experiments strictly conformed to the animal welfare legislation of the Generalitat de Catalunya. All the experiments were approved by the local Research Ethics Committee (Procedure Med 365/16, Clinical Medicine, School of Medicine, University of Barcelona).

3. Results

3.1. Construction of the BCG.HTI$^{2auxo.int}$ Vaccine Strain

In the p2auxo.HTI^{int} *E. coli*-mycobacterial shuttle vector, the heterologous open reading protein expression cassette is under the control of the *Mtb* α-antigen promoter, which is a weak promoter that has been shown to enhance protein stability [37]. The open reading frame of the heterologous protein is initiated by the mycobacterial 19-kDa protein signal sequence, which at its 5′ end was fused to the HTI coding sequence. This enables the localization of the newly synthesized HTI polyprotein to the mycobacterial membrane, and subsequently its secretion, to prevent the internal accumulation of the heterologous protein and enhance protein immunogenicity (Figure 1A). The plasmid contains the *E. coli* origin of replication (*oriE*), attachment sites (*attP*), and the integrase (*int*) genes from the mycobacteriophage L5 [38], and integrates as a single copy into the *attB* region on the BCG chromosome. The plasmid also contains the wild-type glycine A-complementing gene (*glyA*) and lysine A-complementing gene (*lysA5*) for vector selection and maintenance in the auxotrophic *E. coli* and BCG strain, respectively [39,40]. The p2auxo.HTI^{int} was obtained following the methodology previously described [33] and transformed into the glycine auxotrophic *E. coli* M15ΔglyA strain and the lysine auxotrophic BCG Pasteur strain (Δ*lysA5*) [41,42]. The positive recombinant *E. coli* colonies were selected through culture on Minimal M9-D agar plates and the BCG.HTI$^{2auxo.int}$ colonies on Middlebrook agar 7H10 medium without lysine supplementation. Integration of the p2auxo.HTI^{int} plasmid DNA into the mycobacterial genome was assessed by PCR analysis of the *attR* and *attL* DNA insertion regions. The BCG.HTI$^{2auxo.int}$ was used as a template, and bands of 766 bp and 874 bp corresponding to the *attR* and *attL* DNA regions were detected (Figure 1B), demonstrating that p2auxo.HTI^{int} had integrated at the *attB* genomic BCG DNA region. Expression of the full-size chimeric 19-kDa signal sequence-HTI protein was confirmed by Western blot analysis of BCG.HTI$^{2auxo.int}$ lysates (Figure 1C). The selected clones were preserved using the seed-lot system. Clone #3 was selected as the candidate, and Master Seed stocks and Working Vaccine Stocks were prepared for further molecular characterization, immunogenicity, and safety testing in mice.

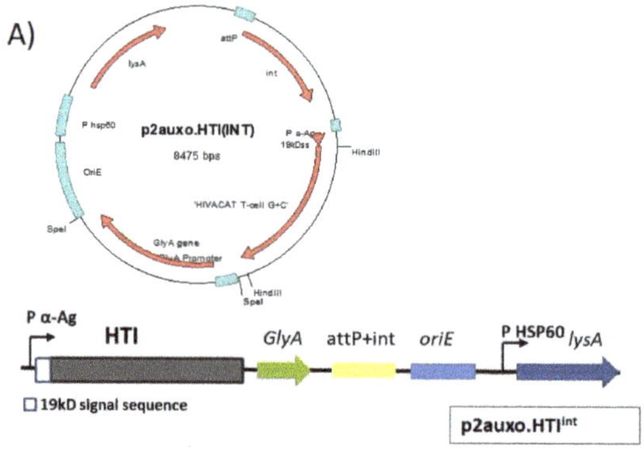

Figure 1. *Cont.*

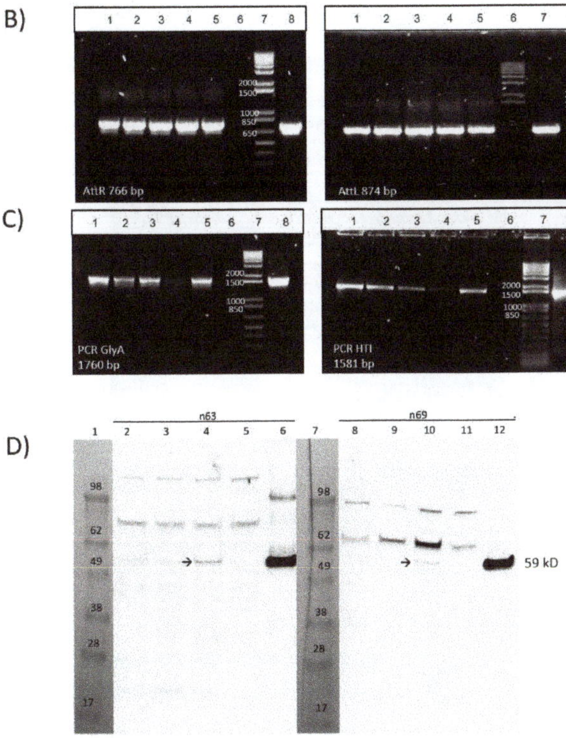

Figure 1. Construction of the recombinant Bacillus Calmette-Guérin HIVACAT T-cell immunogen (BCG.HTI$^{2auxo.int}$) strain. (**A**) The HTI synthetic sequence was BCG codon-optimized and fused to the 19-kDa lipoprotein signal sequence and inserted into the integrative p2auxo.HTI^{int} *E. coli*-mycobacterial shuttle plasmid. This vector contains P α-Ag, which is a *Mycobacterium tuberculosis* α-antigen promoter, PHSP60, which is a heat shock protein 60 gene promoter. The *glyA* and *LysA* complementing genes function as an antibiotic-free selection and maintenance system in the auxotrophic strains of *E. coli* M15Δ*glyA* and BCGΔ*Lys*, respectively; (**B**) PCR analysis of recombinant BCG clones transformed with p2auxo.HTI^{int} for integration sites: "*attR*" (left panel; lanes 1–5; clones 1–5; lane 6: BCG.empty$^{2auxo.int}$; lane 7: molecular weight marker; lane 8: p2auxo.HTI^{int}) and "*attL*" (right panel; lanes 1–5; clones 1–5; lane 6: molecular weight marker; lane 7: p2auxo.HTI^{int}; lane 8: BCG.empty$^{2auxo.int}$), (**C**) PCR analysis using primers specific for *glyA* (left) and HTI (right) on BCG transformed with p2auxo.HTI^{int} lanes 1–5; clones 1–5; lane 6: BCG.empty$^{2auxo.int}$; lane 7: molecular weight marker; lane 8: p2auxo.HTI^{int}. (**D**) Western blot of BCG.HTI$^{2auxo.int}$ lysates; lanes 1 and 7: Molecular weight marker; lanes 2 and 8: Master Seed of BCG.HTI$^{2auxo.int}$ clone 1; lanes 3 and 9: Master seed of BCG.HTI^{2auxoint} clone 3; lanes 4 and 10: Working Vaccine Stock of BCG.HTI$^{2auxo.int}$ clone 3; lanes 5 and 11: BCGwt (negative control); lanes 6 and 12: purified recombinant HTI protein. The HTI proteins were detected using the n63 (left) and n69 (right) mAbs directed against the HTI protein (AELIX Therapeutics, Barcelona, Spain) followed by horseradish peroxidase-goat-anti-mouse and enhanced chemiluminescence (ECL) detection.

3.2. Genetic Identification and Characterization of BCG.HTI$^{2auxo.int}$

To confirm that the identity of the BCG.HTI$^{2auxo.int}$ vaccine strains corresponded to the BCG Pasteur substrain, a multiplex PCR-based method was performed to analyze the BCG regions of difference such as RD1, 2, 8, 14, and 16 and the SenX3-RegX3 regions [35]. Different multiplex profiles obtained by this method allow the differentiation of BCG substrains. A PCR product of 196-bp length was generated using the primers ET1-3, indicating deletions of the RD1 region that were only found in BCG strains, not in the *Mycobacterium bovis* or *Mycobacterium tuberculosis* strains. The presence of the RD8 and RD16 regions was confirmed in the BCG.HTI$^{2auxo.int}$ and the BCG Pasteur substrain, which generated products of 472 bp and 401 bp, respectively. Products of 276 bp representing the SenX3-RegX3 region were also found. The molecular patterns of the BCG Danish, BCG Connaught, and BCG Pasteur substrains (Figure 2A) were consistent with previously published patterns [35].

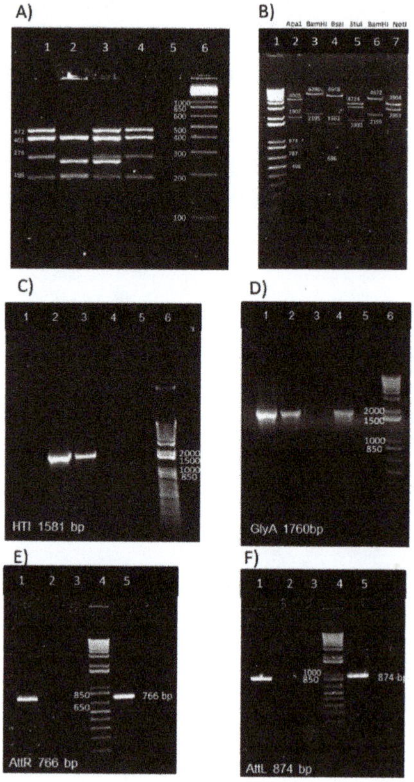

Figure 2. Genetic characterization of the BCG.HTI$^{2auxo.int}$ strain. (**A**) Pasteur substrain identification of BCG.HTI$^{2auxo.int}$ strains by multiplex PCR assay. Lane 1: BCG.HTI^{2auxoint} Working Vaccine Stock giving the bands of 472 bp, 401 bp, 276 bp, and 196 bp; lane 2: BCG Connaught giving the bands of 401 bp, 252 bp, and 196/199 bp; lane 3 BCG Danish with bands of 472 bp, 401 bp, 276 bp, 252 bp, and 196 bp, lane 4: BCG Pasteur with bands of 472 bp, 401 bp, 276 bp, and 196 bp; lane 5: negative control, distilled water; and lane 6: Molecular weight marker. (**B**) Enzymatic restriction analysis of p2auxo.HTI^{int} plasmid DNA purified from transformed *E. coli* M15ΔglyA cultures (pre-BCG transformation). Lane 1: molecular weight marker; Lane 2: *Apa1* digestion of p2auxo.HTI.int; Lane 3: *BamHI* digestion of p2auxo.HTI^{int}; Lane 4: *Bsal* digestion of p2auxo.HTI^{int}; Lane 5: *StuI* digestion of p2auxo.HTI.int; Lane 6: *BamHI* digestion of p2auxo.empty^{int}; Lane 7: *NotI* digestion of p2auxo.empty^{int}. (**C**) PCR detection of the HTI gene in the BCG.HTI$^{2auxo.int}$ WVS; lane 1: H_2O; lane 2: p2auxo.HTI^{int} plasmid; lane 3: working vaccine stock of BCG.HTI$^{2auxo.int}$; lane 4: BCG wt; lane 5: BCG transformed with empty 2auxo.int plasmid; lane 6: molecular weight marker. (**D**) PCR detection of the *GlyA* gene in the BCG.HTI$^{2auxo.int}$ working vaccine stock; lane 1: p2auxo.HTI^{int} plasmid; lane 2: WVS of BCG.HTI$^{2auxo.int}$; lane 3: BCGwt; lane 4: BCG transformed with empty 2auxo.int plasmid; lane 5: water; lane 6: molecular weight marker. PCR for right integration site, *attR* (**E**,**F**) left integration site, *attL* in the BCG.HTI$^{2auxo.int}$ WVS; lane 1 WVS of BCG.HTI$^{2auxo.int}$; lane 2: BCGwt; lane 3: distilled water; lane 4: molecular weight marker; lane 5: positive control, BCG.HIVconsv1$^{2auxo.int}$ Working Vaccine Stock (recombinant BCG expressing the HIVconsv1 immunogen [36,43]).

PCR and enzymatic restriction analysis were performed to characterize the p2auxo.HTI^{int} plasmid DNA. Following transformation of the *E. coli* M15 Δ*glyA* strain, plasmid DNA was purified, and the enzymatic restriction analysis revealed results that were consistent with the predicted enzymatic pattern (Figure 2B): *ApaI* digestion (Lane 2; bands of 4005 bp, 1907 bp, 974 bp, 787 bp, and 498 bp), *BamHI* digestion (Lane 3; bands of 6280 bp and 2195 bp), *BsaI* digestion (lane 4; bands of 4648 bp, 1563 bp, and 686 bp), *StuI* digestion (Lane 5; bands of 4672 bp and 1931 bp). The empty plasmid p2auxo.∅^{INT} restriction enzyme pattern was also consistent with the expected band pattern: *BamHI* (lane 6; 4672 bp and 2195 bp) and *NotI* (lane 7; bands of 3904 bp and 2963 bp). Next, we performed PCR analysis using specific primers for the HTI and E. coli *glyA* DNA coding sequences using the BCG.HTI$^{2auxo.int}$ Working Vaccine Stock as template. Bands of 1581 bp and 1760 bp corresponding to the expected size of HTI (Figure 2C) and the E. coli *glyA* DNA sequence (Figure 2D) were detected. Furthermore, PCR analysis using specific primers designed for 3′ and 5′ HTI ends was employed to confirm integration of the p2auxo.HTI^{int} plasmid DNA into the parental BCGΔ*lysA* strain genome. The BCG.HTI$^{2auxo.int}$ Working Vaccine Stock was used as a template. Bands of 766 bp and 874 bp corresponding to the respective *attR* (Figure 2E) and *attL* (Figure 2F) attachment sites were detected in Working Vaccine Stocks, but not in BCG wt. The HTI DNA coding sequence was detected by PCR in the BCG.HTI$^{2auxo.int}$ after 35 bacterial generations (Appendix A Figure A1).

3.3. Phenotypic Characterization of BCG.HTI$^{2auxo.int}$

To preserve plasmid stability, both in vivo and in vitro, as well as to prevent potential genetic rearrangements, several factors should be considered when constructing mycobacterium-based vaccine candidates. We previously demonstrated that the use of weak promoters (*Mycobacteria spp.* α-antigen promoter) and use of the BCG lysine auxotrophy-complementation system prevent the disruption of gene expression due to genetic rearrangements [33,37]. The lysine auxotrophic BCG strain was used in combination with lysine gene complementation as an antibiotic-free plasmid selection and maintenance system. To phenotypically assess the stability and demonstrate the lack of antibiotic resistance of this system, the BCG.HTI$^{2auxo.int}$ strain was cultured on non-lysine-supplemented agar with and without kanamycin. In line with previous findings, the untransformed lysine auxotrophic BCG strain failed to grow without the presence of lysine and grew upon supplementation with lysine (Figure 3A,B). The BCG.HTI$^{2auxo.int}$ strain, on the other hand, grew on non-lysine supplementation (Figure 3C), and did not grow on agar plates containing kanamycin (Figure 3D).

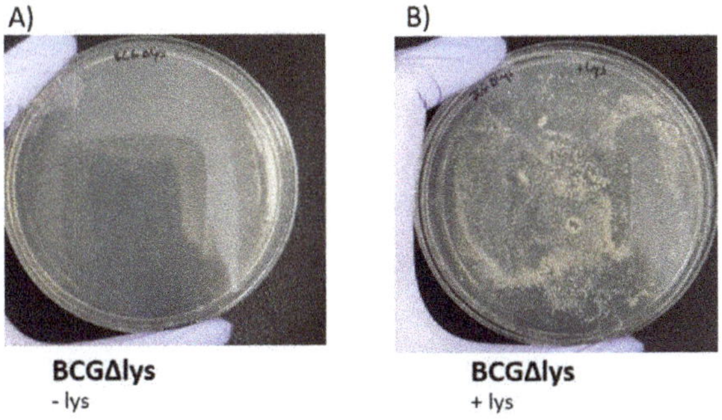

Figure 3. *Cont.*

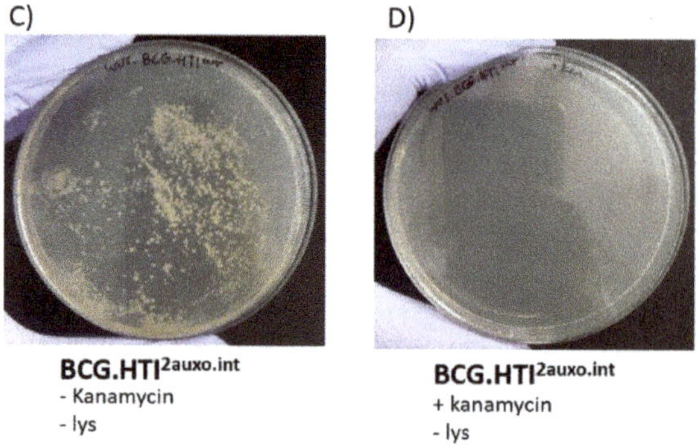

Figure 3. Phenotypic characterization of the BCG.HTI$^{2auxo.int}$ vaccine strain. Phenotype of lysine auxotrophy, lysine complementation, and kanamycin resistance. The BCG lysine auxotroph prior to transformation with p2auxo.HTI^{int} was cultured on non-lysine supplemented 7H10 (**A**) or on lysine supplemented 7H10 (**B**). The BCG.HTI$^{2auxo.int}$ WVS was cultured on 7H10 without lysine or kanamycin supplementation or without lysine but with kanamycin supplementation (**C**,**D**, respectively).

3.4. The BCG.HTI$^{2auxo.int}$ prime-ChAdOx1.HTI Boost Regimen Elicits HIV-1-Specific T-cell Responses

In order to assess the enhancement of cellular immune responses provided by a prime vaccination with BCG.HTI$^{2auxo.int}$, adult mice (seven-week-old, n = 8/group) were immunized with either 10^5 cfu of BCG.HTI$^{2auxo.int}$ (id) and boosted with ChAdOx1.HTI 10^9 viral particles (vp) delivered intramuscularly (im) after five weeks (group A), or with 10^6 BCGwt (id) and boosted with ChAdOx1.HTI (10^9 vp, im) after five weeks (group B), or only immunized with ChAdOx1.HTI (10^9 vp, im) at week five (group C), or left unimmunized (group D). The groups and immunization regimens are illustrated in Figure 4A. A group primed with BCGwt was included to allow comparison of the unspecific adjuvanticity of BCG and the specific priming of BCG expressing HTI. Two weeks post-boost, mice were sacrificed and splenocytes were isolated for an ELISpot analysis of IFN-γ secretion in response to 17 peptide pools spanning the HTI proteome. The total magnitude of IFN-γ secreting cells in response to HTI peptide pools was approximately doubled when priming with BCG.HTI$^{2auxo.int}$ as compared to ChAdOx1.HTI alone; however, the same was observed in BCGwt primed mice (Figure 4B). Overall, priming with BCG.HTI$^{2auxo.int}$ or BCGwt increased responses to peptide pools in the responding mice (Figure 4C–E), although these differences only reached trends when compared with animals only receiving ChAdOx1.HTI. In mice immunized with ChAdOx1.HTI alone, statistically significant differences as compared to naïve mice were only observed in response to one pool representing integrase (int) (pool 2C, Figure 4D). Priming with BCG.HTI$^{2auxo.int}$ induced significantly higher responses as compared to naïve mice in response to five HTI-derived pools (Figure 4: 1E p24; $p = 0.0469$, 1H p24; $p = 0.048$, 1K prot; $p = 0.0004$, 2B RT; $p = 0.0011$, and 2C int; $p = 0.0038$). A similar number was observed for mice primed with BCGwt (Figure 4: 1G p24; $p = 0.0016$, 1K prot; $p = 0.0002$, 2B RT; $p = 0.0004$, and 2C int; $p = 0.0360$). However, the IFN-γ response to pool 1E representing p24 was significantly higher in mice receiving BCG.HTI$^{2auxo.int}$ as compared to those receiving BCGwt (Figure 4C). Both the recombinant and wild-type BCG induced *Mtb*-specific responses (PPD, Figure 4E).

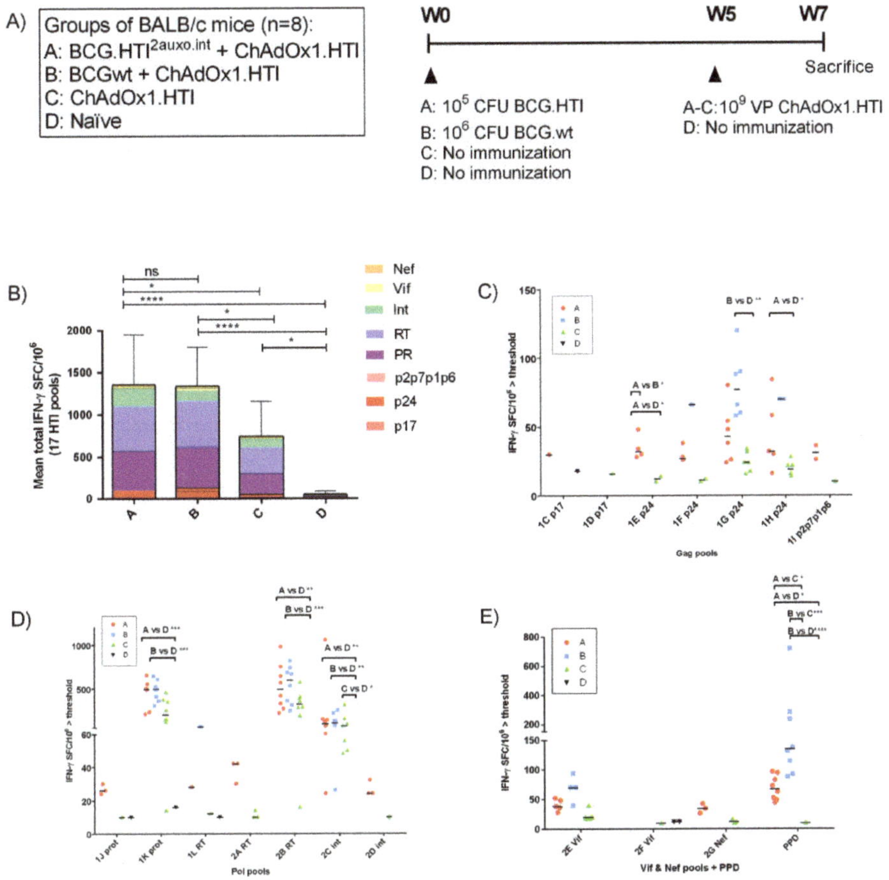

Figure 4. Induction of HIV-1 specific T-cell responses by the BCG.HTI$^{2auxo.int}$ + chimpanzee adenovirus HIVACAT T-cell immunogen (ChAdOx1.HTI) prime-boost regimen in BALB/c mice. Adult mice (seven weeks old, n = 8/group) were immunized with either 10^5 cfu of BCG.HTI$^{2auxo.int}$ (id) and boosted with ChAdOx1.HTI (10^9 vp, im) after five weeks (group A), or with 10^6 BCG.wt (id) and boosted with ChAdOx1.HTI (10^9 vp, im) after five weeks (group B), or only immunized with ChAdOx1.HTI (10^9 vp, im) at week five (group C), or left unimmunized (group D). Groups and the immunization schedule are shown in (**A**). Two weeks post-boost, mice were sacrificed, and splenocytes were isolated for enzyme-linked immune absorbent spot (ELISpot) analysis. (**B**) The total magnitude of HIV-1 specific SFCs/10^6 splenocytes was calculated as sums of the SFCs elicited by the 17 HTI peptide pools, the color-coding represents the HIV-1 gene location of the pools. Data are presented as group means and error bars represent the standard deviation of the total sum of SFC/10^6 splenocytes. Statistics were performed using parametric one-way ANOVA. (C-E) HIV-1 and tuberculosis (TB)-specific T-cell responses interferon-γ (IFN-γ spot-forming cells SFC/10^6 in response to HTI-derived peptide pools representing HIV-1 Gag (**C**), HIV-1 Pol (**D**), and Nef, Vif, and tuberculin purified protein derivative (PPD) (**E**). The data are presented as medians of group responses above the threshold. Statistics were performed using the non-parametric Kruskal–Wallis test adjusted for multiple comparisons, *$p < 0.05$, **$p < 0.01$, ***$p < 0.001$ and ****$p < 0.0001$.

Interestingly, a comparison of the average number of reactive HTI peptide pools in vaccinated mice revealed that the number of reactive pools in BCGwt primed mice was significantly lower than in those primed with BCG.HTI$^{2auxo.int}$ (Figure 5A, p = 0.0262). This indicates a loss of breadth when priming with BCGwt, even though IFN-γ secreting cells in response to HTI peptide pools were similar when compared with BCG.HTI$^{2auxo.int}$ primed mice. No differences between BCG.HTI$^{2auxo.int}$ primed mice as compared to mice only receiving ChAdOx1.HTI (Figure 5A) were observed regarding the number of pools recognized per mouse, although the mean was slightly increased from 7.3 to 7.8 when priming with BCG.HTI$^{2auxo.int}$. The highest number of recognized peptide pools was 13 in both groups. Interestingly, certain mice of the BCG.HTI$^{2auxo.int}$ + ChAdOx1.HTI immunized group reacted to pools less frequently recognized by other groups (Figure 5B: 1E p24, 1F p24, 1J prot, 2D int). On the other hand, lower numbers of mice recognized certain peptide pools (Figure 5B: 1G p24, 1H p24, 2E Vif) when compared to mice only immunized with ChAdOx1.HTI.

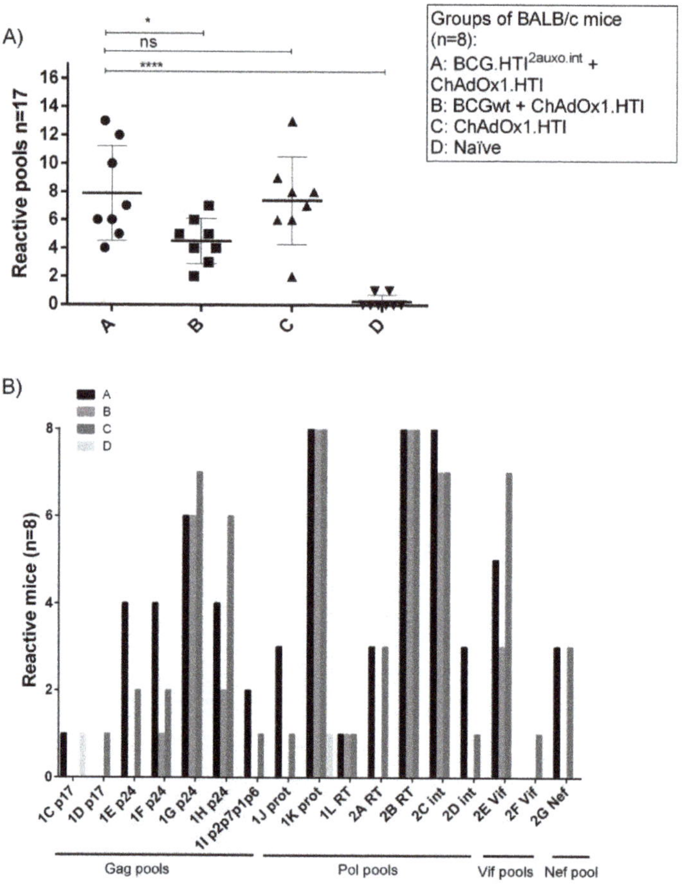

Figure 5. Differential recognition of peptide pools in BCG.HTI$^{2auxo.int}$ + ChAdOx1.HTI immunized BALB/c mice. Adult mice (seven weeks old, $n = 8$/group) were immunized with either 10^5 cfu of BCG.HTI$^{2auxo.int}$ (id) and boosted with ChAdOx1.HTI (10^9 vp, im) after five weeks (group A), or with 10^6 BCG.wt (id) and boosted with ChAdOx1.HTI (10^9 vp, im) after five weeks (group B), or only immunized with ChAdOx1.HTI (10^9 vp, im) at week five (group C), or left unimmunized (group D). Two weeks post-boost, mice were sacrificed, splenocytes were isolated for ELISPOT analysis, and the numbers of reactive peptide pools (total n peptide pools =17) were compared for each mouse. (**A**) The number of reactive pools per mouse. (**B**) The number of reactive mice (eight mice per group) in each group according to peptide pool and HIV-1 gene location. Statistics were performed using parametric one-way ANOVA, $^{*}p < 0.05$, $^{**}p < 0.01$, $^{***}p < 0.001$, $^{****}p < 0.0001$.

3.5. The BCG.HTI$^{2auxo.int}$ + ChAdOx1.HTI Prime-Boost Regimen Is Well Tolerated

Five adult mice per group were either left unimmunized or received 10^6 colony-forming units (cfu) of BCG wt or a total of 10^5 cfu of BCG.HTI$^{2auxo.int}$ intradermally, and five weeks later were boosted with 10^9 vp of ChAdOx1.HTI and their body mass was monitored regularly over time (Figure 6). The body mass curve corresponded to those of the provider (Envigo, Huntington, UK), and there were no statistically significant differences observed between the vaccine recipients and controls at any time point tested (Figure 6). Mice were monitored weekly for signs of malaise. No vaccine-related deaths, no local adverse events, and no associated systemic reactions were observed.

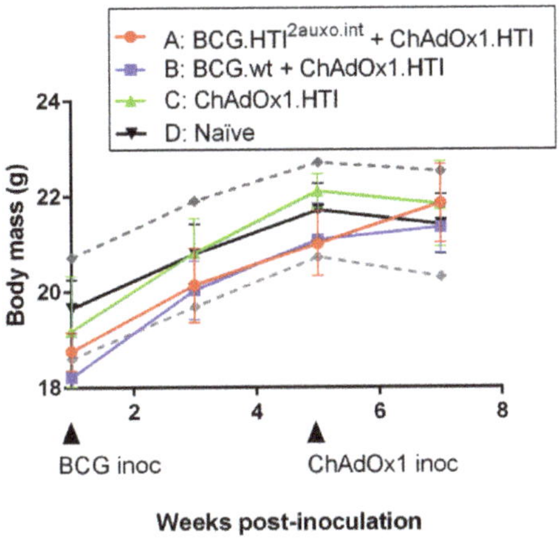

Figure 6. Safety of the BCG.HTI$^{2auxo.int}$ and ChAdOx1.HTI prime-boost regimen in BALB/c mice. Mice in groups of five (female, seven weeks old) were immunized i.d. with 10^5 colony-forming units (CFU) of BCG.HTI$^{2auxo.int}$ or 10^6 CFU BCGwt and boosted with 10^9 VP of ChAdOx1.HTI. Body weights were recorded regularly, and the mean for each group of mice is shown as mean ± SD (n = 5). Data from naive mice are presented as mean ± 2 SD (n = 5) (dashed grey lines).

4. Discussion

Despite the exploration and implementation of numerous HIV-1 prevention strategies, 1.8 million new HIV infections occurred in 2017 [44]. There is an urgent need for the development of an effective, safe, and affordable HIV-1 vaccine. We have constructed an rBCG vaccine candidate expressing the HIVACAT T-cell immunogen, HTI, using the integrative antibiotic-resistance free *E. coli*-mycobacterial shuttle vector, p2auxo.int. The HTI immunogen was designed to target T-cell responses to the most beneficial T-cell targets and the most vulnerable sites of HIV-1. When delivered using DNA and MVA vectors, it has been shown to be capable of inducing broadly and evenly distributed immune responses of high magnitude in mice and monkeys [7]. We have previously demonstrated the in vitro and in vivo stability of the integrative plasmid p2auxo.int for expressing HIV-1 immunogens in BCG [33,43]. Here, we produced the BCG.HTI$^{2auxo.int}$ vaccine candidates under Good Laboratory Practice compatible conditions, and characterized them genotypically and phenotypically, confirming the presence of the HTI gene and protein in the lysates of working vaccine stocks. Furthermore, we demonstrate that the BCG.HTI$^{2auxo.int}$ vaccine in combination with ChAdOx1.HTI induced TB and HIV-1-specific IFN-γ-producing T-cell responses in adult BALB/c mice. The vaccination regimen was well tolerated during the follow-up period, although a longer safety assessment will be necessary, as symptoms related to a lack of attenuation of mycobacteria could take at least 50 days to emerge and impact body mass in the mouse model [45].

BCG is a remarkable live vaccine vehicle due to its capability of delivering antigens to APCs enabling the development of antigen-specific cell-mediated immune responses [24]. Mycobacterial antigens have been shown to be presented to T-cells by non-classical antigen presentation molecules such as CD1a/b/c, Major histocompatibility complex class I-related gene protein (MR1), and Human leukocyte antigen-E (HLA-E). The latter is of specific interest in the context of HIV-1 vaccine development due to the resistance of HLA-E to downregulation by the HIV-1 Nef during infection [46], as well as displaying a low level of allelic variation, with only forty three existing variants as opposed to the thousands of classical HLA class I molecules [47]. Furthermore, BCG-immunized humans elicited HLA-E restricted $CD8^+$ T-cell responses to *Mtb* peptides, which display cytotoxic as well as immunoregulatory activities [48]. One of the most successful HIV-related vaccine trials in animal models has been a Cytomegalovirus (CMV) vectored vaccine against SIV. This vaccine was able to establish persistent, SIV-specific effector memory T-cell responses in rhesus macaques and control pathogenic SIV infection following mucosal challenge [49]. CMV infection is known to upregulate HLA-E expression in humans, and the vaccine regimen in the monkeys induced strong Mamu-E restricted T-cell responses [50]. It is still unknown if BCG can elicit a similar immune response to a heterologous antigen when used as a vaccine vector in humans. However, BCG administered as an oral adjuvant along with inactivated simian immunodeficiency virus (SIV)mac239 particles in Chinese macaques was shown to confer protection to a high-dose SIVmac239 challenge [51]. The protection was attributed to non-cytolytic Major histocompatibility complex (MHC) Ib/E-restricted $CD8^+$ T-regulatory cells that suppressed the activation of SIV-positive $CD4^+$ T-lymphocytes.

As a vector, rBCG shares several traits with plasmid DNA. Both are often used as priming agents in combination with a virally vectored boost [8,24]. A rBCG–DNA prime-boost regimen showed less immunogenicity when explored using the HIVA immunogen, as compared to boosting with viral vectors [28]. On the other hand, a combination regimen of rBCG and DNA expressing HIVA was shown to confer protection in a pathogenic vaccinia–HIVA surrogate challenge model [39]. However, little is known about the advantages for specific immunity to heterologous immunogens upon combining rBCG, DNA, and viral vectors.

Recombinant BCG delivered on its own induces weak transgene-specific immune responses that are difficult to measure. Thus, we have assessed the enhancement of HIV-1 specific cellular immune responses by a prime vaccination with BCG.HTI$^{2auxo.int}$ when delivered with ChAdOx1.HTI in BALB/c mice. The magnitude of the total T-cell response was significantly higher in BCG.HTI$^{2auxo.int}$ primed mice as compared to mice receiving ChAdOx1.HTI alone. A similar magnitude was observed in BCGwt primed mice (Figure 4). The IFN-γ secretion in response to the individual HTI peptide pools was higher in all the assessed pools, although the differences did not reach statistical significance between mice receiving BCG prime and those not. The evident priming effect, even by BCGwt, is in line with the ability of BCG derivatives to act as potent adjuvants for subsequent boosting vaccines. It is known that immunization with BCG not expressing any transgene often can lead to higher vaccine-specific responses when delivered as a prime/adjuvant in combination with a virally vectored vaccine [39,52]. Components of BCG have also been used as an adjuvant for an HIV-1 DNA vaccine [53].

Interestingly, both BCG.HTI$^{2auxo.int}$ primed mice and mice receiving ChAdOx1.HTI alone responded to an average of seven to eight peptide pools, whereas mice primed with BCGwt alone only responded to an average of 4.5 peptide pools. This together suggests that priming with BCG.HTI$^{2auxo.int}$ enhances the HTI-specific immune response when delivered with ChAdOx1.HTI, while maintaining the breadth of the response. Priming with BCGwt appeared to boost the overall magnitude of the response, but ultimately directing responses to fewer peptide pools. The differences in the breadth of immune responses between the BCG.HTI$^{2auxo.int}$ and BCGwt could possibly be related to the strong adjuvant properties of BCG. A possible explanation is its capability of inducing trained immunity. This involves enhanced monocyte function and Natural killer (NK) cell function as reviewed by van der Meer et al. [54]. Macrophages, monocytes, and natural killer cells display enhanced responsiveness following a second encounter with a pathogen. Enhanced monocyte function has been demonstrated in humans three months after BCG vaccination along with increased cytokine production, as well as CD11b and toll-like receptor 4 (TLR-4) expression [17]. This effect could be observed up to one year following immunization [55]. The unspecific immune activation could perhaps be involved in mechanisms enhancing the production of cytokines such as IFN-γ in T-cells, which leads to higher responses in the epitopes, which are more dominant. It is notable that the HTI was designed to avoid useless immunodominant epitopes in humans, but nevertheless, it is inevitable that there will be a hierarchy of epitopes in mice in which cellular immune responses are elicited against. Thus, the higher breadth observed following priming with the BCG.HTI$^{2auxo.int}$ could be related to the priming of responses that are specifically related to the transgene expressed (HTI), whereas the general increase in IFN-γ induced by BCGwt could be related to unspecific or adjuvanticity-related effects on the immune system rather than the specific priming of immune responses directed toward HTI. Previously, C57BL/6 mice immunized with DNA.HTI alone were shown to respond to two to six HTI peptide pools, and following an immunization schedule consisting of three DNA.HTI prime immunizations and one MVA.HTI immunization delivered at three-week intervals, this number was increased to six to 11 peptide pools [7]. Delivering a combination of BCG.HTI$^{2auxo.int}$, DNA, and a viral vector expressing HTI could present a strategy for increasing the number of recognized pools further.

Correlates of protection for HIV-1 vaccines have been discussed following the RV144 trial, such as the IgG Ab response to the variable regions 1 and 2 (V1V2) loops being associated with a reduction in HIV-1 acquisition [56]. However, the translatability of data obtained in small animal models is limited, and pre-clinical design and the evaluation of HIV-1 vaccines remains a challenge. In humans, T-cell responses have also been associated with protection or decreased viral loads following infection. For instance, in the RV144 trial, $CD4^+$ T-cells secreting IL-2, TNF-α, IFN-γ, IL-4, and CD154 in response to HIV-1 envelope peptides were associated with lower infection rates in vaccine recipients [57].

5. Conclusions

We here demonstrate that priming with BCG.HTI$^{2auxo.int}$ significantly increased HTI-specific T-cell responses. Although priming with BCGwt led to a similar enhancement of the magnitude of the response, fewer peptide pools were recognized in BCGwt primed animals. The ability of the BCG.HTI$^{2auxo.int}$ priming immunization to increase T-cell immune responses when combined with ChAdOx1.HTI, while maintaining the breadth of the response, strengthens its applicability as a priming vaccine for the development of an efficacious HIV-1 vaccine. Finally, we demonstrate that in some mice, priming with BCG.HTI$^{2auxo.int}$ can alter the immunodominance profile of the vaccine-induced T-cell response. Further assessments and characterization of the T-cell response by intracellular cytokine staining would provide a more thorough overview of the vaccine-induced immune response and of potential functional differences, depending on the different vaccination regimen.

Author Contributions: Conceptualization, J.J., A.K., and C.B.; methodology, A.K. and N.G.; software, A.K.; validation, A.K., N.S. and A.O.; formal analysis, A.K.; investigation, A.K. and N.S.; resources, J.J., T.H.; data curation, A.K., N.G. and N.S.; writing—original draft preparation, A.K.; writing—review and editing, N.S., J.J. A.O. and C.B.; visualization, A.K.; supervision, N.S. and J.J.; project administration, J.J.; funding acquisition, J.J.", please turn to the CRediT taxonomy for the term explanation. Authorship must be limited to those who have contributed substantially to the work reported.

Funding: This research was funded by the European Union's Horizon 2020 research and innovation program under grant agreement No. 681137 and supported by Instituto de Salud Carlos III FIS PI14/00494. EAVI2020. In addition, it has been supported by the ISCIII, RETIC-RIS RD12/0017, and the HIVACAT Research Program.

Conflicts of Interest: The funders had no role in the design of the study; in the collection, analyses, or interpretation of data; in the writing of the manuscript, or in the decision to publish the results. C. Brander is CSO at AELIX Therapeutics, Barcelona. The remaining authors declare no conflict of interest.

Appendix A

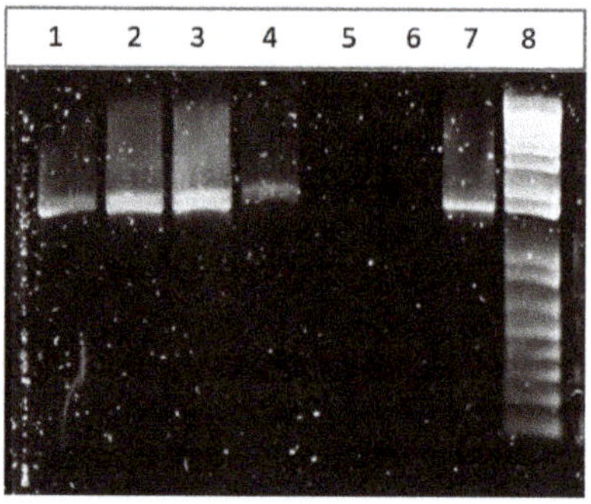

Figure A1. In vitro stability of BCG.HTI^{2auxoint}. *In vitro* stability was assessed by PCR detection of the HTI gene in the BCG.HTI$^{2auxo.int}$ master seeds after five weekly subcultures with and without added lysine; lane 1; BCG.HTI$^{2auxo.int}$ clone 1; lane 2: BCG.HTI$^{2auxo.int}$ clone 3; lane 3: BCG.HTI$^{2auxo.int}$ clone 1 cultured in lysine supplemented medium; lane 4: BCG.HTI$^{2auxo.int}$ clone 3 cultured in lysine supplemented medium; lane 5: BCG.Ø$^{2auxo.int}$; lane 6: distilled water; lane 7: p2auxo.HTI.int plasmid; lane 8: molecular weight marker.

References

1. World Health Organization. Data and Statistics. Available online: https://www.who.int/hiv/data/2017_global_summary_web_v11.pptx (accessed on 5 February 2019).
2. Rowland-Jones, S.L.; Dong, T.; Fowke, K.R.; Kimani, J.; Krausa, P.; Newell, H.; Blanchard, T.; Ariyoshi, K.; Oyugi, J.; Ngugi, E.; et al. Cytotoxic T cell responses to multiple conserved HIV epitopes in HIV-resistant prostitutes in Nairobi. *J. Clin. Investig.* **1998**, *102*, 1758–1765. [CrossRef] [PubMed]
3. Koup, R.A.; Safrit, J.T.; Cao, Y.; Andrews, C.A.; McLeod, G.; Borkowsky, W.; Farthing, C.; Ho, D.D. Temporal association of cellular immune responses with the initial control of viremia in primary human immunodeficiency virus type 1 syndrome. *J. Virol.* **1994**, *68*, 4650–4655. [PubMed]
4. Kuebler, P.J.; Mehrotra, M.L.; McConnell, J.J.; Holditch, S.J.; Shaw, B.I.; Tarosso, L.F.; Leadabrand, K.S.; Milush, J.M.; York, V.A.; Raposo, R.A.S.; et al. Cellular immune correlates analysis of an HIV-1 preexposure prophylaxis trial. *Proc. Natl. Acad. Sci. USA* **2015**, *112*, 8379–8384. [CrossRef] [PubMed]
5. Zuñiga, R.; Lucchetti, A.; Galvan, P.; Sanchez, S.; Sanchez, C.; Hernandez, A.; Sanchez, H.; Frahm, N.; Linde, C.H.; Hewitt, H.S.; et al. Relative dominance of Gag p24-specific cytotoxic T lymphocytes is associated with human immunodeficiency virus control. *J. Virol.* **2006**, *80*, 3122–3125. [CrossRef] [PubMed]
6. Janes, H.; Friedrich, D.P.; Krambrink, A.; Smith, R.J.; Kallas, E.G.; Horton, H.; Casimiro, D.R.; Carrington, M.; Geraghty, D.E.; Gilbert, P.B.; et al. Vaccine-Induced Gag-Specific T Cells Are Associated With Reduced Viremia After HIV-1 Infection. *J. Infect. Dis.* **2013**, *208*, 1231–1239. [CrossRef] [PubMed]
7. Mothe, B.; Hu, X.; Llano, A.; Rosati, M.; Olvera, A.; Kulkarni, V.; Valentin, A.; Alicea, C.; Pilkington, G.R.; Sardesai, N.Y.; et al. A human immune data-informed vaccine concept elicits strong and broad T-cell specificities associated with HIV-1 control in mice and macaques. *J. Transl. Med.* **2015**, *13*, 60. [CrossRef] [PubMed]
8. Iyer, S.S.; Amara, R.R. DNA/MVA Vaccines for HIV/AIDS. *Vaccines* **2014**, *2*, 160–178. [CrossRef] [PubMed]
9. Donnelly, J.J.; Liu, M.A.; Ulmer, J.B. Antigen Presentation and DNA Vaccines. *Am. J. Respir. Crit. Care Med.* **2000**, *162*, S190–S193. [CrossRef] [PubMed]
10. Corr, M.; Lee, D.J.; Carson, D.A.; Tighe, H. Gene vaccination with naked plasmid DNA: Mechanism of CTL priming. *J. Exp. Med.* **1996**, *184*, 1555–1560. [CrossRef]
11. Van Faassen, H.; Dudani, R.; Krishnan, L.; Sad, S. Prolonged antigen presentation, APC-, and CD8+ T cell turnover during mycobacterial infection: Comparison with Listeria monocytogenes. *J. Immunol.* **2004**, *172*, 3491–3500. [CrossRef]

12. Ravn, P.; Boesen, H.; Pedersen, B.K.; Andersen, P. Human T cell responses induced by vaccination with Mycobacterium bovis bacillus Calmette-Guérin. *J. Immunol.* **1997**, *158*, 1949–1955. [PubMed]
13. Averill, L.E.; Cavallo, U.; Wallis, R.S.; Boom, W.H.; Bona, M.; Mincek, M.; Pascopella, L.; Jacobs, W.R.; Ellner, J.J. Screening of a cosmid library of Mycobacterium bovis BCG in Mycobacterium smegmatis for novel T-cell stimulatory antigens. *Res. Microbiol.* **1993**, *144*, 349–362. [CrossRef]
14. World Health Organization. BCG Vaccine. Available online: http://www.who.int/biologicals/areas/vaccines/bcg/en/ (accessed on 6 September 2018).
15. Roth, A.; Gustafson, P.; Nhaga, A.; Djana, Q.; Poulsen, A.; Garly, M.-L.; Jensen, H.; Sodemann, M.; Rodriques, A.; Aaby, P. BCG vaccination scar associated with better childhood survival in Guinea-Bissau. *Int. J. Epidemiol.* **2005**, *34*, 540–547. [CrossRef] [PubMed]
16. Post, C.L.; Victora, C.G.; Valente, J.G.; Leal, M.d.C.; Niobey, F.M.; Sabroza, P.C. Prognostic factors of hospital mortality from diarrhea or pneumonia in infants younger than 1 year old. A case-control study. *Rev. Saude Publica* **1992**, *26*, 369–378. [CrossRef] [PubMed]
17. Kleinnijenhuis, J.; Quintin, J.; Preijers, F.; Joosten, L.A.B.; Ifrim, D.C.; Saeed, S.; Jacobs, C.; van Loenhout, J.; de Jong, D.; Stunnenberg, H.G.; et al. Bacille Calmette-Guerin induces NOD2-dependent nonspecific protection from reinfection via epigenetic reprogramming of monocytes. *Proc. Natl. Acad. Sci. USA* **2012**, *109*, 17537–17542. [CrossRef] [PubMed]
18. Kilpeläinen, A.; Maya-Hoyos, M.; Saubí, N.; Soto, C.Y.; Joseph Munne, J. Advances and challenges in recombinant Mycobacterium bovis BCG-based HIV vaccine development: Lessons learned. *Expert Rev. Vaccines* **2018**, *17*, 1005–1020. [CrossRef]
19. Melancon-Kaplan, J.; Hunter, S.W.; McNeil, M.; Stewart, C.; Modlin, R.L.; Rea, T.H.; Convit, J.; Salgame, P.; Mehra, V.; Bloom, B.R. Immunological significance of Mycobacterium leprae cell walls. *Proc. Natl. Acad. Sci. USA* **1988**, *85*, 1917–1921. [CrossRef] [PubMed]
20. Oiso, R.; Fujiwara, N.; Yamagami, H.; Maeda, S.; Matsumoto, S.; Nakamura, S.; Oshitani, N.; Matsumoto, T.; Arakawa, T.; Kobayashi, K. Mycobacterial trehalose 6,6′-dimycolate preferentially induces type 1 helper T cell responses through signal transducer and activator of transcription 4 protein. *Microb. Pathog.* **2005**, *39*, 35–43. [CrossRef]
21. Fujita, Y.; Naka, T.; Doi, T.; Yano, I. Direct molecular mass determination of trehalose monomycolate from 11 species of mycobacteria by MALDI-TOF mass spectrometry. *Microbiology* **2005**, *151*, 1443–1452. [CrossRef]
22. Brightbill, H.D.; Libraty, D.H.; Krutzik, S.R.; Yang, R.B.; Belisle, J.T.; Bleharski, J.R.; Maitland, M.; Norgard, M.V.; Plevy, S.E.; Smale, S.T.; et al. Host defense mechanisms triggered by microbial lipoproteins through toll-like receptors. *Science* **1999**, *285*, 732–736. [CrossRef]
23. Gheorghiu, M.; Lagrange, P.H.; Fillastre, C. The stability and immunogenicity of a dispersed-grown freeze-dried Pasteur BCG vaccine. *J. Biol. Stand.* **1988**, *16*, 15–26. [CrossRef]
24. Matsuo, K.; Yasutomi, Y. Mycobacterium bovis Bacille Calmette-Guérin as a Vaccine Vector for Global Infectious Disease Control. *Tuberc. Res. Treat.* **2011**, *2011*, 9.
25. Joseph, J.; Saubi, N.; Pezzat, E.; Gatell, J.M. Progress towards an HIV vaccine based on recombinant Bacillus Calmette–Guérin: Failures and challenges. *Expert Rev. Vaccines* **2006**, *5*, 827–838. [CrossRef] [PubMed]
26. World Health Organization BCG vaccine. WHO position paper. *Relev. Epidemiol. Hebd.* **2004**, *79*, 27–38.
27. Hopkins, R.; Bridgeman, A.; Joseph, J.; Gilbert, S.C.; McShane, H.; Hanke, T. Dual neonate vaccine platform against HIV-1 and M. tuberculosis. *PLoS ONE* **2011**, *6*, e20067. [CrossRef] [PubMed]
28. Hopkins, R.; Bridgeman, A.; Bourne, C.; Mbewe-Mvula, A.; Sadoff, J.C.; Both, G.W.; Joseph, J.; Fulkerson, J.; Hanke, T. Optimizing HIV-1-specific CD8+ T-cell induction by recombinant BCG in prime-boost regimens with heterologous viral vectors. *Eur. J. Immunol.* **2011**, *41*, 3542–3552. [CrossRef]
29. Chapman, R.; Stutz, H.; Jacobs, W.; Shephard, E.; Williamson, A.L.L. Priming with Recombinant Auxotrophic BCG Expressing HIV-1 Gag, RT and Gp120 and Boosting with Recombinant MVA Induces a Robust T Cell Response in Mice. *PLoS ONE* **2013**, *8*, 8. [CrossRef]
30. Hart, B.E.; Asrican, R.; Lim, S.Y.; Sixsmith, J.D.; Lukose, R.; Souther, S.J.R.; Rayasam, S.D.G.; Saelens, J.W.; Chen, C.J.; Seay, S.A.; et al. Stable Expression of Lentiviral Antigens by Quality-Controlled Recombinant Mycobacterium bovis BCG Vectors. *Clin. Vaccine Immunol.* **2015**, *22*, 726–741. [CrossRef]
31. Yu, J.S.; Peacock, J.W.; Jacobs, W.R., Jr.; Frothingham, R.; Letvin, N.L.; Liao, H.X.; Haynes, B.F. Recombinant Mycobacterium bovis Bacillus Calmette-Guérin Elicits Human Immunodeficiency Virus Type 1 Envelope-Specific T Lymphocytes at Mucosal Sites. *Clin. Vaccine Immunol.* **2007**, *14*, 886. [CrossRef]

32. Ami, Y.; Izumi, Y.; Matsuo, K.; Someya, K.; Kanekiyo, M.; Horibata, S.; Yoshino, N.; Sakai, K.; Shinohara, K.; Matsumoto, S.; et al. Priming-boosting vaccination with recombinant Mycobacterium bovis bacillus Calmette-Guérin and a nonreplicating vaccinia virus recombinant leads to long-lasting and effective immunity. *J. Virol.* **2005**, *79*, 12871–12879. [CrossRef]
33. Mahant, A.; Saubi, N.; Eto, Y.; Guitart, N.; Gatell, J.M.; Hanke, T.; Joseph, J. Preclinical development of BCG.HIVA2auxo.int, harboring an integrative expression vector, for a HIV-TB Pediatric vaccine. Enhancement of stability and specific HIV-1 T-cell immunity. *Hum. Vaccines Immunother.* **2017**, *13*, 1798–1810. [CrossRef]
34. Kanekiyo, M.; Matsuo, K.; Hamatake, M.; Hamano, T.; Ohsu, T.; Matsumoto, S.; Yamada, T.; Yamazaki, S.; Hasegawa, A.; Yamamoto, N.; et al. Mycobacterial Codon Optimization Enhances Antigen Expression and Virus-Specific Immune Responses in Recombinant Mycobacterium bovis Bacille Calmette-Guerin Expressing Human Immunodeficiency Virus Type 1 Gag. *J. Virol.* **2005**, *79*, 8716–8723. [CrossRef]
35. Bedwell, J.; Kairo, S.K.; Behr, M.A.; Bygraves, J.A. Identification of substrains of BCG vaccine using multiplex PCR. *Vaccine* **2001**, *19*, 2146–2151. [CrossRef]
36. Ondondo, B.; Murakoshi, H.; Clutton, G.; Abdul-Jawad, S.; Wee, E.G.T.; Gatanaga, H.; Oka, S.; McMichael, A.J.; Takiguchi, M.; Korber, B.; et al. Novel Conserved-region T-cell Mosaic Vaccine With High Global HIV-1 Coverage Is Recognized by Protective Responses in Untreated Infection. *Mol. Ther.* **2016**, *24*, 832–842. [CrossRef]
37. Joseph, J.; Fernández-Lloris, R.; Pezzat, E.; Saubi, N.; Cardona, P.J.; Mothe, B.; Gatell, J.M. Molecular characterization of heterologous HIV-1gp120 gene expression disruption in mycobacterium bovis BCG host strain: A critical issue for engineering Mycobacterial based-vaccine vectors. *J. Biomed. Biotechnol.* **2010**, *2010*, 1–10. [CrossRef]
38. Chapman, R.; Chege, G.; Shephard, E.; Stutz, H.; Williamson, A.L. Recombinant Mycobacterium bovis BCG as an HIV vaccine vector. *Curr. HIV Res.* **2010**, *8*, 282–298. [CrossRef]
39. Im, E.J.; Saubi, N.; Virgili, G.; Sander, C.; Teoh, D.; Gatell, J.M.; McShane, H.; Joseph, J.; Hanke, T. Vaccine platform for prevention of tuberculosis and mother-to-child transmission of human immunodeficiency virus type 1 through breastfeeding. *J. Virol.* **2007**, *81*, 9408–9418. [CrossRef]
40. Saubi, N.; Gea-Mallorquí, E.; Ferrer, P.; Hurtado, C.; Sánchez-Úbeda, S.; Eto, Y.; Gatell, J.M.; Hanke, T.; Joseph, J. Engineering new mycobacterial vaccine design for HIV-TB pediatric vaccine vectored by lysine auxotroph of BCG. *Mol. Ther. Methods Clin. Dev.* **2014**, *1*, 14017. [CrossRef]
41. Pavelka, M.S.; Jacobs, W.R. Comparison of the construction of unmarked deletion mutations in Mycobacterium smegmatis, Mycobacterium bovis bacillus Calmette-Guerin, and Mycobacterium tuberculosis H37RV by allelic exchange. *J. Bacteriol.* **1999**, *181*, 4780–4789.
42. Lee, M.H.; Pascopella, L.; Jacobs, W.R.; Hatfull, G.F. Site-specific integration of mycobacteriophage L5: Integration-proficient vectors for Mycobacterium smegmatis, Mycobacterium tuberculosis, and bacille Calmette-Guérin. *Proc. Natl. Acad. Sci. USA* **1991**, *88*, 3111–3115. [CrossRef]
43. Kilpeläinen, A.; Saubi, N.; Guitart, N.; Moyo, N.; Wee, E.G.; Hanke, T.H.; Joseph, J. Priming with recombinant BCG expressing novel HIV-1 mosaic immunogens and boosting with recombinant ChAdOx1 is safe, stable and elicits HIV-1-specific T-cell responses in BALB/c mice. *Front. Immunol.* **2019**, *10*, 923. [CrossRef]
44. World Health Organization. Global HIV & AIDS Statistics—2018 Fact Sheet UNAIDS. Available online: http://www.unaids.org/en/resources/fact-sheet (accessed on 8 October 2018).
45. Segueni, N.; Tritto, E.; Bourigault, M.L.; Rose, S.; Erard, F.; Le Bert, M.; Jacobs, M.; Di Padova, F.; Stiehl, D.P.; Moulin, P.; et al. Controlled Mycobacterium tuberculosis infection in mice under treatment with anti-IL-17A or IL-17F antibodies, in contrast to TNFα neutralization. *Sci. Rep.* **2016**, *6*, 36923. [CrossRef]
46. Cohen, G.B.; Gandhi, R.T.; Davis, D.M.; Mandelboim, O.; Chen, B.K.; Strominger, J.L.; Baltimore, D. The selective downregulation of class I major histocompatibility complex proteins by HIV-1 protects HIV-infected cells from NK cells. *Immunity* **1999**, *10*, 661–671. [CrossRef]
47. Institute, A.N.R. HLA Class I and Class II Sequence Alignments. Updates. Available online: http://www.ebi.ac.uk/ipd/imgt/hla/ (accessed on 10 July 2019).
48. Joosten, S.A.; van Meijgaarden, K.E.; van Weeren, P.C.; Kazi, F.; Geluk, A.; Savage, N.D.L.; Drijfhout, J.W.; Flower, D.R.; Hanekom, W.A.; Klein, M.R.; et al. Mycobacterium tuberculosis Peptides Presented by HLA-E Molecules Are Targets for Human CD8+ T-Cells with Cytotoxic as well as Regulatory Activity. *PLoS Pathog.* **2010**, *6*, e1000782. [CrossRef]

49. Hansen, S.G.; Ford, J.C.; Lewis, M.S.; Ventura, A.B.; Hughes, C.M.; Coyne-Johnson, L.; Whizin, N.; Oswald, K.; Shoemaker, R.; Swanson, T.; et al. Profound early control of highly pathogenic SIV by an effector memory T-cell vaccine. *Nature* **2011**, *473*, 523–527. [CrossRef]
50. Tomasec, P.; Braud, V.M.; Rickards, C.; Powell, M.B.; McSharry, B.P.; Gadola, S.; Cerundolo, V.; Borysiewicz, L.K.; McMichael, A.J.; Wilkinson, G.W. Surface expression of HLA-E, an inhibitor of natural killer cells, enhanced by human cytomegalovirus gpUL40. *Science* **2000**, *287*, 1031. [CrossRef]
51. Andrieu, J.M.; Chen, S.; Lai, C.; Guo, W.; Lu, W. Mucosal SIV Vaccines Comprising Inactivated Virus Particles and Bacterial Adjuvants Induce CD8+ T-Regulatory Cells that Suppress SIV-Positive CD4+ T-Cell Activation and Prevent SIV Infection in the Macaque Model. *Front. Immunol.* **2014**, *5*, 297. [CrossRef]
52. Jongwe, T.I.; Chapman, R.; Douglass, N.; Chetty, S.; Chege, G.; Williamson, A.L. HIV-1 Subtype C Mosaic Gag Expressed by BCG and MVA Elicits Persistent Effector T Cell Responses in a Prime-Boost Regimen in Mice. *PLoS ONE* **2016**, *11*, e0159141. [CrossRef]
53. Sun, J.; Hou, J.; Li, D.; Liu, Y.; Hu, N.; Hao, Y.; Fu, J.; Hu, Y.; Shao, Y. Enhancement of HIV-1 DNA vaccine immunogenicity by BCG-PSN, a novel adjuvant. *Vaccine* **2013**, *31*, 472–479. [CrossRef]
54. Van der Meer, J.W.M.; Joosten, L.A.B.; Riksen, N.; Netea, M.G. Trained immunity: A smart way to enhance innate immune defence. *Mol. Immunol.* **2015**, *68*, 40–44. [CrossRef]
55. Kleinnijenhuis, J.; Quintin, J.; Preijers, F.; Joosten, L.A.B.; Jacobs, C.; Xavier, R.J.; van der Meer, J.W.M.; van Crevel, R.; Netea, M.G. BCG-induced trained immunity in NK cells: Role for non-specific protection to infection. *Clin. Immunol.* **2014**, *155*, 213–219. [CrossRef]
56. Haynes, B.F.; Gilbert, P.B.; McElrath, M.J.; Zolla-Pazner, S.; Tomaras, G.D.; Alam, S.M.; Evans, D.T.; Montefiori, D.C.; Karnasuta, C.; Sutthent, R.; et al. Immune-correlates analysis of an HIV-1 vaccine efficacy trial. *N. Engl. J. Med.* **2012**, *366*, 1275–1286. [CrossRef]
57. Lin, L.; Finak, G.; Ushey, K.; Seshadri, C.; Hawn, T.R.; Frahm, N.; Scriba, T.J.; Mahomed, H.; Hanekom, W.; Bart, P.A.; et al. COMPASS identifies T-cell subsets correlated with clinical outcomes. *Nat. Biotechnol.* **2015**, *33*, 610–616. [CrossRef]

vaccines

Review

Cytolytic Perforin as an Adjuvant to Enhance the Immunogenicity of DNA Vaccines

Ashish C. Shrestha *, Danushka K. Wijesundara, Makutiro G. Masavuli, Zelalem A. Mekonnen, Eric J. Gowans and Branka Grubor-Bauk *

Virology Laboratory, Discipline of Surgery, Basil Hetzel Institute for Translational Health Research and University of Adelaide, Adelaide 5011, Australia; danushka.wijesundara@adelaide.edu.au (D.K.W.); makutiro.masavuli@adelaide.edu.au (M.G.M.); zelalem.mekonnen@adelaide.edu.au (Z.A.M.); eric.gowans@adelaide.edu.au (E.J.G.)

* Correspondence: ashish.shrestha@adelaide.edu.au (A.C.S.); branka.grubor@adelaide.edu.au (B.G.-B.); Tel.: +61-8-8222-6590 (A.C.S.); +61-8-8222-7368 (B.G.-B.)

Received: 8 March 2019; Accepted: 25 April 2019; Published: 30 April 2019

Abstract: DNA vaccines present one of the most cost-effective platforms to develop global vaccines, which have been tested for nearly three decades in preclinical and clinical settings with some success in the clinic. However, one of the major challenges for the development of DNA vaccines is their poor immunogenicity in humans, which has led to refinements in DNA delivery, dosage in prime/boost regimens and the inclusion of adjuvants to enhance their immunogenicity. In this review, we focus on adjuvants that can enhance the immunogenicity of DNA encoded antigens and highlight the development of a novel cytolytic DNA platform encoding a truncated mouse perforin. The application of this innovative DNA technology has considerable potential in the development of effective vaccines.

Keywords: DNA vaccine; adjuvants; vaccine delivery; plasmid; cytolytic; perforin; bicistronic; HCV; HIV

1. Introduction

Vaccines represent an effective strategy in the fight against infectious diseases and recent estimates suggest that vaccination prevents 2–3 million deaths every year [1]. The need for rapid and large scale vaccine production during epidemics against emerging pathogens is a major challenge in vaccine development [2], including effective vaccines for antigenically diverse and versatile pathogens that successfully subvert host immunity such as human immunodeficiency virus (HIV), hepatitis C virus (HCV), and malaria [3–5].

DNA vaccines can overcome some of these challenges, as it is relatively easy to produce large number of doses within a short period of time, and they are stable at ambient temperature and do not require cold chain transportation. They are also consistent between lots and have an excellent safety profile allowing for safety evaluations by regulatory authorities and distribution in a large scale [6,7]. Importantly, DNA vaccines can induce both humoral and cell-mediated responses in the vaccinated host [8–10]. Although they are safe and well tolerated, they are often poorly immunogenic and inefficacious in humans [11]. Therefore, recent studies on the advancements of DNA vaccines are focused on effective delivery and increasing the immunogenicity of the encoded antigen/s of interest [12,13].

Effective immunization with DNA vaccines requires efficient transfection of host cells which is highly dependent on the delivery route and use of devices. Conventional delivery routes to introduce the DNA vaccine include intramuscular, intradermal, subcutaneous and oral routes [12]. The preferred delivery route depends on the requirement to activate specific immune cells. The skin is rich in immune cells including local dendritic cells (DCs) and natural killer (NK) cells, and is therefore likely to be a more favorable site for vaccine delivery [14,15]. Attempts to improve DNA delivery have been made through other physical methods with the use of 'gene guns' or electroporation, which transiently permeabilizes the cell membrane to efficiently transfer the DNA resulting in increased vaccine uptake by skin and muscle cells [16]. Although these methods have shown to increase DNA uptake [17,18], they require optimization to achieve increased efficiency and acceptance for clinical use. An alternative approach to improve transfection efficiency includes formulation of DNA with liposomes or nanoparticles [19]. Liposomal delivery can be affected by pre-systemic (epithelial) and systemic barriers (enzymatic degradation, binding, and opsonization) [20]. Encapsulation of DNA with nanoparticles has been reported to increase DNA uptake or transfection efficiency [21,22]. Some of the challenges in the use of nanoparticles with DNA include encapsulation inefficiency, endocytosis by target cells and toxicity [23].

The use of genetic adjuvants is one approach to enhance the immunogenicity of the antigen and can be used to complement other strategies (e.g., DNA delivery) also designed to improve the immunogenicity of DNA vaccines. Upon immunization with a DNA vaccine, the target cells uptake DNA by endocytosis [24] and the transfected cells express the DNA-encoded protein antigen(s). When antigen-presenting cells (APCs) are directly transfected, the intracellular proteins are processed and immunogenic epitopes are then presented by MHC Class I molecules, which can directly stimulate naïve $CD8^+$ T cells [12,25]. The protein immunogen released from transfected cells can be endocytosed and/or phagocytosed by other APCs and are presented by MHC class II molecules to activate naive $CD4^+$ T cells [25,26]. If the proteins are expressed by stromal cells like keratinocytes, APCs can also indirectly capture secreted antigens and cross-present by MHC Class I molecules to further stimulate $CD8^+$ T cells [27]. After DNA vaccination, $CD8^+$ T cells specific to the vaccine antigen undergo expansion, acquire effector functions and differentiates into memory $CD8^+$ T cells [28,29]. The memory cells differentiate into effector memory T cells upon re-exposure to the antigen [29,30]. The ability of a DNA vaccine to elicit T cell immunity is thus dependent on activating APCs to present antigen: MHC complexes to T cells [31] and adjuvants can serve as an important costimulatory factor to enhance this process.

In this brief review, based on our experience, we discuss the progress in the development of DNA vaccines, approaches to improve delivery and genetic adjuvants used to enhance immunogenicity. We focus on an innovative cytolytic DNA technology developed and patented in our laboratory.

2. DNA Vaccine Adjuvants

The immunogenicity of DNA vaccines is enhanced by CpG motifs present in the plasmid backbone, which can activate APC via toll like receptors (TLR9) [32–34]. Unmethylated CpG motifs have been reported to induce B cell proliferation and secretion of immunoglobulin in vitro and in vivo [33]. Activation of macrophages and DCs results in upregulation of antigen presentation and costimulatory molecules, and secretion of cytokines (IL-12 and IL-18) involved in helper T cells (Th1) response [34]. Thus, CpG motifs in DNA plasmids serve as a 'natural adjuvant' for DNA vaccines. Plasmid DNA can be designed to encode additional adjuvants with the antigen(s) of interest. Molecular adjuvants such as fusion proteins including heat shock protein 70 (HSP70), and vesicular stomatitis virus (VSVG) have been developed and used to enhance vaccine immunogenicity [35–37]. The gene encoding such proteins as adjuvants is either fused with the gene encoding the vaccine antigen to produce a fusion protein driven by a same promoter or as separate proteins driven by different promoters in the same or different plasmid. Co-encoding of genes creates a suitable cellular micro environment such as sustained antigen release and/or upregulation of cytokines, enhancing the immunogenicity of DNA vaccines [38].

A majority of the studies on experimental DNA vaccines with genetic adjuvants have been studied in animal models such as mice (Table 1), and very few of these have been clinically tested (Table 2). Limited published data on clinical trials pose difficulty to compare efficacy between adjuvants in animals and humans.

Table 1. Molecular adjuvants and immunogenicity of DNA vaccines in animals.

Adjuvants	Antigens	Delivery	Host	Responses	Ref.
		Costimulatory molecules			
CD80, CD86	HIV-1 (Env, Gag, Pol)	DC, IM	Mouse Chimpanzee	+CMI	[39]
CD40 LT	beta-gal	DC, SC	Mouse	+Ab, +CMI	[40]
ICAM-1	HIV-1 (Env)	DC, IM	Mouse	+CMI	[41]
		Cytokines			
IL-2, IFN-γ	HIV-1 (Env, Gag, Pol)	DC, IM	Mouse	+Ab, +CMI	[42]
IL-6	Influenza (HA)	DC, GG	Mouse	+Ab	[43]
IL-2,12, IFN-γ	HBV	DC, IM	Mouse	+CMI	[44]
TNF-α, IL-15	HIV (Env, Gag, Pol)	DC, IM	Mouse	+CMI	[45]
		Toll like receptor adaptor/signaling molecules			
TRIF	Influenza (HA), tumor E7	BC, IM/EP	Mouse	+CMI	[46]
MyD88	Influenza (HA), tumor E7	BC, IM/EP	Mouse	+Ab	[46]
FliC	Influenza A (Np)	DC, ID	Mouse	+Ab, +CMI	[47]
IRF 1,3, 7	Influenza virus (HA, Np)	DC/BC, IM	Mouse	+Ab, +CMI	[48]
TBK-1	P. f (SE36)	DC, IM	Mouse	+Ab, +CMI	[49]
HMGB1	HIV-1 (Gag, Env)	DC, IM/EP	Mouse	+Ab, +CMI	[50]
DAI	Survivin	DC, ID	Mouse	+CMI	[51]
chMDA5	Influenza (HA)	DC, IM	Chicken	+Ab	[52]
Ii	P. f (ME)	FC, IM	Mouse	+CMI	[53]
		Toxins/Viral proteins			
FrC	Sc-fv	FC, IM	Mouse	+Ab	[54]
DTa	HIV (Gag)	BC, ID	Mouse	−CMI	[55]
NSP4	HCV NS3	BC, ID	Mouse	+/−CMI	[56]
VSVG	HIV (Gag)	DC, ID	Mouse	+CMI	[37]
	NS3	BC, ID	Mouse	+/−CMI	[57]
		Heat shock proteins			
Calreticulin	mucin 1	DC	Mouse	+CMI	[58]
	HPV-16 E7	FC, GG	Mouse	+CMI	[59]
HSP70	HIV (Gag)	BC, ID	Mouse	+CMI	[60]
		Complement inhibitor			
IMX313	HIV (Tat)	FC, ID	Mouse	+Ab, +CMI	[36]
		Cytolytic protein			
PRF	HIV (Gag)	BC, ID	Mouse	+CMI	[55]
	HCV (NS3)	BC, ID	Mouse, Pig	+CMI	[26]
	HCV (NS345B)	BC, ID	Mouse	+CMI	[57]

Adjuvants: LT: ligand/trimer, IL: Interleukin, TNF: Tumor necrosis factor, TRIF: Toll-interleukin-1 receptor domain-containing adaptor-inducing beta interferon, MyD88: myeloid differentiation primary response, FliC: phase-1 flagellin, IRF: Interferon regulatory factor, TBK-1: TANK-binding kinase 1, HMGB1: High-mobility group box 1 protein, DAI: DNA-dependent activator of interferon (IFN) regulatory factors, chMDA5: melanoma differentiation-associated gene 5 product, FrC: Fragment C of tetanus toxin, DTa: Diphtheria toxin subunit A, NSP4: Nonstructural protein 4, li: MHC class II invariant chain, HSP: Heat shock protein, VSVG: Vesicular stomatitis virus, PRF: Perforin; **Antigens:** HIV: Human immunodeficiency virus, Env: Envelope, GAG: Group antigens, Pol: Reverse transcriptase, beta-gal: beta galactosidase, FMDV: Foot and Mouth Disease Virus, VP1: Virus protein 1, HBV: Hepatitis B virus, HA: Haemagglutinin, Sc-fv: Single chain fragment variable, Np: Nucleoprotein, P.f: *Plasmodium falciparum*, SE36: serine repeat antigen 36, HCV: Hepatitis C virus, NS3: Nonstructural protein 3, ME: Multiepitope string fused to the native *P. falciparum* T9/96 strain,NS345B: Nonstructural proteins 3, 4, 5B; **Delivery:** DC: Different constructs, BC: Bicistronic construct, FC: Fusion protein/single construct, IM: Intra muscular, SC: Subcutaneous, GG: Gene gun, EP: Electroporation, ID: Intradermal; Responses: +: Increase, −: Decrease, +/−: No significant change, CMI: T cell responses, Ab: Humoral responses; **Ref.:** References.

Table 2. Molecular adjuvants tested with DNA vaccines in humans.

Adjuvants	Antigens	Delivery	Responses	Trial Phase	Ref.
IL-12, IL-15	HIV-1 (Gag)	DC, IM	+/−Ab, +/−CMI	I	[61]
GM-CSF, IL-2	Her2	RP, IM	+Ab, +CMI	I	[62]
GM-CSF	CEA	RP, ID	+Ab, +CMI	I	[63]
IL-2/Ig	HIV-1 Gag/Pol/Nef/Env	BC, IM	+Ab, +CMI	I	[64]
IL-12	HIV (MAG-Gag, Pol, Env, Nef, Tat, Vif)	DC, IM/EP	−Ab, +CMI	I	[65,66]
IL-12	HIV-1 (Env, Gag, Pol)	DC, IM/EP	+CMI	I	[67]
GM-CSF	PAP	RPID	−Ab, +CMI	I/IIa	[68]
HSP70	HPV16 (E7)	FC, IM	−Ab, +/−CMI	I	[69]

Adjuvants: IL: Interleukin, GM-CSF: Granulocyte/macrophage colony-stimulating factor; **Antigens:** HIV: Human immunodeficiency virus, Gag: Group antigens, Her2: Human epidermal growth factor receptor 2, CEA: Human carcinoembryonic antigen, MAG: Multi antigen, Env: Envelope, Pol: Reverse transcriptase, Nef: N-terminally myristoylated protein, Tat: Transactivator of transcription, Vif: viral infectivity factor, PAP: Prostatic Acid Phosphatase, HSP: Heat shock protein, HPV: Human Papilloma Virus; **Delivery:** DC: Different constructs, BC: Bicistronic construct, FC: Fusion protein/single construct, RP: Adjuvant as recombinant protein, IM: Intramuscular, ID: Intradermal; Responses: +: Increase, −: Decrease, +/−: No significant change, Ab: Humoral responses, CMI: T cell responses; **Ref.:** References.

2.1. Cytokines

Different cytokines, such as interleukins (IL-2, IL-6, IL-12), chemokines, granulocyte/macrophage colony-stimulating factor (GM-CSF), costimulatory molecules (CD40, CD80, and CD86), and signaling molecules (Interferon regulatory factor -3) have been used as genetic adjuvants with DNA vaccines [39,40,42–44,48,68]. Genes expressing IFN-γ IL-2, IL-12, IL-15, and IL-18 have been used to stimulate Th1 responses [44,45,70], and IL-4, IL-6, IL-10, IL-13, for Th2 stimulation [42,43,71–73]. The inclusion of genes encoding cytokines, like IL-2 or IL-12, as adjuvants for HIV-1 DNA vaccines is known to increase cell mediated immunity (CMI) [74,75]. However, a bicistronic HIV DNA encoding gp120 and IL-2 elicited weaker specific immune response than monocistronic HIV-1 gp120 DNA [76]. Combinations of genetic adjuvants like IL-2 and IL-15 with HIV-1 DNA vaccine have also been used but no synergistic effect on the level of total antibody to HIV-1 antigen was reported [77]. A phase I/IIa trial showed that coadministration of DNA vaccine encoding prostatic acid phosphatase (PAP) with GM-CSF elicited PAP-specific $CD4^+$ and/or $CD8^+$ T cell responses [68]. However, GM-CSF was administered as a recombinant protein.

2.2. Heat Shock Proteins

HSP70, a class of molecular chaperone, is known to induce maturation of DCs and activation of the Th1 pathway [78–80]. A fusion vaccine for multiple myeloma termed hDKK1-hHSP70 was shown to be effective in inhibiting the targeted tumor and increased survival of vaccinated mice by eliciting tumor-specific humoral and cellular immune responses [80]. However, a DNA vaccine encoding HPV16E7 fused with HSP70, targeting HPV16 and cervical intraepithelial neoplasia 2/3 failed to enhance significant T cell responses in a Phase I clinical trial [69]. A bicistronic DNA encoding HSP70 as a membrane bound or secreted protein has been used to improve the immunogenicity of a HIV Gag [60]. In this case, HSP70 expression was driven by a weaker SV40 promoter and HIV Gag by a stronger CMV promoter. Such a vaccine design enhanced Gag-specific T cell responses, providing greater protection in mice challenged with EcoHIV [60]. EcoHIV is a chimeric virus containing the envelope protein gp 80 of mouse leukemia virus rather than HIV gp 120 that can replicate in mouse leukocytes in vivo, thus representing a viable mouse challenge model for early assessment of HIV vaccines [81]. The proposed mechanism of HSP70 as an adjuvant is that TLR 2/4 on DCs interacts with secreted or bound HSP70, further attracting DCs to the site of antigen expression. This is followed by DC maturation, presentation of antigens by MHC molecules and secretion of cytokines and costimulatory molecules [82], thus enhancing T cell immune responses against the vaccine antigen.

2.3. Chicken Complement Inhibitor

A chimeric version of the oligomerization domain from the chicken complement inhibitor (C4bp) was used to produce an oligomeric form of vaccine antigens [35,83]. This protein, termed IMX313, forms a heptameric structure of the vaccine protein. This has been used to develop DNA vaccines for tuberculosis, malaria and HIV to enhance humoral and/or cellular responses [35,36,84]. Vaccination with a DNA vaccine encoding secreted HIV Tat (TPA-Tat IMX313) induced higher humoral and cellular responses and improved protection against EcoHIV challenge in mice [36]. A phase I clinical trial of tuberculosis vaccine MVA85A-IMX313 evaluated the vaccine to be safe and immunogenic, but cellular (Ag85A-specific IFN- Y) and humoral (MVA-specific IgG) responses were not significant [85]. Thus, the ability of such an adjuvant to enhance immunogenicity of DNA vaccines in humans is still debated.

2.4. Viral Fusion Protein

VSV G is a type III viral fusion envelope protein, which mediates fusion of the virus envelope and the host cell membrane [86]. The use of fusogenic membrane glycoprotein (FMG) gene from VSV in a DNA vaccine encoding the H7 protein of human papillomavirus type 16 was shown to enhance $CD8^+$ T cell responses and effectively control growth of tumors [87]. The VSV G protein was also shown to induce a T-response at low doses or a T-independent response at higher doses [88]. FMG fuses cells into large multinucleated syncytia, which are then killed by a nonapoptotic mechanism [89]. Syncytiosomes are released from the membrane and present antigens efficiently to DCs [90]. FMGs can thus act as an adjuvant for any antigen expressed by a DNA vaccine. Vaccination of mice with the hepatitis C virus (HCV) nonstructural protein 3 (NS3) together with VSVG resulted in increased frequency of IFN- γ, but not TNF-α- or IL-2-producing CD3+ CD44+ CD8+ effector memory T (T_{EM}) cells [57]. This DNA vaccine was constructed in a bicistronic vector with VSVG co-encoded in the same plasmid with HCV NS3. VSVG expression was driven by a weaker SV40 promoter and NS3 by a stronger CMV promoter [57]. However, others have also reported an increase in the specific CMI when the immunogen and VSVG were expressed from different plasmids [37,87].

2.5. Cytolytic Protein

Perforin (PRF) is a pore forming protein released by immune cells including NK cells and cytotoxic T lymphocytes (CTL) [91]. The 67-kilodalton PRF protein oligomerizes to form pores that serve as a channel to release granzyme into the cytosol of target cells [92]. Suicide genes inducing apoptosis of target cells have been used for cancer therapies, and the role of apoptotic cell death in vaccination, whether immune-stimulatory or immune-suppressive, is debated [93]. Recently, a novel DNA technology has been developed—-termed cytolytic DNA technology—in which a truncated mouse PRF is incorporated in a bicistronic DNA vector to act as a vaccine adjuvant [55–57,94].

3. Cytolytic DNA Vaccines

Cytolytic DNA vaccines are based on a bicistronic DNA plasmid constructed on a pVax backbone (Invitrogen) with a Cytomegalovirus (CMV) promoter and a Simian Virus (SV40) promoter [55]. The gene encoding the protein of interest as an immunogen is inserted downstream of the CMV promoter and the gene encoding a truncated version of mouse PRF downstream of the SV40 promoter (Figure 1). The SV40 is a weaker promoter compared to CMV and has been shown to result in 10-fold lower protein expression in transfected HEK293T cells in vitro [55,95].

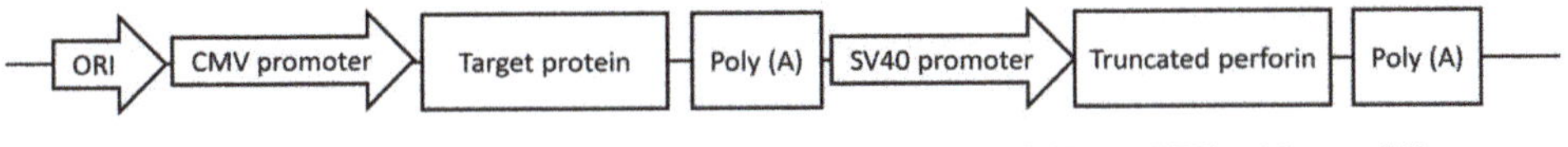

Figure 1. Schematic diagram of cytolytic bicistronic DNA plasmid (rDNA-PRF) with two different promoters and encoding protein of interest (immunogen) and truncated perforin.

The PRF gene was modified to express a truncated version of PRF (~60KDa) lacking the final 12 amino acid residues of the C terminus (unstructured region of PRF) [56,57,94] in order for PRF to become cytolytic [96]. The final 12 C-terminal amino acids are required to export PRF protein from the endoplasmic reticulum (ER) to the Golgi, from where glycosylated PRF is then transported to secretory granules [96]. Removal of the C-terminal abrogates the export of PRF from the ER and its subsequent accumulation in the ER is cytotoxic to the host cell [96,97].

3.1. Mechanism

Different recombinant cytolytic DNA-PRF vaccines (rDNA-PRF) have been shown to elicit immune responses higher than those elicited by canonical DNA vaccines (without PRF) and the mechanism underlying this has been established [94]. A previous study showed that coexpression of HCV NS3 and PRF elicited nonapoptotic cell death in transfected cells, whilst immunization with NS3-PRF DNA vaccine increased NS3-specific T cell mediated responses as evidenced by increased NS3-specific IFN-γ responses in an ELISpot assay and increased numbers of polyfunctional $CD8^+$ T_{EM} cells that simultaneously secreted IFN-γ, IL-2, and TNF-α [56]. Cytolytic DNA platform where the expression of immunogen is driven by a stronger promoter allows for sufficient antigen expression and accumulation within the target cells followed by nonapoptotic cell death due to lesser expression of PRF driven by a weaker SV40 promoter; thus, balancing the level of antigen expression with the timing of cell death [94].

Necrosis is considered as the mechanism of cell death by PRF as evidenced by release of lactate dehydrogenase (LDH) and low caspase activity [55,56,94]. LDH release occurs after the rupture of cell membrane during secondary necrosis [98,99]. In contrast, LDH was not released by cells treated with doxorubicin (a proapoptotic drug) or cells transfected with NS3 wild type PRF or NS3 12del483A PRF (mutant and nontoxic PRF) [94]. Expression of PRF from a cytolytic DNA, e.g., NS3 PRF vaccine, thus results in necrotic cell death mediated by receptor-interacting protein-1 kinase activity, as evidenced by detection of uncleaved cytokeratin 18 in Huh-7 cells [56]. Necrosis releases damage associated molecular patterns (DAMPs) which in turn activate DCs to migrate to the site of vaccination [100,101].

When purified DCs including the $CD8\alpha^+$ subset from naïve C57BL/6 mice were exposed to HEK293T cells (transfected with Ovalbumin-PRF), it resulted in upregulation of costimulatory molecules (CD80/CD86), indicating maturation of the immune cells with the cytolytic DNA [94]. A significant increase in $CD11c^+$ DCs and cross-presenting $CD8a^+$ DCs, and upregulation of CD80 has been reported in mice vaccinated with a cytolytic DNA HIV 1 Gag PRF compared to a canonical DNA vaccine [55]. Local and migrated DCs at the site of inflammation can take up antigens by endocytosis and are also exposed to DAMPs. Activated and matured DCs can then prime naïve $CD8^+$ T cells (Figure 2). Antigen cross-presentation by DCs to $CD8^+$ T cells has been shown to increase the number of proliferating $CD8^+$ T cells by ~2-fold with cytolytic DNA compared to the noncytolytic PRF DNA [94]. Thus, a cytolytic DNA vaccine has an inbuilt adjuvant to enhance the immunogenicity of the vaccine immunogen. Whereas, the immunogenicity of canonical DNA vaccines mostly depends on direct transfection of DCs and to a lesser extent cross-presentation of antigens shed from transfected cells and/or derived from transfected cells that have undergone spontaneous cell death [94].

Several studies have established that DCs exposed to necrotic or lytic cells expressing antigens mature and cross-present more efficiently than DCs exposed to antigens derived from a cellular milieu that comprise of apoptotic cells [102–106]. Comparative studies evaluating the ability of proapoptotic (e.g., rotavirus nonstructural protein 4 (NSP4) and diphtheria toxin subunit A (DTa)) and necrotic proteins (e.g., truncated PRF) to enhance the immunogenicity of DNA when encoded in plasmid DNA vaccines showed that truncated PRF is the most effective for this purpose [55–57]. However, a caveat is that vaccine-encoded antigens need to accumulate significantly inside the cell before necrosis occurs following expression of truncated PRF in order to activate DCs to cross-present vaccine-encoded antigens [55,94].

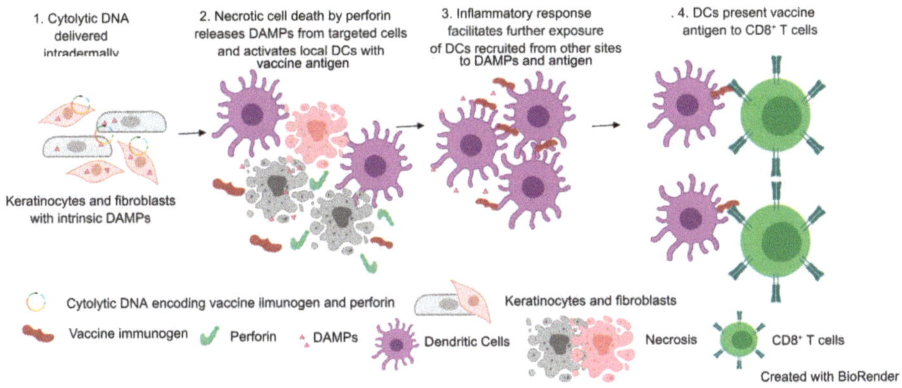

Figure 2. Mechanism of rDNA-PRF immunogenicity.

3.2. Cytolytic HIV and HCV DNA Vaccines

rDNA-PRF technology has been used in the development of HIV and HCV DNA vaccines [55,57,107]. Direct comparison of the effects of the cytolytic PRF and the apoptotic protein DTa on the immunogenicity of the HIV-1 Gag protein showed that PRF activated DCs more efficiently, as evidenced by the increase in frequency of cross-presenting DCs and upregulation of activation marker (CD80) [55]. In both DNA vaccines, PRF and DTa were driven by SV40 promoter. Immunization of mice with a DNA vaccine encoding proapoptotic DTa as an adjuvant in a HIV Gag DTa vaccine resulted in decreased DC activation, suggesting that DTa-induced apoptosis attenuated immune response [55]. Furthermore, improved protection in the mouse EcoHIV challenge model was achieved with rDNA-PRF encoding HIV Gag compared to protection levels in mice vaccinated with a canonical Gag DNA vaccine [57]. A rDNA-PRF vaccine encoding the HCV NS3 protein coexpressed with PRF was shown to increase NS3-specific CMI in mice and pigs, compared to NS3 coexpression with a proapoptotic protein, the rotavirus NSP4 protein [56]. NSP4 is an enterotoxin that elicits a proapoptotic effect by disrupting the mitochondrial membrane and activating caspase-3, -8, and -9 [108,109]. This study showed that PRF coexpression induced cell death by necrosis, and thus enhanced NS3-specific immune responses, whereas, proapoptotic NSP4 reduced NS3-specific response [56]. Importantly, HCV NS3 PRF was more immunogenic than the canonical NS3 vaccine in pigs, demonstrating the translational potential of the cytolytic DNA vaccines in human clinical trials [56]. Likewise, we have shown that a multi-antigenic HCV DNA vaccine encoding genotype 3a proteins NS3, NS4A, NS4B, and NS5B coexpressed with PRF induced robust CMI against the range of HCV NS proteins, compared to coexpression with VSVG [57]. We also showed that multi-antigenic and multigenotypic (HCV genotype 1 and 3a) DNA cocktail vaccines encoding PRF can significantly increase the magnitude and breadth of CMI responses to NS3 and NS5B against both genotypes compared to those elicited by a single-genotype vaccine [107].

4. Conclusions

DNA vaccines are still a promising option in the development of novel vaccination strategies. Although they have many advantages, the ability to induce effective immune responses in humans required for protection has been challenging. These challenges include ineffective delivery and poor uptake of DNA. Consequently, a recent focus has been in the development of delivery methods and/or inclusion of genetic adjuvants. Such genetic adjuvants are generally coexpressed with the antigen of interest or delivered through different plasmids. In the quest to develop and identify effective genetic adjuvants, a range of adjuvants was tested (HSP70, VSVG, IMX313, DTa, and PRF) and a novel and promising cytolytic DNA vaccine strategy has been developed. This cytolytic DNA vaccine is unique as it is based on a bicistronic plasmid with the ability to coexpress antigen and PRF in a balanced mechanism causing necrosis of vaccine-transduced cells, followed by increased activation of immune cells and cross presentation of vaccine immunogen. Cytolytic DNA vaccines encoding nonstructural proteins of HCV have been tested to enhance immunogenicity of vaccine antigen in mice [57,107] and in a large preclinical animal model, the pig [56]. Likewise, increased immunogenicity and improved protection against EcoHIV challenge in mice with HIV Gag PRF [60] demonstrate the effectiveness of cytolytic DNA vaccines.

Adjuvants that provide effective costimulation for immune responses with specific immunogens may not have a similar effect with other immunogens, and therefore these need to be tested for their efficacy. Use of a genetic adjuvant such as PRF produces a suitable microenvironment for multiple/different immunogens and thus improves the delivery, immunogenicity and effectiveness of DNA vaccines. This strategy has considerable potential in the development of DNA-based vaccines against a range of infectious agents.

Author Contributions: Writing—concept and original draft preparation: A.C.S.; concept, review, and editing: B.G.-B., E.J.G., and D.K.W.; section contributions and review: M.G.M. and Z.A.M.

Funding: Cytolytic DNA vaccines developed in our laboratory and reviewed in this manuscript have been supported by the grants received from the National Health and Medical Research Council, Australian Centre for HIV and Hepatitis Virology Research, the National Foundation for Medical Research and Innovation, and The Hospital Research Foundation (THRF).

Acknowledgments: We thank THRF and the donor community for supporting the development of our novel DNA vaccines. Ashish C. Shrestha and Danushka K. Wijesundara are recipients of Early Career Fellowships from THRF.

Conflicts of Interest: The authors declare no conflict of interest.

References

1. World Health Organisation. 10 Facts on Immunization. Available online: https://www.who.int/features/factfiles/immunization/en/ (accessed on 20 December 2018).
2. Plotkin, S.; Robinson, J.M.; Cunningham, G.; Iqbal, R.; Larsen, S. The complexity and cost of vaccine manufacturing—An overview. *Vaccine* **2017**, *35*, 4064–4071. [CrossRef]
3. Li, S.; Plebanski, M.; Smooker, P.; Gowans, E.J. Editorial: Why Vaccines to HIV, HCV, and Malaria Have So Far Failed-Challenges to Developing Vaccines Against Immunoregulating Pathogens. *Front. Microbiol.* **2015**, *6*, 1318. [CrossRef]
4. Wilhelm, J. HIV, Tuberculosis, and Malaria. Available online: https://www.sabin.org/sites/sabin.org/files/wilhelm_v2.pdf (accessed on 19 February 2019).
5. Rappuoli, R.; Aderem, A. A 2020 vision for vaccines against HIV, tuberculosis and malaria. *Nature* **2011**, *473*, 463–469. [CrossRef] [PubMed]
6. Whalen, R.G. DNA vaccines for emerging infectious diseases: What if? *Emerg. Infect. Dis.* **1996**, *2*, 168–175. [CrossRef] [PubMed]
7. Suschak, J.J.; Williams, J.A.; Schmaljohn, C.S. Advancements in DNA vaccine vectors, non-mechanical delivery methods, and molecular adjuvants to increase immunogenicity. *Hum. Vaccin. Immunother.* **2017**, *13*, 2837–2848. [CrossRef] [PubMed]
8. Seok, H.; Noh, J.Y.; Lee, D.Y.; Kim, S.J.; Song, C.S.; Kim, Y.C. Effective humoral immune response from a H1N1 DNA vaccine delivered to the skin by microneedles coated with PLGA-based cationic nanoparticles. *J. Controlled Release* **2017**, *265*, 66–74. [CrossRef]
9. Hurtado-Melgoza, M.L.; Ramos-Ligonio, A.; Álvarez-Rodríguez, L.M.; Meza-Menchaca, T.; López-Monteon, A. Differential humoral and cellular immunity induced by vaccination using plasmid DNA and protein recombinant expressing the NS3 protein of dengue virus type 3. *J. Biomed. Sci.* **2016**, *23*, 85. [CrossRef]
10. Maslow, J.N. Vaccines for emerging infectious diseases: Lessons from MERS coronavirus and Zika virus. *Hum. Vaccin. Immunother.* **2017**, *13*, 2918–2930. [CrossRef]
11. Ferraro, B.; Morrow, M.P.; Hutnick, N.A.; Shin, T.H.; Lucke, C.E.; Weiner, D.B. Clinical applications of DNA vaccines: Current progress. *Clin. Infect. Dis.* **2011**, *53*, 296–302. [CrossRef]

12. Hobernik, D.; Bros, M. DNA Vaccines—How Far From Clinical Use? *Int. J. Mol. Sci.* **2018**, *19*. [CrossRef]
13. Wahren, B.; Liu, M.A. DNA Vaccines: Recent Developments and the Future. *Vaccines* **2014**, *2*, 785–796. [CrossRef]
14. Kenney, R.T.; Frech, S.A.; Muenz, L.R.; Villar, C.P.; Glenn, G.M. Dose sparing with intradermal injection of influenza vaccine. *N. Engl. J. Med.* **2004**, *351*, 2295–2301. [CrossRef]
15. Fehres, C.; Garcia-Vallejo, J.J.; Unger, W.; Van Kooyk, Y. Skin-Resident Antigen-Presenting Cells: Instruction Manual for Vaccine Development. *Front. Immunol.* **2013**, *4*, 157. [CrossRef] [PubMed]
16. Gothelf, A.; Gehl, J. What you always needed to know about electroporation based DNA vaccines. *Hum. Vaccin. Immunother.* **2012**, *8*, 1694–1702. [CrossRef]
17. Aihara, H.; Miyazaki, J. Gene transfer into muscle by electroporation in vivo. *Nat. biotechnol.* **1998**, *16*, 867–870. [CrossRef] [PubMed]
18. Young, J.L.; Dean, D.A. Electroporation-mediated gene delivery. *Adv. Genet.* **2015**, *89*, 49–88. [CrossRef]
19. Schwendener, R.A. Liposomes as vaccine delivery systems: A review of the recent advances. *Ther. Adv. Vaccines* **2014**, *2*, 159–182. [CrossRef] [PubMed]
20. Saffari, M.; Moghimi, H.R.; Dass, C.R. Barriers to Liposomal Gene Delivery: from Application Site to the Target. *Iran. J. Pharm. Res.* **2016**, *15*, 3–17.
21. Gvili, J.; Machluf, M. 544. PLGA Nanoparticles for DNA Vaccination–Waiving Complexity and Increasing Efficiency. *Mol. Ther.* **2006**, *13*, S209. [CrossRef]
22. Penumarthi, A.; Parashar, D.; Abraham, A.N.; Dekiwadia, C.; Macreadie, I.; Shukla, R.; Smooker, P.M. Solid lipid nanoparticles mediate non-viral delivery of plasmid DNA to dendritic cells. *J. Nanoparticle Res.* **2017**, *19*, 210. [CrossRef]
23. Chen, J.; Guo, Z.; Tian, H.; Chen, X. Production and clinical development of nanoparticles for gene delivery. *Mol. Ther. Methods. Clin. Dev.* **2016**, *3*, 16023. [CrossRef]
24. Seternes, T.; Tonheim, T.C.; Løvoll, M.; Bøgwald, J.; Dalmo, R.A. Specific endocytosis and degradation of naked DNA in the endocardial cells of cod (*Gadus morhua* L.). *J. Exp. Biol.* **2007**, *210*, 2091. [CrossRef]
25. Elnekave, M.; Furmanov, K.; Nudel, I.; Arizon, M.; Clausen, B.E.; Hovav, A.-H. Directly Transfected Langerin$^+$ Dermal Dendritic Cells Potentiate CD8$^+$; T Cell Responses following Intradermal Plasmid DNA Immunization. *J. Immunol.* **2010**, *185*, 3463. [CrossRef]
26. Greenland, J.R.; Letvin, N.L. Chemical adjuvants for plasmid DNA vaccines. *Vaccine* **2007**, *25*, 3731–3741. [CrossRef]
27. Coban, C.; Kobiyama, K.; Jounai, N.; Tozuka, M.; Ishii, K.J. DNA vaccines. *Hum. Vaccin. Immunother.* **2013**, *9*, 2216–2221. [CrossRef]
28. Badovinac, V.P.; Harty, J.T. Programming, demarcating, and manipulating CD8+ T-cell memory. *Immunol. Rev.* **2006**, *211*, 67–80. [CrossRef]
29. Hovav, A.-H.; Panas, M.W.; Rahman, S.; Sircar, P.; Gillard, G.; Cayabyab, M.J.; Letvin, N.L. Duration of Antigen Expression In Vivo following DNA Immunization Modifies the Magnitude, Contraction, and Secondary Responses of CD8$^+$ T Lymphocytes. *J. Immunol.* **2007**, *179*, 6725. [CrossRef]
30. Jabbari, A.; Harty, J.T. Secondary memory CD8$^+$ T cells are more protective but slower to acquire a central–memory phenotype. *J. Exp. Med.* **2006**, *203*, 919. [CrossRef]
31. Mahanty, S.; Prigent, A.; Garraud, O. Immunogenicity of infectious pathogens and vaccine antigens. *BMC Immunol.* **2015**, *16*, 31. [CrossRef]
32. Ahmad-Nejad, P.; Häcker, H.; Rutz, M.; Bauer, S.; Vabulas, R.M.; Wagner, H. Bacterial CpG-DNA and lipopolysaccharides activate Toll-like receptors at distinct cellular compartments. *Eur. J. Immunol.* **2002**, *32*, 1958–1968. [CrossRef]
33. Krieg, A.M.; Yi, A.-K.; Matson, S.; Waldschmidt, T.J.; Bishop, G.A.; Teasdale, R.; Koretzky, G.A.; Klinman, D.M. CpG motifs in bacterial DNA trigger direct B-cell activation. *Nature* **1995**, *374*, 546. [CrossRef]
34. Dalpke, A.; Zimmermann, S.; Heeg, K. CpG-Oligonucleotides in Vaccination: Signaling and Mechanisms of Action. *Immunobiology* **2001**, *204*, 667–676. [CrossRef]
35. Li, Y.; Leneghan, D.B.; Miura, K.; Nikolaeva, D.; Brian, I.J.; Dicks, M.D.; Fyfe, A.J.; Zakutansky, S.E.; de Cassan, S.; Long, C.A.; et al. Enhancing immunogenicity and transmission-blocking activity of malaria vaccines by fusing Pfs25 to IMX313 multimerization technology. *Sci. Rep.* **2016**, *6*, 18848. [CrossRef]

36. Tomusange, K.; Wijesundara, D.; Gummow, J.; Garrod, T.; Li, Y.; Gray, L.; Churchill, M.; Grubor-Bauk, B.; Gowans, E.J. A HIV-Tat/C4-binding protein chimera encoded by a DNA vaccine is highly immunogenic and contains acute EcoHIV infection in mice. *Sci. Rep.* **2016**, *6*, 29131. [CrossRef]
37. Marsac, D.; Loirat, D.; Petit, C.; Schwartz, O.; Michel, M.L. Enhanced Presentation of Major Histocompatibility Complex Class I-Restricted Human Immunodeficiency Virus Type 1 (HIV-1) Gag-Specific Epitopes after DNA Immunization with Vectors Coding for Vesicular Stomatitis Virus Glycoprotein-Pseudotyped HIV-1 Gag Particles. *J. Virol.* **2002**, *76*, 7544. [CrossRef]
38. Awate, S.; Babiuk, L.A.; Mutwiri, G. Mechanisms of action of adjuvants. *Front. Immunol.* **2013**, *4*, 114. [CrossRef]
39. Kim, J.J.; Nottingham, L.K.; Wilson, D.M.; Bagarazzi, M.L.; Tsai, A.; Morrison, L.D.; Javadian, A.; Chalian, A.A.; Agadjanyan, M.G.; Weiner, D.B. Engineering DNA vaccines via co-delivery of co-stimulatory molecule genes. *Vaccine* **1998**, *16*, 1828–1835. [CrossRef]
40. Yang, B.; Jeang, J.; Yang, A.; Wu, T.C.; Hung, C.F. DNA vaccine for cancer immunotherapy. *Hum. Vaccin. Immunother.* **2014**, *10*, 3153–3164. [CrossRef]
41. Kim, J.J.; Tsai, A.; Nottingham, L.K.; Morrison, L.; Cunning, D.M.; Oh, J.; Lee, D.J.; Dang, K.; Dentchev, T.; Chalian, A.A.; et al. Intracellular adhesion molecule-1 modulates beta-chemokines and directly costimulates T cells in vivo. *J. Clin. Invest.* **1999**, *103*, 869–877. [CrossRef]
42. Kim, J.J.; Yang, J.S.; Montaner, L.; Lee, D.J.; Chalian, A.A.; Weiner, D.B. Coimmunization with IFN-gamma or IL-2, but not IL-13 or IL-4 cDNA can enhance Th1-type DNA vaccine-induced immune responses in vivo. *J. Interferon Cytokine Res.* **2000**, *20*, 311–319. [CrossRef]
43. Larsen, D.L.; Dybdahl-Sissoko, N.; McGregor, M.W.; Drape, R.; Neumann, V.; Swain, W.F.; Lunn, D.P.; Olsen, C.W. Coadministration of DNA encoding interleukin-6 and hemagglutinin confers protection from influenza virus challenge in mice. *J. Virol.* **1998**, *72*, 1704–1708.
44. Chow, Y.H.; Chiang, B.L.; Lee, Y.L.; Chi, W.K.; Lin, W.C.; Chen, Y.T.; Tao, M.H. Development of Th1 and Th2 populations and the nature of immune responses to hepatitis B virus DNA vaccines can be modulated by codelivery of various cytokine genes. *J. Immunol.* **1998**, *160*, 1320–1329.
45. Kim, J.J.; Trivedi, N.N.; Nottingham, L.K.; Morrison, L.; Tsai, A.; Hu, Y.; Mahalingam, S.; Dang, K.; Ahn, L.; Doyle, N.K.; et al. Modulation of amplitude and direction of in vivo immune responses by co-administration of cytokine gene expression cassettes with DNA immunogens. *Eur. J. Immunol.* **1998**, *28*, 1089–1103. [CrossRef]
46. Takeshita, F.; Tanaka, T.; Matsuda, T.; Tozuka, M.; Kobiyama, K.; Saha, S.; Matsui, K.; Ishii, K.J.; Coban, C.; Akira, S.; et al. Toll-like receptor adaptor molecules enhance DNA-raised adaptive immune responses against influenza and tumors through activation of innate immunity. *J. Virol.* **2006**, *80*, 6218–6224. [CrossRef]
47. Applequist, S.E.; Rollman, E.; Wareing, M.D.; Liden, M.; Rozell, B.; Hinkula, J.; Ljunggren, H.G. Activation of innate immunity, inflammation, and potentiation of DNA vaccination through mammalian expression of the TLR5 agonist flagellin. *J. Immunol.* **2005**, *175*, 3882–3891. [CrossRef]
48. Sasaki, S.; Amara, R.R.; Yeow, W.-S.; Pitha, P.M.; Robinson, H.L. Regulation of DNA-raised immune responses by cotransfected interferon regulatory factors. *J. Virol.* **2002**, *76*, 6652–6659. [CrossRef]
49. Coban, C.; Kobiyama, K.; Aoshi, T.; Takeshita, F.; Horii, T.; Akira, S.; Ishii, K.J. Novel strategies to improve DNA vaccine immunogenicity. *Curr. Gene Ther.* **2011**, *11*, 479–484. [CrossRef]
50. Muthumani, G.; Laddy, D.J.; Sundaram, S.G.; Fagone, P.; Shedlock, D.J.; Kannan, S.; Wu, L.; Chung, C.W.; Lankaraman, K.M.; Burns, J.; et al. Co-immunization with an optimized plasmid-encoded immune stimulatory interleukin, high-mobility group box 1 protein, results in enhanced interferon-gamma secretion by antigen-specific CD8 T cells. *Immunology* **2009**, *128*, e612–e620. [CrossRef]
51. Lladser, A.; Mougiakakos, D.; Tufvesson, H.; Ligtenberg, M.A.; Quest, A.F.; Kiessling, R.; Ljungberg, K. DAI (DLM-1/ZBP1) as a genetic adjuvant for DNA vaccines that promotes effective antitumor CTL immunity. *Mol. Ther.* **2011**, *19*, 594–601. [CrossRef]
52. Liniger, M.; Summerfield, A.; Ruggli, N. MDA5 can be exploited as efficacious genetic adjuvant for DNA vaccination against lethal H5N1 influenza virus infection in chickens. *PLoS ONE* **2012**, *7*, e49952. [CrossRef]
53. Halbroth, B.R.; Sebastian, S.; Poyntz, H.C.; Bregu, M.; Cottingham, M.G.; Hill, A.V.S.; Spencer, A.J. Development of a Molecular Adjuvant to Enhance Antigen-Specific CD8(+) T Cell Responses. *Sci. Rep.* **2018**, *8*, 15020. [CrossRef]

54. King, C.A.; Spellerberg, M.B.; Zhu, D.; Rice, J.; Sahota, S.S.; Thompsett, A.R.; Hamblin, T.J.; Radl, J.; Stevenson, F.K. DNA vaccines with single-chain Fv fused to fragment C of tetanus toxin induce protective immunity against lymphoma and myeloma. *Nat. Med.* **1998**, *4*, 1281–1286. [CrossRef]
55. Gargett, T.; Grubor-Bauk, B.; Garrod, T.; Yu, W.; Miller, D.; Major, L.; Wesselingh, S.; Suhrbier, A.; Gowans, E. Induction of antigen-positive cell death by the expression of Perforin, but not DTa, from a DNA vaccine enhances the immune respons. *Immunol. Cell Biol.* **2014**, *92*, 359–367. [CrossRef]
56. Grubor-Bauk, B.; Yu, W.; Wijesundara, D.; Gummow, J.; Garrod, T.; Brennan, A.J.; Voskoboinik, I.; Gowans, E.J. Intradermal delivery of DNA encoding HCV NS3 and perforin elicits robust cell-mediated immunity in mice and pigs. *Gene Ther.* **2016**, *23*, 26–37. [CrossRef]
57. Gummow, J.; Li, Y.; Yu, W.; Garrod, T.; Wijesundara, D.; Brennan, A.J.; Mullick, R.; Voskoboinik, I.; Grubor-Bauk, B.; Gowans, E.J. A Multiantigenic DNA Vaccine That Induces Broad Hepatitis C Virus-Specific T-Cell Responses in Mice. *J. Viro.l* **2015**, *89*, 7991–8002. [CrossRef]
58. Wang, J.; Gao, Z.P.; Qin, S.; Liu, C.B.; Zou, L.L. Calreticulin is an effective immunologic adjuvant to tumor-associated antigens. *Exp. Ther. Med.* **2017**, *14*, 3399–3406. [CrossRef]
59. Peng, S.; Ji, H.; Trimble, C.; He, L.; Tsai, Y.-C.; Yeatermeyer, J.; Boyd, D.A.K.; Hung, C.-F.; Wu, T.C. Development of a DNA Vaccine Targeting Human Papillomavirus Type 16 Oncoprotein E6. *J. Virol.* **2004**, *78*, 8468. [CrossRef]
60. Garrod, T.J.; Grubor-Bauk, B.; Gargett, T.; Li, Y.; Miller, D.S.; Yu, W.; Major, L.; Burrell, C.J.; Wesselingh, S.; Suhrbier, A.; et al. DNA vaccines encoding membrane-bound or secreted forms of heat shock protein 70 exhibit improved potency. *Eur. J. Immunol.* **2014**, *44*, 1992–2002. [CrossRef]
61. Kalams, S.A.; Parker, S.; Jin, X.; Elizaga, M.; Metch, B.; Wang, M.; Hural, J.; Lubeck, M.; Eldridge, J.; Cardinali, M.; et al. Safety and immunogenicity of an HIV-1 gag DNA vaccine with or without IL-12 and/or IL-15 plasmid cytokine adjuvant in healthy, HIV-1 uninfected adults. *PLoS ONE* **2012**, *7*, e29231. [CrossRef]
62. Norell, H.; Poschke, I.; Charo, J.; Wei, W.Z.; Erskine, C.; Piechocki, M.P.; Knutson, K.L.; Bergh, J.; Lidbrink, E.; Kiessling, R. Vaccination with a plasmid DNA encoding HER-2/neu together with low doses of GM-CSF and IL-2 in patients with metastatic breast carcinoma: a pilot clinical trial. *J. Transl. Med.* **2010**, *8*, 53. [CrossRef]
63. Staff, C.; Mozaffari, F.; Haller, B.K.; Wahren, B.; Liljefors, M. A Phase I safety study of plasmid DNA immunization targeting carcinoembryonic antigen in colorectal cancer patients. *Vaccine* **2011**, *29*, 6817–6822. [CrossRef]
64. Baden, L.R.; Blattner, W.A.; Morgan, C.; Huang, Y.; Defawe, O.D.; Sobieszczyk, M.E.; Kochar, N.; Tomaras, G.D.; McElrath, M.J.; Russell, N.; et al. Timing of plasmid cytokine (IL-2/Ig) administration affects HIV-1 vaccine immunogenicity in HIV-seronegative subjects. *J. Infect. Dis.* **2011**, *204*, 1541–1549. [CrossRef]
65. Elizaga, M.L.; Li, S.S.; Kochar, N.K.; Wilson, G.J.; Allen, M.A.; Tieu, H.V.N.; Frank, I.; Sobieszczyk, M.E.; Cohen, K.W.; Sanchez, B.; et al. Safety and tolerability of HIV-1 multiantigen pDNA vaccine given with IL-12 plasmid DNA via electroporation, boosted with a recombinant vesicular stomatitis virus HIV Gag vaccine in healthy volunteers in a randomized, controlled clinical trial. *PLoS ONE* **2018**, *13*, e0202753. [CrossRef]
66. Li, S.S.; Kochar, N.K.; Elizaga, M.; Hay, C.M.; Wilson, G.J.; Cohen, K.W.; De Rosa, S.C.; Xu, R.; Ota-Setlik, A.; Morris, D.; et al. DNA Priming Increases Frequency of T-Cell Responses to a Vesicular Stomatitis Virus HIV Vaccine with Specific Enhancement of CD8+ T-Cell Responses by Interleukin-12 Plasmid DNA. *Clin. Vaccin. Immunol.* **2017**, *24*. [CrossRef]
67. Kalams, S.A.; Parker, S.D.; Elizaga, M.; Metch, B.; Edupuganti, S.; Hural, J.; De Rosa, S.; Carter, D.K.; Rybczyk, K.; Frank, I.; et al. Safety and comparative immunogenicity of an HIV-1 DNA vaccine in combination with plasmid interleukin 12 and impact of intramuscular electroporation for delivery. *J. Infect. Dis.* **2013**, *208*, 818–829. [CrossRef]
68. McNeel, D.G.; Dunphy, E.J.; Davies, J.G.; Frye, T.P.; Johnson, L.E.; Staab, M.J.; Horvath, D.L.; Straus, J.; Alberti, D.; Marnocha, R.; et al. Safety and Immunological Efficacy of a DNA Vaccine Encoding Prostatic Acid Phosphatase in Patients With Stage D0 Prostate Cancer. *J. Clin. Oncol.* **2009**, *27*, 4047–4054. [CrossRef]
69. Trimble, C.L.; Peng, S.; Kos, F.; Gravitt, P.; Viscidi, R.; Sugar, E.; Pardoll, D.; Wu, T.C. A phase I trial of a human papillomavirus DNA vaccine for HPV16+ cervical intraepithelial neoplasia 2/3. *Clin. Cancer Res.* **2009**, *15*, 361–367. [CrossRef]

70. Kim, J.J.; Nottingham, L.K.; Tsai, A.; Lee, D.J.; Maguire, H.C.; Oh, J.; Dentchev, T.; Manson, K.H.; Wyand, M.S.; Agadjanyan, M.G.; et al. Antigen-specific humoral and cellular immune responses can be modulated in rhesus macaques through the use of IFN-gamma, IL-12, or IL-18 gene adjuvants. *J. Med. Primatol.* **1999**, *28*, 214–223. [CrossRef]
71. Scheerlinck, J.-P.Y. Genetic adjuvants for DNA vaccines. *Vaccine* **2001**, *19*, 2647–2656. [CrossRef]
72. Okada, E.; Sasaki, S.; Ishii, N.; Aoki, I.; Yasuda, T.; Nishioka, K.; Fukushima, J.; Miyazaki, J.; Wahren, B.; Okuda, K. Intranasal immunization of a DNA vaccine with IL-12- and granulocyte-macrophage colony-stimulating factor (GM-CSF)-expressing plasmids in liposomes induces strong mucosal and cell-mediated immune responses against HIV-1 antigens. *J. immunol.* **1997**, *159*, 3638–3647.
73. Kim, J.J.; Simbiri, K.A.; Sin, J.I.; Dang, K.; Oh, J.; Dentchev, T.; Lee, D.; Nottingham, L.K.; Chalian, A.A.; McCallus, D.; et al. Cytokine molecular adjuvants modulate immune responses induced by DNA vaccine constructs for HIV-1 and SIV. *J. Interferon Cytokine Res.* **1999**, *19*, 77–84. [CrossRef]
74. Xin, K.Q.; Hamajima, K.; Sasaki, S.; Honsho, A.; Tsuji, T.; Ishii, N.; Cao, X.R.; Lu, Y.; Fukushima, J.; Shapshak, P.; et al. Intranasal administration of human immunodeficiency virus type-1 (HIV-1) DNA vaccine with interleukin-2 expression plasmid enhances cell-mediated immunity against HIV-1. *Immunology* **1998**, *94*, 438–444. [CrossRef]
75. Tsuji, T.; Hamajima, K.; Fukushima, J.; Xin, K.Q.; Ishii, N.; Aoki, I.; Ishigatsubo, Y.; Tani, K.; Kawamoto, S.; Nitta, Y.; et al. Enhancement of cell-mediated immunity against HIV-1 induced by coinnoculation of plasmid-encoded HIV-1 antigen with plasmid expressing IL-12. *J. Immunol.* **1997**, *158*, 4008–4013.
76. Barouch, D.H.; Santra, S.; Steenbeke, T.D.; Zheng, X.X.; Perry, H.C.; Davies, M.E.; Freed, D.C.; Craiu, A.; Strom, T.B.; Shiver, J.W.; et al. Augmentation and suppression of immune responses to an HIV-1 DNA vaccine by plasmid cytokine/Ig administration. *J. Immunol.* **1998**, *161*, 1875–1882.
77. Xin, K.Q.; Hamajima, K.; Sasaki, S.; Tsuji, T.; Watabe, S.; Okada, E.; Okuda, K. IL-15 expression plasmid enhances cell-mediated immunity induced by an HIV-1 DNA vaccine. *Vaccine* **1999**, *17*, 858–866. [CrossRef]
78. Wang, L.; Rollins, L.; Gu, Q.; Chen, S.Y.; Huang, X.F. A Mage3/Heat Shock Protein70 DNA vaccine induces both innate and adaptive immune responses for the antitumor activity. *Vaccine* **2009**, *28*, 561–570. [CrossRef]
79. Feder, M.E.; Hofmann, G.E. Heat-shock proteins, molecular chaperones, and the stress response: evolutionary and ecological physiology. *Annu. Rev. Physiol.* **1999**, *61*, 243–282. [CrossRef]
80. Liu, T.-T.; Wu, Y.; Niu, T. Human DKK1 and human HSP70 fusion DNA vaccine induces an effective anti-tumor efficacy in murine multiple myeloma. *Oncotarget* **2017**, *9*, 178–191. [CrossRef]
81. Potash, M.J.; Chao, W.; Bentsman, G.; Paris, N.; Saini, M.; Nitkiewicz, J.; Belem, P.; Sharer, L.; Brooks, A.I.; Volsky, D.J. A mouse model for study of systemic HIV-1 infection, antiviral immune responses, and neuroinvasiveness. *Proc. Natl. Acad. Sci. USA* **2005**, *102*, 3760–3765. [CrossRef]
82. Garrod, T.; Grubor-Bauk, B.; Yu, S.; Gargett, T.; Gowans, E.J. Encoded novel forms of HSP70 or a cytolytic protein increase DNA vaccine potency. *Hum. Vaccin. Immunother.* **2014**, *10*, 2679–2683. [CrossRef]
83. Spencer, A.J.; Hill, F.; Honeycutt, J.D.; Cottingham, M.G.; Bregu, M.; Rollier, C.S.; Furze, J.; Draper, S.J.; Sogaard, K.C.; Gilbert, S.C.; et al. Fusion of the Mycobacterium tuberculosis antigen 85A to an oligomerization domain enhances its immunogenicity in both mice and non-human primates. *PLoS ONE* **2012**, *7*, e33555. [CrossRef]
84. Ogun, S.A.; Dumon-Seignovert, L.; Marchand, J.B.; Holder, A.A.; Hill, F. The oligomerization domain of C4-binding protein (C4bp) acts as an adjuvant, and the fusion protein comprised of the 19-kilodalton merozoite surface protein 1 fused with the murine C4bp domain protects mice against malaria. *Infect. Immun.* **2008**, *76*, 3817–3823. [CrossRef]
85. Minhinnick, A.; Satti, I.; Harris, S.; Wilkie, M.; Sheehan, S.; Stockdale, L.; Manjaly Thomas, Z.R.; Lopez-Ramon, R.; Poulton, I.; Lawrie, A.; et al. A first-in-human phase 1 trial to evaluate the safety and immunogenicity of the candidate tuberculosis vaccine MVA85A-IMX313, administered to BCG-vaccinated adults. *Vaccine* **2016**, *34*, 1412–1421. [CrossRef]
86. Ci, Y.; Yang, Y.; Xu, C.; Shi, L. Vesicular stomatitis virus G protein transmembrane region is crucial for the hemi-fusion to full fusion transition. *Sci Rep* **2018**, *8*, 10669. [CrossRef]
87. Mao, C.-P.; Hung, C.-F.; Kang, T.H.; He, L.; Tsai, Y.-C.; Wu, C.-Y.; Wu, T.C. Combined administration with DNA encoding vesicular stomatitis virus G protein enhances DNA vaccine potency. *J. Virol.* **2010**, *84*, 2331–2339. [CrossRef]

88. Freer, G.; Burkhart, C.; Ciernik, I.; Bachmann, M.F.; Hengartner, H.; Zinkernagel, R.M. Vesicular stomatitis virus Indiana glycoprotein as a T-cell-dependent and -independent antigen. *J. Virol.* **1994**, *68*, 3650.
89. Bateman, A.; Bullough, F.; Murphy, S.; Emiliusen, L.; Lavillette, D.; Cosset, F.-L.; Cattaneo, R.; Russell, S.J.; Vile, R.G. Fusogenic Membrane Glycoproteins As a Novel Class of Genes for the Local and Immune-mediated Control of Tumor Growth. *Cancer Res.* **2000**, *60*, 1492.
90. Bateman, A.R.; Harrington, K.J.; Kottke, T.; Ahmed, A.; Melcher, A.A.; Gough, M.J.; Linardakis, E.; Riddle, D.; Dietz, A.; Lohse, C.M.; et al. Viral Fusogenic Membrane Glycoproteins Kill Solid Tumor Cells by Nonapoptotic Mechanisms That Promote Cross Presentation of Tumor Antigens by Dendritic Cells. *Cancer Res.* **2002**, *62*, 6566.
91. Chiang, S.C.C.; Theorell, J.; Entesarian, M.; Meeths, M.; Mastafa, M.; Al-Herz, W.; Frisk, P.; Gilmour, K.C.; Ifversen, M.; Langenskiöld, C.; et al. Comparison of primary human cytotoxic T-cell and natural killer cell responses reveal similar molecular requirements for lytic granule exocytosis but differences in cytokine production. *Blood* **2013**, *121*, 1345. [CrossRef]
92. Law, R.H.; Lukoyanova, N.; Voskoboinik, I.; Caradoc-Davies, T.T.; Baran, K.; Dunstone, M.A.; D'Angelo, M.E.; Orlova, E.V.; Coulibaly, F.; Verschoor, S.; et al. The structural basis for membrane binding and pore formation by lymphocyte perforin. *Nature* **2010**, *468*, 447–451. [CrossRef]
93. Leitner, W.W.; Restifo, N.P. DNA vaccines and apoptosis: to kill or not to kill? *J. Clin. Investig.* **2003**, *112*, 22–24. [CrossRef]
94. Wijesundara, D.K.; Yu, W.; Quah, B.J.C.; Eldi, P.; Hayball, J.D.; Diener, K.R.; Voskoboinik, I.; Gowans, E.J.; Grubor-Bauk, B. Cytolytic DNA vaccine encoding lytic perforin augments the maturation of- and antigen presentation by- dendritic cells in a time-dependent manner. *Sci. Rep.* **2017**, *7*, 8530. [CrossRef]
95. Qin, J.Y.; Zhang, L.; Clift, K.L.; Hulur, I.; Xiang, A.P.; Ren, B.-Z.; Lahn, B.T. Systematic comparison of constitutive promoters and the doxycycline-inducible promoter. *PLoS ONE* **2010**, *5*, e10611. [CrossRef]
96. Brennan, A.J.; Chia, J.; Browne, K.A.; Ciccone, A.; Ellis, S.; Lopez, J.A.; Susanto, O.; Verschoor, S.; Yagita, H.; Whisstock, J.C.; et al. Protection from endogenous perforin: Glycans and the C terminus regulate exocytic trafficking in cytotoxic lymphocytes. *Immunity* **2011**, *34*, 879–892. [CrossRef]
97. Lopez, J.A.; Susanto, O.; Jenkins, M.R.; Lukoyanova, N.; Sutton, V.R.; Law, R.H.; Johnston, A.; Bird, C.H.; Bird, P.I.; Whisstock, J.C.; et al. Perforin forms transient pores on the target cell plasma membrane to facilitate rapid access of granzymes during killer cell attack. *Blood* **2013**, *121*, 2659–2668. [CrossRef]
98. Zhan, Y.; van de Water, B.; Wang, Y.; Stevens, J.L. The roles of caspase-3 and bcl-2 in chemically-induced apoptosis but not necrosis of renal epithelial cells. *Oncogene* **1999**, *18*, 6505. [CrossRef]
99. Fink, S.L.; Cookson, B.T. Apoptosis, pyroptosis, and necrosis: mechanistic description of dead and dying eukaryotic cells. *Infect. Immun.* **2005**, *73*, 1907–1916. [CrossRef]
100. Matzinger, P. Tolerance, danger, and the extended family. *Annu. Rev. Immunol.* **1994**, *12*, 991–1045. [CrossRef]
101. Kono, H.; Rock, K.L. How dying cells alert the immune system to danger. *Nat. Rev. Immunol.* **2008**, *8*, 279–289. [CrossRef]
102. Melcher, A.; Todryk, S.; Hardwick, N.; Ford, M.; Jacobson, M.; Vile, R.G. Tumor immunogenicity is determined by the mechanism of cell death via induction of heat shock protein expression. *Nat. Med.* **1998**, *4*, 581–587. [CrossRef]
103. Gallucci, S.; Lolkema, M.; Matzinger, P. Natural adjuvants: endogenous activators of dendritic cells. *Nat. Med.* **1999**, *5*, 1249–1255. [CrossRef] [PubMed]
104. Sauter, B.; Albert, M.L.; Francisco, L.; Larsson, M.; Somersan, S.; Bhardwaj, N. Consequences of cell death: exposure to necrotic tumor cells, but not primary tissue cells or apoptotic cells, induces the maturation of immunostimulatory dendritic cells. *J. Exp. Med.* **2000**, *191*, 423–434. [CrossRef] [PubMed]
105. Basu, S.; Binder, R.J.; Suto, R.; Anderson, K.M.; Srivastava, P.K. Necrotic but not apoptotic cell death releases heat shock proteins, which deliver a partial maturation signal to dendritic cells and activate the NF-kappa B pathway. *Int. Immunol.* **2000**, *12*, 1539–1546. [CrossRef] [PubMed]
106. Joffre, O.P.; Segura, E.; Savina, A.; Amigorena, S. Cross-presentation by dendritic cells. *Nat. Rev. Immunol.* **2012**, *12*, 557–569. [CrossRef]
107. Wijesundara, D.K.; Gummow, J.; Li, Y.; Yu, W.; Quah, B.J.; Ranasinghe, C.; Torresi, J.; Gowans, E.J.; Grubor-Bauk, B. Induction of Genotype Cross-Reactive, Hepatitis C Virus-Specific, Cell-Mediated Immunity in DNA-Vaccinated Mice. *J. Virol.* **2018**, *92*, e02133-17. [CrossRef] [PubMed]

108. Bhowmick, R.; Halder, U.C.; Chattopadhyay, S.; Chanda, S.; Nandi, S.; Bagchi, P.; Nayak, M.K.; Chakrabarti, O.; Kobayashi, N.; Chawla-Sarkar, M. Rotaviral enterotoxin nonstructural protein 4 targets mitochondria for activation of apoptosis during infection. *J. Biol. Chem.* **2012**, *287*, 35004–35020. [CrossRef]
109. Ma, Z.; Wang, Y.; Zhao, H.; Xu, A.T.; Wang, Y.; Tang, J.; Feng, W.H. Porcine reproductive and respiratory syndrome virus nonstructural protein 4 induces apoptosis dependent on its 3C-like serine protease activity. *PLoS ONE* **2013**, *8*, e69387. [CrossRef]

vaccines

MDPI

Article

Long-Lasting Mucosal and Systemic Immunity against Influenza A Virus Is Significantly Prolonged and Protective by Nasal Whole Influenza Immunization with Mucosal Adjuvant N3 and DNA-Plasmid Expressing Flagellin in Aging In- and Outbred Mice

Jorma Hinkula [1,*], Sanna Nyström [2], Claudia Devito [3], Andreas Bråve [4] and Steven E. Applequist [2]

1 Division of Molecular Virology, Department of Clinical and Experimental Medicine, University of Linköping, SE-581 83 Linköping, Sweden
2 Center for Infectious Medicine, F59, Department of Medicine, Karolinska Institutet, Karolinska University Hospital Huddinge, SE-141 86 Stockholm, Sweden
3 Division of Immunology, HD Immunity, 126 25 Stockholm, Sweden
4 Public Health Agency of Sweden, 171 82 Stockholm, Sweden
* Correspondence: Jorma.Hinkula@liu.se; Tel.: +46-1328-2846

Received: 1 April 2019; Accepted: 11 July 2019; Published: 16 July 2019

Abstract: *Background*: Vaccination is commonly used to prevent and control influenza infection in humans. However, improvements in the ease of delivery and strength of immunogenicity could markedly improve herd immunity. The aim of this pre-clinical study is to test the potential improvements to existing intranasal delivery of formalin-inactivated whole Influenza A vaccines (WIV) by formulation with a cationic lipid-based adjuvant (N3). Additionally, we combined WIV and N3 with a DNA-encoded TLR5 agonist secreted flagellin (pFliC(-gly)) as an adjuvant, as this adjuvant has previously been shown to improve the effectiveness of plasmid-encoded DNA antigens. *Methods*: Outbred and inbred mouse strains were intranasally immunized with unadjuvanted WIV A/H1N1/SI 2006 or WIV that was formulated with N3 alone. Additional groups were immunized with WIV and N3 adjuvant combined with pFliC(-gly). Homo and heterotypic humoral anti-WIV immune responses were assayed from serum and lung by ELISA and hemagglutination inhibition assay. Homo and heterotypic cellular immune responses to WIV and Influenza A NP were also determined. *Results*: WIV combined with N3 lipid adjuvant the pFliC(-gly) significantly increased homotypic influenza specific serum antibody responses (>200-fold), increased the IgG2 responses, indicating a mixed Th1/Th2-type immunity, and increased the HAI-titer (>100-fold). Enhanced cell-mediated IFNγ secreting influenza directed $CD4^+$ and $CD8^+$ T cell responses (>40-fold) to homotypic and heterosubtypic influenza A virus and peptides. Long-term and protective immunity was obtained. *Conclusions*: These results indicate that inactivated influenza virus that was formulated with N3 cationic adjuvant significantly enhanced broad systemic and mucosal influenza specific immune responses. These responses were broadened and further increased by incorporating DNA plasmids encoding FliC from *S. typhimurum* as an adjuvant providing long lasting protection against heterologous Influenza A/H1N1/CA09pdm virus challenge.

Keywords: influenza; immunization; intranasal; adjuvant; lipid; flagellin

1. Introduction

250,000–500,000 people die from influenza or bacterial infections every year following influenza infection (www.who.int/influenza/en/). Viral spread also results in considerable days of illness and the loss of millions of work days annually. Influenza A virus is an RNA virus with a segmented genome of eight genes. The two surface proteins hemagglutinin (HA) and neuraminidase (NA) are the main targets for the neutralizing antibodies. The combination of these two antigens (20 different serotypes of HA [HA1 to HA20] and eleven NA in [NA1 to NA11]) with the two most recent bat influenzas identified, greatly determines the variability between the influenza virus strains [1]. Human vaccination using these immunodominant antigens is a primary method of influenza prevention that is used to control both seasonal and pandemic influenza strains [2]. When unchecked, seasonal and pandemic influenza both strongly affect the elderly who are especially sensitive to complications following influenza infection. Furthermore, existing influenza vaccines are less effective in the elderly when compared to younger people. The development of mucosally administered live or killed inactivated adjuvanted vaccines would be one way to create vaccines that are more conveniently delivered efficiently to the elderly [3].

It would be highly desirable to develop influenza vaccines that provide broader influenza-specific immune responses than what can be obtained with the currently available commercial inactivated flu-vaccines. If stronger and more long-lasting, cell-mediated and humoral flu-specific immunity could be obtained, it would be more likely that the obtained immunity could better protect against disease in future epidemics. In preclinical models, it has been reported that the killed formalin-inactivated influenza vaccines nasally given induce immunity almost equally with or without adjuvants [4–6]. Nevertheless, it would be advantageous to broaden the often elicited homosubtypic immunity into a heterosubtypic immune response recognizing more divergent influenza virus strains. Several recent preclinical studies in mice suggest that this is possible [7–10] by using virus-like particle vaccines [11]. It seems clear that both arms of the humoral adaptive immune system will need to be employed to broaden vaccine immunity, with influenza A neutralizing serum IgG, and also preferably with mucosal immunity consisting of secretory IgA towards the outer envelope proteins HA and NA [12]. This should then be combined with a systemic cell-mediated immunity as the second line of defense, which consists of CD8+ T cells recognizing conserved internal influenza virus epitopes [13], as well as a broad repertoire of memory CD4+ Th cells, which are critical to the maintenance of long-lasting humoral and CD8+ T cell immunity [14–16].

A new pandemic would probably be more rapidly spread and extensive than the Spanish flu of 1918–1919 when considering growing human populations and ease of international travel [17]. Indeed, these factors appear to have facilitated the emergence of the recent A/H1N1/"Swine" influenza, which appears to be a mixture of influenza viruses previously not seen in man, such as three triple reassorted genes from north American swine and human, three genes from classical swine influenza, and two genes from Eurasian swine [18]. When another pandemic appears, there will be many challenges to overcome in order to rapidly develop an effective vaccine against influenza, especially if they evolve from complex reassorted gene mixtures, as seen with the 2009 Swine-origin 2009 A (H1N1) influenza viruses. The time it takes to produce influenza vaccines needs to be decreased as well as issues of immunogenicity, quality control, and safety. Development and testing of vaccines while using new technologies are to be lauded. However, they can introduce unquantified risk in the development chain slowing vaccine development. Finding ways to improve upon existing technologies may be a way of mitigating development risk, while at the same time improving immunogenicity, safety, and production speed. The aim of this study was to use a licensed, existing whole formalin-inactivated influenza A virus (WIV) as a source of antigen and improve upon its ability to elicit immune responses by the addition of adjuvants. WIV vaccines are well known to induce poor cellular immune responses, unless combined with adjuvants [19]. This study investigated how additon lipid and genetic adjuvant(s) could be formulated to contain several critical components that cooperate to provide both a strong humoral, systemic and mucosal, as well as systemic cell-mediated heterosubtypic immune response, in both inbred mice (C57BL/6) and the outbred NMRI mice. Flagellin is an agonist of TLR5, but it is also directly recognized by the cytosolic Nod-like receptor family member Naip5, which signals through NLRC4 to form an inflammasome. Soluble flagellin has been shown to be a potent adjuvant in numerous studies and triggers numerous immune responses [20]. In previous studies, the presence and uptake of the bacterial flagellin proteins by CD103+ dendritic cells (DC) have resulted in their increased presence in mesenteric lymphnodes. Further, the flagellin-proteins have been shown to increase B-cells to switsch into IgA secreting cells, thereby enhancing the mucosal B and T cell responses against antigenic proteins [21]. However, there are few studies on the adjuvant effects of DNA-encoded flagellin [19]. The novelty of the present vaccination design of inactivated influenza A virus is the combination of previously never studied combined adjuvants. Thus, the adjuvants, the cationic lipid N3 alone, or N3 lipid mixed with DNA-plasmid expressing the TLR5-agonistic, de-glycosylated flagellin C-protein mixed with the WIV/Salomon Island/2006 A/H1N1-antigen prepared as an emulsion for nasal mucosal administration in two strains of aging mice.

The reasons for proposing mucosal administration would be to obtain mucosal immunity in the nasal and respiratory organs, where respiratory viral infections enter the body, to provide mucosal first-line barrier immunity. Furthermore, the immunization protocol aimed to study the long-term protective effect in an aging target-group of elderly individuals of mice reaching 22–23 months of age (representing human ages 60–70 yrs), where the influenza specific systemic and mucosal Th1/Th2-type immune pattern responses were followed and they could be correlated with different vaccination designs and levels of heterologous influenza A virus protection.

Here, we evaluated the potential benefits of combining the WIV vaccine with an experimental mucosal cationic oleic oil-based adjuvant alone and with a DNA-plasmid expressing a secreted form of flagellin from *Salmonella typhimurium*.

2. Materials and Methods

2.1. Inactivated Viral Vaccine, Lipid Adjuvants, and Formulations

Whole inactivated viral (WIV) vaccines are whole viral particles that are inactivated with formalin [22]. The influenza strain A/H1N1/Salomon Island/2006 (A/H1N1/SI) was used as a model vaccine candidate. The adjuvant N3 is based on a natural human fatty acid (L3) that is composed of: oleic acid 92%, linoleic acid 6%, and saturated monoolein 2% [23], and modified by coupling an amine-group to obtain a charged cationic molecule, N3 [24].

2.2. DNA Expression Adjuvant Constructs and Immunizations

pFliC-Tm(-gly) *S. typhimurium* has been described previously [25]. pFliC-Tm(-gly) was subjected to site-directed mutagenesis to insert two in-frame translational stop-codons after AA 459 of FliC(-gly) to generate a secreted version of FliC(-gly) (AA numbering is based on GenBank Accession #D13689). Changes were confirmed by DNA sequencing. The immunizations were intranasaly performed (i.n.) as previously described (Table 1) with five groups of outbred female NMRI mice and five groups of inbred female C57BL/6J mice. Briefly, mice were sedated with isoflurane (4% in air) and given WIV vaccine 5 μL/nostril (total volume 10 μL/mouse, 1.5 μg HA antigen/mouse or a total of 25 μg protein/mouse). In groups where the N3 adjuvant was used, a 1% concentration was intranasally given, 6 uL/nostril. Female mice of the NMRI strain were purchased from ScanBur, Sollentuna, Sweden, and C57BL/6 mice were purchased from Charles River, Dortmund, Germany. The animals were kept until 13 (±1) months before immunizations were initiated in accordance with ethical guidelines and permissions at the AF animal facility at the Karolinska Institutet, Stockholm, Sweden under specific pathogen free conditions [26].

Table 1. Study design and nasal immunization of NMRI and C57BL/6 mice against formalin-inactivated Influenza A/H1N1/Salomon Island/2006.

Immunization Schedule					
Group	n	Immunization Days	Dose and Immunogen	Adjuvant	Mouse Strain
1	32	0, 60	1.5 µg HA in whole intact inactivated H1N1	None	NMRI
2	32	0, 60	1.5 µg HA in whole intact inactivated H1N1	N3	NMRI
3	16	0, 60	1.5 µg HA in whole intact inactivated H1N1	pFliC(-gly)	NMRI
4	32	0, 60	1.5 µg HA in whole intact inactivated H1N1	N3 + pFliC(-gly)	NMRI
5	30	0, 60	Saline	N3 + pFliC(-gly)	NMRI
6	32	0, 56	1.5 µg HA in whole intact inactivated H1N1	None	C57BL/6
7	32	0, 56	1.5 µg HA in whole intact inactivated H1N1	N3	C57BL/6
8	12	0, 56	1.5 µg HA in whole intact inactivated H1N1	pFliC(-gly)	C57BL/6
9	32	0, 56	1.5 µg HA in whole intact inactivated H1N1	N3 + pFliC(-gly)	C57BL/6
10	24	0, 56	Saline	N3 + pFliC(-gly)	C57BL/6

Abbreviations: HA = Hemagglutinine protein from influenza A, pFliC(-gly) = Plasmid encoding secreted Flagellin type C of *Salmonella typhimurium* with mammalian glycosylation signal sequences removed.

2.3. ELISA Detection of Anti-Influenza A IgG, IgG isotypes, and IgA

IgG and ELISA measured IgA responses to influenza A in samples, as described [26]. The plates were coated with inactivated influenza A antigen (Swedish Institute for Communicable Disease Control, Solna, Sweden and Solvay Pharmaceuticals, BV, Weesp, Holland and recombinant HA/influenza A/H1N1/CA09pdm or NP Protein BioSciences, CT, USA) that was diluted to 2 µg/mL in sodium carbonate buffer pH 9.5–9.7 before 100 µL was added to each well. Influenza A positive mouse serum and naïve mouse serum were used as the controls for mouse anti-influenza A reactivity. The coated plates were washed with phosphate buffer saline (PBS)/0.05% Tween 20 (Sigma-Aldrich, S:t Louis, MO, USA) and then blocked with PBS/5% dry milk at 37 °C for 1 h followed by one wash. Mouse sera was diluted in PBS (pH 7.4)/0.5% bovine serum albumine (BSA, Boehring Mannheim, Mannheim, Germany)/0.05% Tween 20, and 100 µL of serial dilutions (1/50–1/5,000,000) were added to each well and then incubated at 37 °C for 90 min. After incubation, the plates were washed and 100 µL of HRP-conjugated goat-anti mouse IgG (BioRad, Richmond, VA, USA) or HRP-conjugated anti-mouse IgA (Southern Biotechnologies, Birmingham, AL, USA) (1:1000) diluted in 2.5% dry milk/0.05% Tween 20 (1:2000) was added to each well. The plate was incubated for 1 h at 37 °C and then washed. Ortho-phenylene diamine (OPD, Sigma) substrate was prepared by solving OPD-tablets 2 mg/mL in 0.1 M citrate buffer/0.003% H_2O_2. 100 µL was added to each well and the plate was then covered and incubated at room temperature for 30 min. The reaction was stopped by adding 100 µL 2.5M H_2SO_4 to each well and the absorbance was measured at OD 490 nm (24). The avidity index (AI) was determined by using the 8M urea wash procedure against the influenza antigens. IgG isotype reactivity to WIV was tested while using the ISO-2 ELISA reagent kit (Sigma), as recommended by the manufacturer. Isotype calculations of IgG1/IgG2a or 2c-ratios were calculated by dividing the OD 490 nm values for each subclass at dilution 1/100 or 1/1000. Inter-group ratio comparisons were made while using unpaired two-tailed, student t test. The ratio comparisons within each group were made using Pearsons correlation coefficient r.

2.4. Total IgA Quantification and Detection of Lung Anti-Influenza A IgA Responses

Lung-washes were harvested by flushing the lungs with PBS that was supplemented with protease inhibitors (Complete Mini, Roche, Mannheim, Germany) and then subjected to total IgA isolation while using the Kaptive IgA/IgE reagents (Biotech IgG, Copenhagen, Denmark) as recommended by the manufacturer. Total isolated IgA quantities were determined using an in-house murine IgA capture ELISA. Briefly, purified lung-wash IgA and standard mouse IgA (1 mg/mL, Sigma) was diluted ten-fold (PBS/5% dry-milk/0.05% Tween 20). 100 µL/per dilution was added to a 96-microwell plate that was precoated with rabbit anti-murine IgA (Dakopatts AB, Copenhagen, Denmark) and then incubated at 37 °C for 1 h. The plates were washed four times with PBS/0.05% Tween 20 before 100 µL HRP-conjugated goat anti-murine IgA was added to each well (Southern Biotechnologies) (1:1000). After 1 h incubation at 37 °C plates were washed and bound conjugate was detected by using OPD, as described above. The reactions were terminated using 100 µL/well 2.5M H_2SO_4 and the absorbance was measured at OD 490 nm. Total IgA was determined by comparing the OD-values of the test samples with the IgA standard. Detection of anti-influenza A IgA in total lung-wash IgA was done as with IgA from serum (above).

2.5. *Hemagglutination Inhibition Assay*

The hemagglutination inhibition assay (HAI) was used to quantify the antibodies against viral influenza A particles in serum from individual mice, as described previously [27]. An HI titre ≥ 40 was defined as a protective amount of serum antibodies [28]. Briefly, serum from individual mice were treated with receptor-destroying enzyme (RDE) overnight at 37 °C to remove the non-specific serum HAI inhibitors [29]. RDE was inactivated by incubation at 56 °C for 30 min., followed by the addition of 350 µL NaCl 0.9%. The HAI assay was initiated by adding 25 µL PBS to each well of a microtitre plate, followed by the addition of 50 µL of RDE treated serum. Serum was diluted in two-fold serial dilutions. 25 µL of influenza A/H1N1/SI or A/H1N1/CA09pdm containing four haemagglutinating units (HU) was added to each well. The plate was shaken, covered, and incubated at 20–25 °C for 15 min. Subsequently, 50 µL guinea pig erythrocytes were added, mixed, and followed by incubation for one hour at 4 °C. Thereafter, the plate was evaluated for hemagglutination and the degree of hemagglutination inhibition (HAI).

2.6. *T-Cell Responses to Influenza A Antigens*

T cell analysis was performed, as described here. Briefly, the splenocytes were isolated by physical disruption of the spleens, followed by Ficoll purification and washed twice with PBS. The depletion of $CD8^+$ T cells was performed while using Dynabeads (Dynal Biotech, Oslo, Norway), according to the manufacturer's instructions. The efficiency of $CD8^+$ cell depletion was confirmed by flow cytometry. On average, 98% ± 2.4% of the $CD8^+$ cells were removed. Total and CD8+ T cell depleted splenocytes from individual animals were suspended in RPMI 1640 (Sigma) supplemented with penicillin/streptomycin (Invitrogen) and 10% fetal calf serum (FCS, Sigma) and then subjected to anti-Interferon-γ (IFNγ) (Mabtech, Nacka, Sweden) antibody coated 96-well polyvinylidene fluoride (PVDF) bottomed plates (MAIPN 4510, Millipore Corporation, Bedford, MA, USA). WIV antigen restimulation was performed while using influenza A/H1N1/2006/SI or A/H3N2/1995/Wuhan at 100 TCID50. Peptide restimulations were performed using the H-2Kd binding NP peptides TYQRTRALV (147-156/aa), RLIQNSLTIERMVLS (55-69/aa) and the H-1Kb binding NP peptide ASNENMDAM (366-374/aa) at 1 µM final concentration (GenScript, Piscataway, NJ, USA). Concanavalin A (1 µg/well, Sigma) was used as a positive control to test cell activation and medium alone was used as the negative control. Spot-forming cells were quantified after 24 h incubation and then counted by an AID ELISPOT reader (AutoImmun Diagnostika, Strassberg, Germany). The results are given as cytokine-producing spot-forming cells (SFC) per million plated cells. The total and $CD8^+$ depleted splenocytes (10^6) were stained for 30 min. at 4 °C with FITC conjugated anti CD4 antibodies and with PerCP conjugated anti-CD8α antibodies (BD Pharmingen, Stockholm, Sweden). IL-5 production was determined by ELISA after restimulation of total splenocytes from individual mice with WIV A/H1N1/SI (1 µg total), as determined by the manufacturer (Omninvest, Budapest, Hungary) after 48 h from C57BL/6 samples and 72 h from the NMRI samples. The different time points chosen for the two mouse strains were determined in an in vitro pre-study influenza/ConA stimulation of spleen cells, and the optimal time point for highest levels of IL-5 secretion in elderly animals was chosen. Furthermore, IL-5 secretion was shown to be secreted at higher amounts for a longer period than IL-4 in vitro (or possibly consumed less rapidly) in aged mice, thus making IL-5 easier to use as a Th2-biomarker than IL-4, as shown by McDonald et al. 2017.

2.7. *Influenza Challenge*

To obtain information regarding tge longevity of heterologous influenza A-directed protective immunity mice were kept for up to 270 days after final booster immunization. Thereafter, at day 180 and at day 270, the influenza vaccinated and unvaccinated mice were intranasally challenged with influenza A/H1N1/2009pdm virus (10× LD50/mouse). Mice were monitored daily for four weeks post challenge, and when body weight loss was 20% or more the mice were sacrificed according with animal guidelines. Mice reaching this time point of sacrifice were sedated with isoflurane and blood and spleens were collected for the final immune analysis post-challenge.

2.8. *Data Analysis and Statistics*

Data was analyzed while using Prism v5.0d (GraphPad Inc.La Jolla, CA, USA). Confidence levels (95.0%) and the differences between the groups and doses of vaccines (nonparametric Mann–Whitney U test) (Table 2) were calculated using Prism. A significant difference was considered when a p-value of <0.05 was obtained. Inter-vaccination group ratio comparisons of IgG isotypes were made using unpaired two-tailed, student t test. IgG isotype ratio comparisons within each vaccination group were made while using Pearsons correlation coefficient r.

Table 2. Humoral IgG subclass IgG1/IgG2a or IgG2c immune responses to Influenza A after nasal immunization of NMRI and C57BL/6 mice.

Immunization Schedule			Humoral Anti-Influenza Specific Immune Responses					
	Dose and Immunogen	Adjuvant	Day 21		Subclass IgG 1/2a Ratio	Day 90		Subclass IgG 1/2a Ratio
			IgG1	IgG2a	Day 21	IgG1	IgG2a	Day 90
1	1.5 µg HA in whole intact inactivated H1N1	None	0.421 (0.179–0.624)	0.266 (0.094–0.419)	1.67	1.025 (0.306–1.131)	0.225 (0.099–0.279)	4.6
2	1.5 µg HA in whole intact inactivated H1N1	N3	1.091 (0.883–1.212)	0.360 (0.198–0.444)	3.02 **	2.313 (1.818–2.466)	0.707 (0.611–1.127)	3.3
3	1.5 µg HA in whole intact inactivated H1N1	pFliC(-gly)	0.231 (0.089–0.166)	0.259 (0.141–0.202)	0.82 *	0.305 (0.239–0.404)	0.273 (0.179–0.375)	1.11 **
4	1.5 µg HA in whole intact inactivated H1N1	N3 + pFliC(-gly)	1.343 (0.863–1.803)	1.909 (1.725–2.454)	0.7 ***	2.544 (2.161–2.707)	2.007 (1.933–2.414)	0.79 ***
5	None	N3 + pFliC(-gly)	0.029 (0.016–0.035)	0.026 (0.022–0.033)	n.a.	0.031 (0.019–0.035)	0.022 (0.017–0.028)	n.a.
			IgG1	IgG2c	Subclass IgG1/2c Ratio Day 21	IgG1	IgG2c	Subclass IgG1/2c Ratio Day 90
6	1.5 µg HA in whole intact inactivated H1N1	None	0.244 (0.202–0.302)	0.130 (0.079–0.143)	1.88	0.353 (0.277–0.421)	0.092 (0.056–0.141)	3.84
7	1.5 µg HA in whole intact inactivated H1N1	N3	0.701 (0.599–0.801)	0.625 (0.406–0.777)	1.12 **	2.007 (1.799–2.105)	1.138 (0.455–1.506)	1.76 *
8	1.5 µg HA in whole intact inactivated H1N1	pFliC(-gly)	0.102 (0.088–0.245)	0.223 (0.206–0.365)	0.45 *	0.259 (0.191–0.295)	0.301 (0.280–0.338)	0.86 **
9	1.5 µg HA in whole intact inactivated H1N1	N3 + pFliC(-gly)	0.728 (0.524–1.005)	1.126 (1.021–1.514)	0.65 **	2.489 (2.290–2.501)	2.796 (2.611–3.096)	0.9
10	Saline	N3 + pFliC(-gly)	0.019 (0.016–0.022)	0.015 (0.011–0.020)	n.a.	0.017 (0.015–0.021)	0.019 (0.015–0.022)	n.a.

Abbreviations. * = $p \leq 0.05$, ** = $p \leq 0.01$, *** = $p \leq 0.001$, n.a = Not analysed. Median OD490 nm values are shown for each group of mice (n = 6–8 mice/test day and group). Values in parenthesis show OD range.

3. Results

3.1. Serum IgG and IgA Antibody Responses

The anti-influenza serum IgG and IgA titers in NMRI mice were significantly higher than baseline in animals receiving WIV combined with N3 adjuvant or N3 combined with FliC-DNA adjuvant already at day 21 after a single immunization (Figure 1A,C).

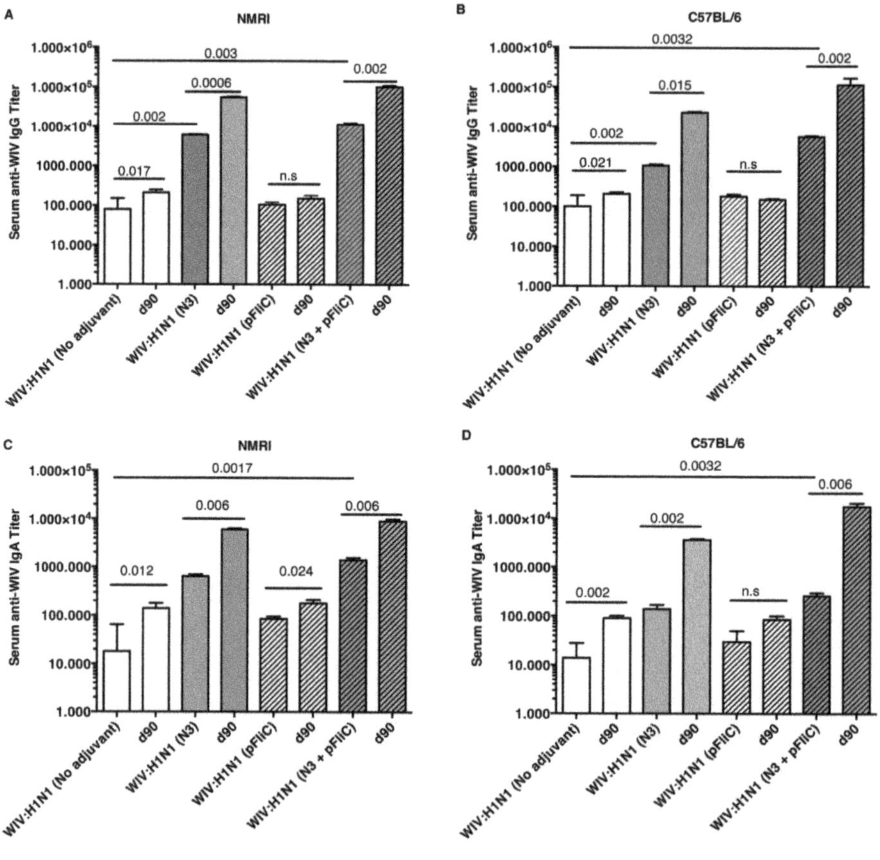

Figure 1. Influenza A H1N1/WIV/SI specific serum IgG and IgA titers. NMRI mice (**A**) and C57BL/6 mice (**B**) IgG titers 3 weeks (day 21) after one immunization and 4 weeks (day 90) after the booster immunization shown for each group. Each bar shows geometric mean (GMT) serum titer, and error-bars show 95% confidence interval values for each study group. Influenza A H1N1 specific serum IgA titers in NMRI mice (**C**) and C57BL/6 mice (**D**) three weeks (day 21) after one immunization and four weeks (day 90) after the booster immunization shown for each group. Bars show geometric mean (GMT) serum titer, and error-bars show 95% confidence interval values for each study group. Significant differences are indicated by nonparametric Mann–Whitney U analysis p-values. n.s. = not significant.

WIV given with pFliC(-gly) DNA did not result in significantly higher serum IgG titers then seen in mice that were immunized with only WIV demonstrating the important contribution of N3 to the effect of pFliC(-gly). The highest serum IgG titers were seen when both N3 and pFliC-DNA were combined with WIV with 100–140-fold increased titers. Booster immunizations at day 60 resulted in further elevation of the IgG and IgA titers (Figure 1A,C). Three weeks after booster immunization, the serum IgG in non-adjuvanted WIV immunized animals increased two-fold and IgA-titers increased five-fold. However, with WIV immunizations containing N3, a 100-fold serum IgG and 50-fold IgA increase was seen over WIV alone. Similar increases were also observed in mice receiving WIV with N3 and pFliC(-gly). Thus, the humoral influenza-specific immune responses between mice receiving WIV with N3 or N3 and FliC-DNA were not significantly different when analyzed by ELISA. Thus, binding antibodies alone may provide a misleading immune pattern from a functional point of view, as can be seen in the more detailed assays, such as subclass IgG ELISA (Figures 2–4) or functional antiviral assays, such as in virus-inhibition assays (Figure 5). IgG isotype comparisons revealed a correlation with the use of pFliC-DNA and the appearance of stronger IgG2a responses (Table 2).

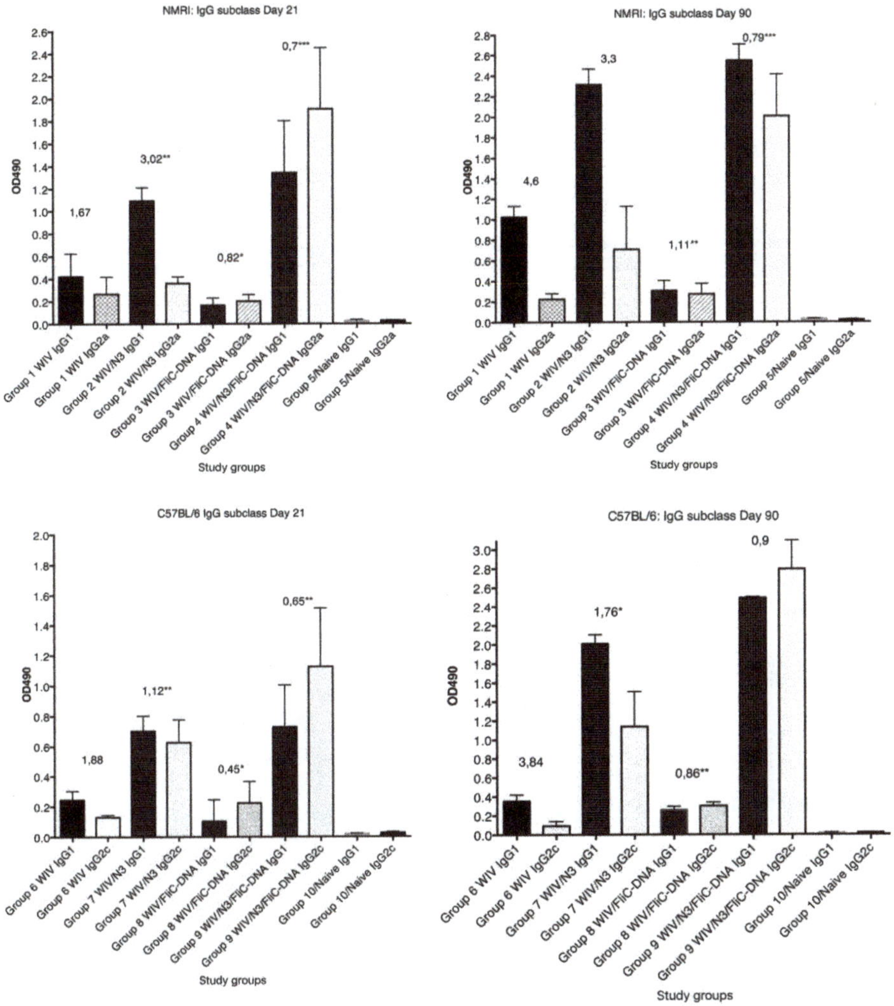

Figure 2. The anti-influenza A/H1N1/SI whole inactivated viral (WIV) specific serum IgG1 and IgG2a/2c subclass reactivity OD490 reactivity in serum collected at 21 days post primary immunization and 30 days post booster immunization (day 90). The median and range OD490 reactivity is shown for each study group (n = 6–8 animals/group), illustrating the results that are shown in Table 2. Significance. * = $p \leq 0.05$, ** = $p \leq 0.01$, *** = $p \leq 0.001$.

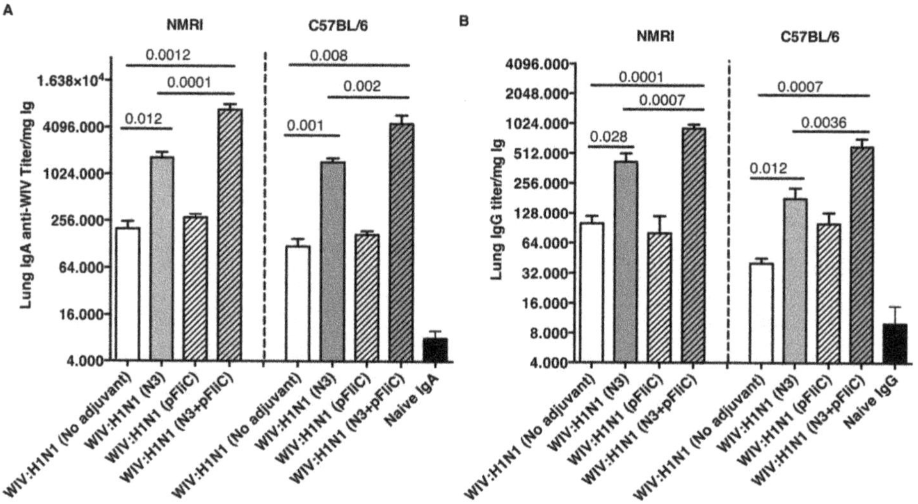

Figure 3. Influenza A H1N1 specific lung wash IgA and IgG. IgA anti-WIV titer in NMRI and C57BL/6 mice four weeks after booster immunization (day 90) (**A**). IgG anti-WIV titer in NMRI and C57BL/6 mice four weeks after booster immunization (day 90) (**B**). Titers presented are as anti-WIV titer/mg total IgA or IgG. Bars show GMT, and error-bars show 95% confidence intervals for each study group. Significant differences are indicated by Mann–Whitney U analysis p-values.

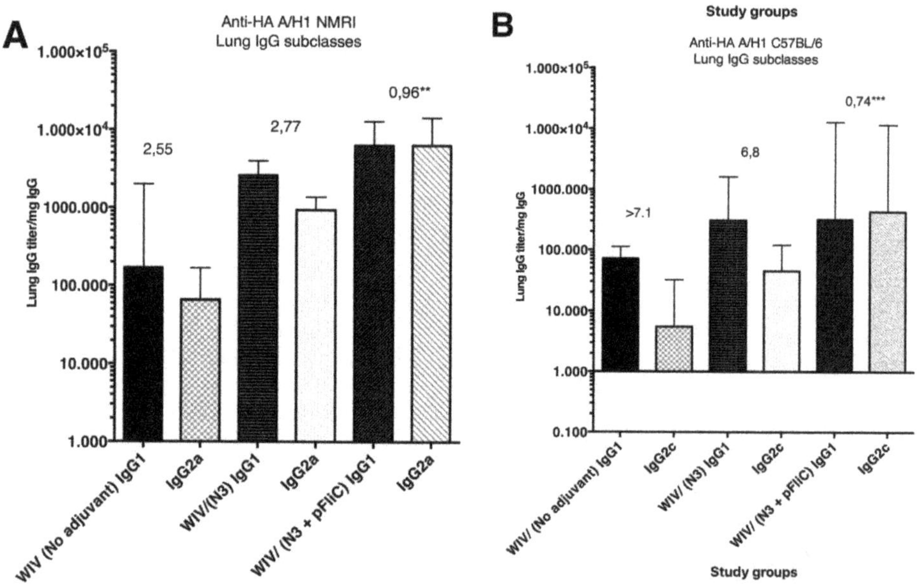

Figure 4. Anti-influenza A/H1N1/2009pdm rHA in lung-wash subclass IgG1 and IgG2a/IgG2c ELISA reactivity seen in three study groups at day 90 post primary immunization. (**A**) show IgG1 and IgG2a median subclass ELISA reactivity (and range) in lungs wash samples collected from outbread NMRI mice. The value given on top of each pair of bars indicates the median IgG1/IgG2a ratio in the group. (**B**) show IgG1 and IgG2c median subclass ELISA reactivity (and range) in lungs wash samples collected from inbread C57BL/6 mice. The value given on top of each pair of bars indicates the median IgG1/IgG2c ratio in the group. * = $p \leq 0.05$, ** = $p \leq 0.01$, *** = $p \leq 0.001$.

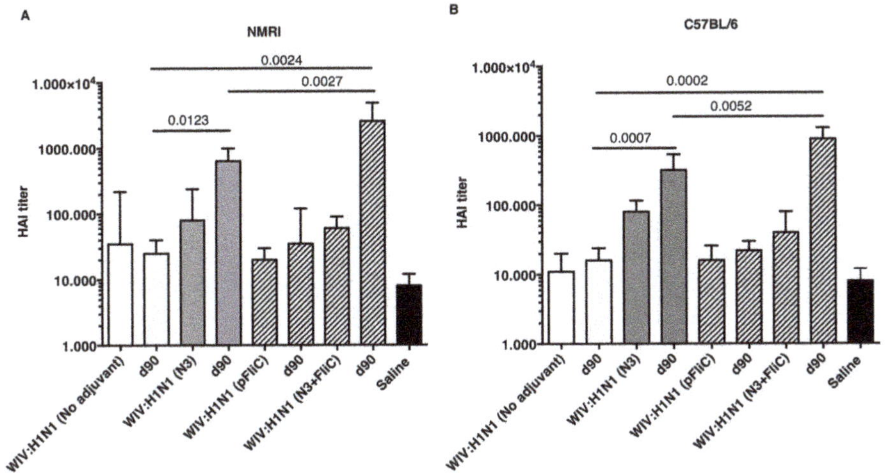

Figure 5. Influenza A H1N1/SI specific serum HAI titers. Titers in NMRI mice (**A**) three weeks after one immunization (day 21) and 4 weeks after the booster immunization (day 90) for each group of mice. Titers in C57BL/6 mice (**B**) three weeks after one immunization and four weeks after the booster immunization for each group of mice. Bars show GMT serum titer, and error-bars show 95% confidence intervals for each study group. Significant differences are indicated by nonparametric Mann–Whitney U analysis *p*-values.

The most pronounced effect on the IgG1/IgG2a ratio was seen after the primary immunization with WIV in animals receiving N3 with pFliC-DNA ($p < 0.01$) in contrast to WIV alone or WIV with only N3 or pFliC-DNA alone. Both the IgG1 and IgG2a serum titers increased after the booster immunization, but the IgG1 titers increased more than IgG2a titers. In all groups of influenza vaccine immunized mice receiving WIV with all adjuvants both subclasses IgG1 and IgG2a responses were seen, which indicated a mixed Th1/Th2 immune response. Nevertheless, the inclusion of pFliC(-gly) skewed the response away from Th2.

In C57BL/6 mice, significant serum IgG and IgA titer increase over baseline was only seen when the influenza vaccine and N3 adjuvant was used alone or when N3 was combined with pFliC(-gly) (Figure 1B,D). Similar to NMRI mice, when WIV was given with N3 or N3 and pFliC(-gly), a 10-fold and 20-40-fold increased serum IgG was observed, respectively. As observed in the NMRI mice, WIV given with pFliC(-gly) DNA did not result in significantly higher serum IgG titers than that seen in mice that were only immunized with WIV. After a booster-immunization serum, the IgG titers were doubled and IgA titers increased four-fold in vaccinated non-adjuvanted C57BL/6 mice. However, mice receiving booster WIV immunization with N3 increased the serum IgG titers 100-fold and 1000-fold when N3 was combined with pFliC(-gly) as compared to WIV alone. When compared to mice receiving WIV alone, serum IgA titers increased 20 to 100-fold with the use of N3 or N3 with pFliC(-gly). Similar to NMRI mice, C57BL/6 mice receiving WIV and pFliC(-gly) immunizations did not have significant increases in antigen-specific IgG or IgA responses at either day 21 or 90. IgG isotype comparisons revealed a higher Th1-like response in mice that were given WIV with N3 and pFliC-DNA (Table 2). Booster immunization induced a mixed Th1/Th2-type immune response with increases in the titer of both IgG subclasses. As with the NMRI mice, after the booster immunization both the IgG1 and IgG2c serum titers increased, but the IgG1 titers increased more than the IgG2c titers. The inclusion of pFliC(-gly) also skewed responses to a Th1-like IgG isotype.

3.2. *Mucosal IgA and IgG Responses*

Lung washes were collected after booster immunization to study the presence of influenza A specific immunoglobulins in the airways. Lung IgA and low levels of IgG specific for Influenza A were seen in all groups of immunized mice (Figure 3). The highest IgA titers were obtained in both mouse strains, where WIV was given together with N3 or N3 and pFliC(-gly) (Figure 3A).

No significant differences were seen between WIV immunized non-adjuvanted mice and mice receiving WIV with pFliC(-gly) alone. Similar trends were observed in the lung IgG titers (Figure 3B), and both subclasses IgG1 and IgG2a were detected. The highest lung IgA and IgG titers were seen in the groups where WIV was given with N3 and pFliC(-gly).

The subclass IgG pattern seen in lung washes that were collected after the booster immunization (Figure 4) show a significantly different pattern in the animals nasally immunized with WIV with N3 and FliC (-gly) DNA that was seen in animals receiving WIV or WIV/N3 adjuvant. In the N3/FliC-DNA groups of both outbred NMRI and inbred C57BL/6 a significantly stronger influenza-specific IgG2-response was detectable in lung washes, which suggested a more balanced Th2/Th1 immunresponse against the H1 hemagglutinine antigen.

3.3. *Hemagglutination Inhibition*

Although increases in serum HAI titers were observed at day 21 when comparing WIV to WIV and adjuvant groups, significantly increased HAI titers were only detectable after booster immunizations (Figure 5).

Booster immunization of both mouse strains with WIV with N3 or N3 and pFliC(-gly) significantly raised their HAI titer against A/H1N1/SI virus between four- and 32-fold. In mice receiving WIV immunization alone or WIV with pFliC(-gly), at best a non-significant doubling of HAI titer was seen. However, when combined with N3, pFliC(-gly) was able to promote a significant increase in HAI over WIV with N3 alone. None of the tested mice from any of the groups showed HAI titers against the A/H3N2/Wuhan strain. In general, the C57BL/6 mice developed lower serum HAI titers. These results indicate that the immune responses that were elicited by WIV together combined with N3 and N3 with pFliC(-gly) adjuvants were able to elicit clear increases in HAI titer that were well above the benchmark level of ≥40. Among the NMRI mice, all of the influenza immunized groups had animals that developed HAI-serum titer of 40 or more. The most significant responses were seen in groups where N3 and N3 combined with FliC-DNA was used as adjuvants, where all animals/group developed HAI antibody titers and the highest serum titers reached 65,000 at day 90. Among C57BL/6 mice, only animals in the two groups where N3 adjuvant was used with influenza antigen responded with HAI titers over 40. The highest HAI titers were seen in the group receiving N3 and FliC-DNA as adjuvant, with the highest HAI titers of 2560 being obtained at day 90 post-immunization.

3.4. *Interleukin-5 Release Responses*

A significantly higher amount of Interleukin-5 (IL-5) secretion was produced from animals immunized with WIV combined with adjuvants when the spleen cells at day 90 were stimulated in vitro with WIV Influenza A virus (A/H1N1/SI) (Figure 6).

The highest average amounts were observed in NMRI mice (Figure 6A) in WIV with N3 adjuvant as compared to WIV alone. The addition of pFliC(-gly) to WIV led to lower IL-5 production, however this difference was not significant. However, NMRI mice receiving WIV and N3 with pFliC(-gly) had a significantly lower secretion of IL-5 production after influenza antigen restimulation. In naïve mice only given adjuvant, no IL-5 secretion was seen when stimulated with WIV. Restimulated spleen cells from C57BL/6 mice produced, on average, one-third of the IL-5 amounts that were observed in NMRI mice (Figure 6B). Cells from all mice immunized with WIV and adjuvant produced significantly higher IL-5 amounts than WIV alone immunized mice. However, no significant difference in IL-5 production was observed between the WIV and N3 vaccinated mice and those that were given WIV and pFliC(-gly) or WIV with N3 and pFliC(-gly). Together, these results demonstrate that WIV immunization with N3 leads to cellular immune responses that were capable of IL-5 production, which can be attenuated by the addition of pFliC(-gly).

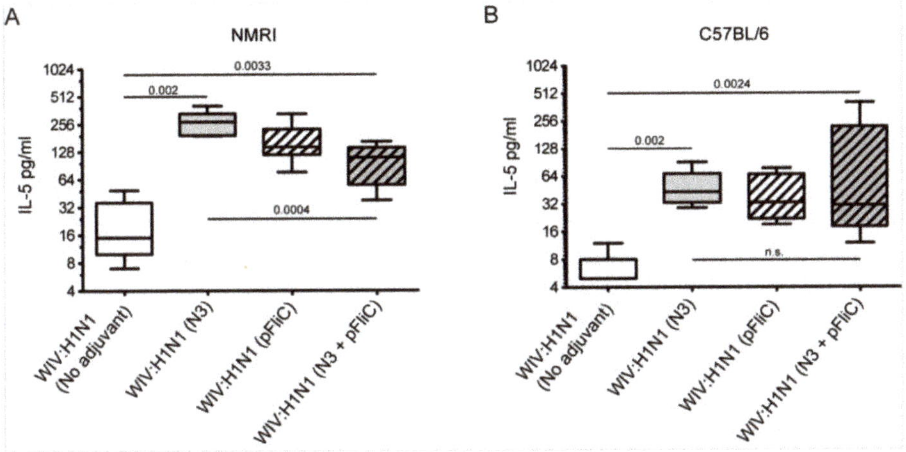

Figure 6. Splenocyte IL-5 release in response to Influenza A recall. (**A**) Influenza A specific IL-5 secretion (median pg/mL) million spleen cells at 48 h in NMRI mice, four weeks after booster immunization. (**B**) Influenza A specific IL-5 secretion (median pg/mL) million spleen cells at 72 h in C57BL/6 mice, four weeks after booster immunization. Block figures show median culture medium IL-5 concentrations after in vitro stimulation with WIV A/H1N1/SI, and error-bars show maximum and minimum values for each study group. The different time points chosen for the two mouse strains were determined in an in vitro pre-study influenza/ConA stimulation of spleen cells, and the optimal time point for highest levels of IL-5 secretion in spleen cells of adjuvant-vaccinated aged animals was chosen. Significant differences are indicated by nonparametric Mann–Whitney U test *p*-values.

3.5. Systemic Cell-Mediated Immunity

T cell-mediated immune responses to influenza A/H1N1/SI, NP-peptides, and A/H3N2/Wuhan virus showed significantly higher IFNγ spot reactivity in animals that were immunized with WIV with N3 and pFliC(-gly) adjuvant. Already, after one immunization (Figure 7A, day 21) IFNγ secreting spleen cells responding to A/H1N1/SI were significantly increased in NMRI and C57BL/6 mice that were immunized with WIV and N3 or WIV with N3 and pFliC(-gly) adjuvants.

After one booster immunization, IFNγ responses to A/H1N1/SI in both strains of mice were significantly increased in the WIV immunized groups if adjuvant was used (Figure 7B, day 90) as compared to non-adjuvanted immunizations.

Peptides from the conserved nucleoprotein (NP) from influenza A were selected to characterize the responses to a defined CTL-epitope. A H2d NP (aa 147-156) binding peptide was chosen to restimulate NMRI mice, and NP (aa 55-64) was chosen to restimulate H2b C57BL/6 mice. Mice in the groups given WIV with N3 responded by developing significantly higher numbers of IFNγ secreting cells than animals receiving WIV alone (Figure 7C). Adjuvant effects were further enhanced in WIV with N3 groups by the addition of pFliC(-gly).

A significant reduction in IFNγ ELIspot reactivity was only observed animals in groups where pFliC(-gly) was used as adjuvant when CD8+ T cell depletions were performed (Figure 7D). These results reveal the proportion of responses that are derived from CD8+ cells, but also indicate that all of the influenza responding mice develop IFNγ secreting CD4+ T cells against influenza. In all experiments, mice that were immunized with WIV alone developed no or very few IFNγ ELIspot secreting cells

(7–55 spots/spleen million cells), which was not significantly higher than influenza naïve control mice (Figure 7A–D).

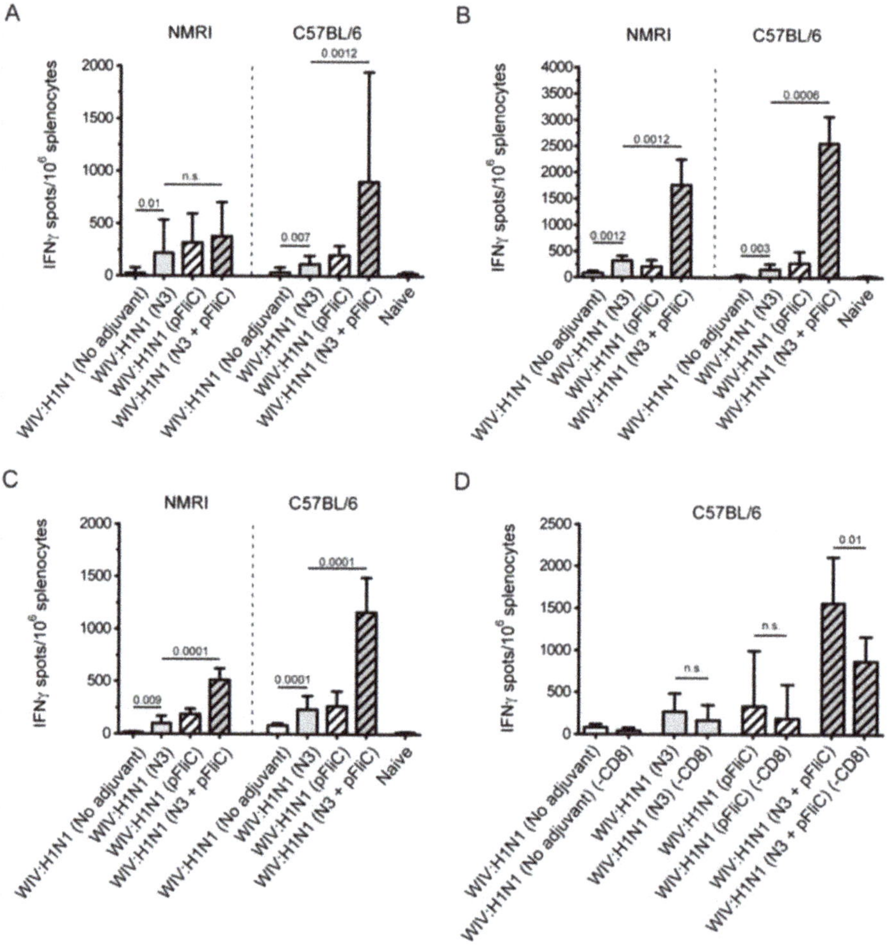

Figure 7. Splenocyte anti-Interferon-γ (IFNγ) producing cell frequency (ELIspot) in response to Influenza A antigen recall. (**A**) Influenza A/H1N1/SI specific IFNγ producing spleen cells in NMRI mice (left side) and C57BL/6 mice (right side), three weeks after primary immunization. (**B**) Influenza A/H1N1/SI specific IFNγ producing spleen cells in NMRI mice (left side) and C57BL/6 mice (right side), four weeks after booster immunization. (**C**) Influenza A/NP-peptide specific IFNγ producing spleen cells in NMRI mice (left side) (against peptide; NP147-156/aa TYQRTRALV) and C57BL/6 mice (right side) (against peptide, NP 366-374 aa ASNENMDAM), four weeks after booster immunization. (**D**) Influenza A/H1N1/SI specific IFNγ producing CD8-depleted spleen cells in C57BL/6 mice, four weeks after booster immunization. Bar-height shows geometric mean (GMT) spots/million cells, and error-bars show 95% confidence intervals for each study group. Significant differences are indicated by nonparametric Mann-Whitney U analysis p-values.

Heterosubtypic cell-mediated IFN-γ secreting immunity was tested while using A/H3N2/Wuhan influenza as a recall antigen (Figure 8).

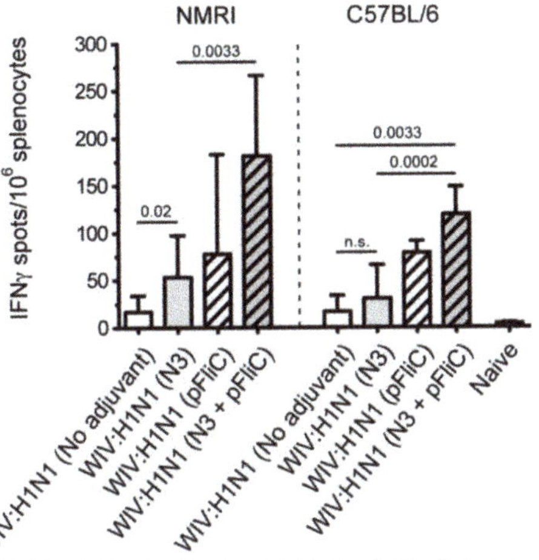

Figure 8. Splenocyte IFNγ producing cell frequency (ELIspot) in response to influenza A/H3N2/Wuhan stimulation. Influenza A/H3N2/Wuhan specific IFNγ spleen cells in NMRI mice (left side) and C57BL/6 mice (right side), 4 weeks after booster immunization. Bar-height shows geometric mean (GMT) spots/million cells, and error-bars show 95% confidence intervals for each study group. Significant differences are indicated by nonparametric Mann–Whitney U analysis p-values.

In general, the total numbers of IFNγ secreting cells were two-fold lower than those that were elicited by the homologous influenza strain (H1N1). Among the NMRI mice, all groups of immunized with WIV and N3 adjuvant developed significantly higher numbers of IFNγ secreting cells than the mice receiving WIV alone. A similar trend was observed among the C57BL/6 mice. The addition of the pFliC(-gly) adjuvant lead to even greater numbers of IFNγ secreting cells responding to H3N2.

Together, these results demonstrate that the addition of N3 adjuvant significantly elicits splenic T cell responses to homotypic whole influenza A after just one vaccination and after a single boost enhances the responses even further. The addition of pFliC(-gly) to a WIV and N3 immunization was, in nearly all cases, able to greatly enhance the immune responses when compared to WIV and N3 alone. Analysis of T cell responses after WIV and N3 boosting also revealed an ability to respond to conserved Class I T cell epitopes, as well as heterotypic influenza A strains. The addition of pFliC(-gly) to WIV and N3 immunizations were also able to greatly enhance these responses, but the analysis of specific T cell populations additionally revealed that a significant portion of immune reactivity came from both CD8 as well as CD4-expressing cells.

Summarizing the cell-mediated immune responses that were obtained at day 90, prior to influenza virus challenge, suggest that the used adjuvants were all capable of supporting both influenza-antigen stimulated IFN-γ secreting and IL-5 secreting immunity in vitro. The highest levels of IFN-γ secreting responses were detectable in the animals (of both strains of mice) given WIV and FliC-DNA/N3 adjuvant, of which around 50% seem to be from CD8+ T cells against the tested NP-epitope in the spleen of C57BL/6 animals (Figure 7D) and with cross-reactivity towards influenza A/H3N2 virus antigen (Figure 8). Thus, the most pronounced and broad influenza-specific immune responses were obtained through the combination of WIV A/H1N1/SI with FliC (-gly) and N3 adjuvant administered twice nasally.

The potential correlates of protective immunity on long-term periods were tested after in vivo challenge with a heterologous influenza A strain (California H1N1/2009pdm strain) and systemically analyzed in spleen cells, and in mucosal samples from lung wash samples.

Nasal challenge with influenza A virus resulted in significantly better survival in mice immunized with Influenza A vaccine and adjuvants N3 and N3 + FliC(-gly) DNA. This was seen in both strains of mice (Figure 9A–D).

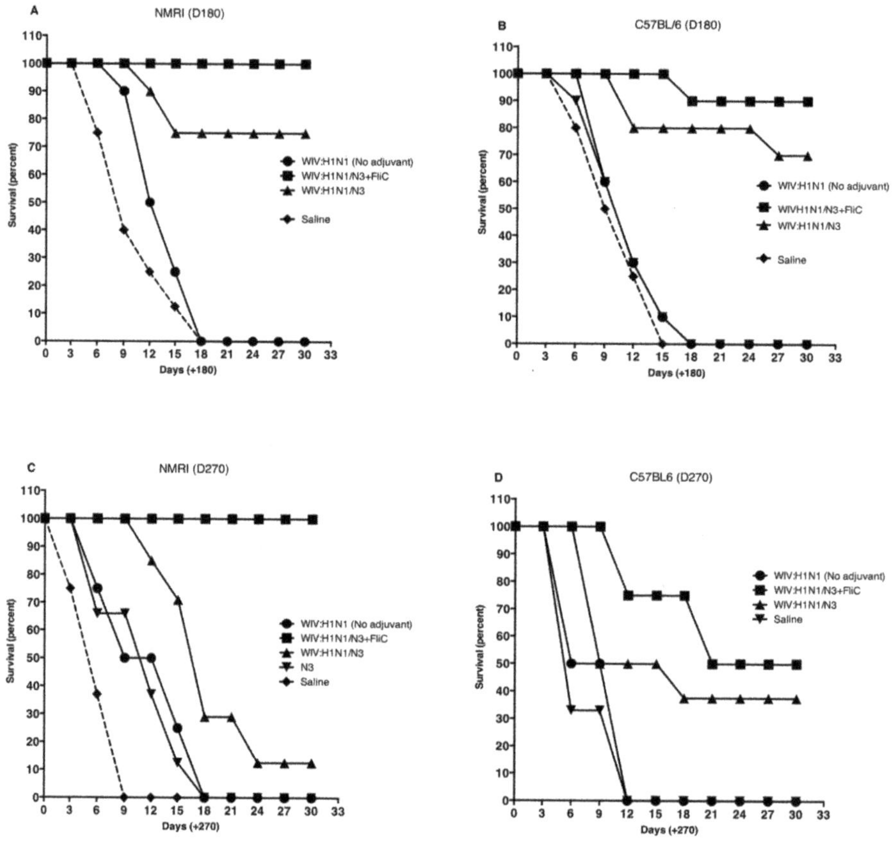

Figure 9. Kaplan-Meier graphs from day 180 post challenge show significantly better survival (100% to 87.5%) in NMRI mice (**A**) and in C57Bl/6 mice (**B**) if the WIV influenza vaccine was combined with N3 and FliC-DNA. as adjuvant and 80–75% survival when WIV with N3 adjuvant was used. (**C**,**D**). Kaplan-Meier graphs from day 270 post-challenge show significantly better survival (100% to 50%) in NMRI mice (**C**) and in C57Bl/6 mice (**D**) if the WIV influenza vaccine was combined with N3 and FliC-DNA. as adjuvant and 20–37.5% survival when WIV with N3 adjuvant was used.

Interestingly, the group survival data in both in- and outbred animals fit well with the pre-immunization immune responses that were measured, where especially elevated IFN-gamma levels after influenza-peptide stimulation in vitro and subclass IgG pattern with higher influenza-antigen ELISA binding IgG2 levels, seem to be associated with increased survival. In this study, the number of survivors post challenge was prolonged with at least three months in comparison with the inbred C57BL/6 mice. N3 with FliC-DNA plasmids provided the most elevated levels of both Th1 and Th2 type immune signaling, since almost all the studied immune parameters in the study (humoral responses: influenza virus specific HAI (Table 3). lung-IgG and IgA ELISA binding antibodies, subclass IgG pattern in serum and lung wash and IFNgamma ELIspot and cytokine release pattern in vitro) show that the adjuvant combination. The data may indicate that all of these immune parameters may need to be activated in elderly animals, since, in groups immunized with single adjuvant, obtaining good Th2-type humoral immune responses, at a higher age were not as efficiently protected when challenged with pathogenic influenza virus nasally.

Table 3. Serum antibody reactivity in blood samples collected at day of sacrifice in influenza A/H1N1/California/2009 challenged mice. Serum was tested for their hemagglutination inhibition assay (HAI) titer against the challenge influenza and by IgG ELISA titration against the challenge virus in samples collected two weeks prior to challenge and in serum collected at day of sacrifice post-challenge.

Serum Reactivity Against Influenza A/H1N1/Ca09pdm GMT and (Range) Pre- and Post-Challenge						
			HAI		ELISA Titers	(rHA/H1N1/09pdm)
Group	Antigen	Adjuvant	Titer Pre-Challenge	Titer Post-Challenge	Pre-Chall. IgG Titer	Post-Chall. IgG Titer
NMRI						
1	1.5 μg HA	No	<10	<10	140 (<50–180)	200 (60–240)
2	1.5 μg HA	N3	<10	10 (<10–30)	2220 (1600–4850)	5880 (3800–11240)
4	1.5 μg HA	N3 + FliC	<10	30 (20–60)	26770 (13,800–38,550)	106800 (46,560–224,450)
5	Saline	No	<10	<10	<100	<100
C57BL/6						
6	1.5 μg HA	No	<10	<10	<50 (<50–80)	75 (50–90)
7	1.5 μg HA	N3	<10	<10	1820 (480–3130)	4240 (3330–1550)
9	1.5 μg HA	N3 + FliC	<10	20 (<10–20)	5980 (5000–8690)	38820 (24,450–88,580)
10	Saline	No	<10	<10	<100	<100

There is a variable test sample timepoint difference between the animals that are presented in Figures 9–11. Animals from groups that more rapidly became ill after nasal influenza challenge where spleen cells were collected at day 9 to 15, at the day when they had to be sacrificed due to pathogenicity. From the groups where animals better resisted the influenza virus challenge (among NMRI mice groups 2 and 4 and C57BL/6 mice groups 7 and 9), the spleens were collected at day 29–30.

The IFN-gamma ELIspot analyses in splenocytes that were collected from mice challenged with heterologous A/H1N1/pdm09 virus without a FluA vaccination with potent Th1-type enhancing adjuvant illustrate that, if mice are allowed to reach old age, their cell-mediated immunity responds to slowly to protect from disease. Even though they have previously responded with a substantial influenza A neutralizing (HAI) response and at least a detectable influenza-antigen binding serum and mucosal IgG and IgA ELISA response, with time due, to aging on poor stimulation the levels may drop to low levels. This seems to be the case both for in- and outbred mouse strains.

Avidity Index (AI) against the recombinant HA of A/H1N1/Ca09pdm was significantly higher in the serum samples that were collected from mice immunized with N3 + FliC-DNA adjuvant (Groups 4 and 9, $p < 0.01$). Prior to challenge, the median AI in group 4 was 0.97 (0.86–1.11) and in group 9 median AI 0.86 (0.78–0.91) in comparison with the other influenza vaccinated groups with median AI 0.34 (0.09–0.46).

An attempt to perform mucosal influenza A/H1N1neutralization assays was performed against the challenge virus. However, the amount of IgA was quite low in each individual washing solution, so to perform the assay pooling and the concentration of samples was needed. Thus, we obtained one single pool from each study group for a single assay effort. The obtained results showed a HAI titer of 40, and only in the lung wash pool from the group of NMRI mice that were immunized with the N3 and FliC-DNA adjuvant.

It seems clear that the analyzed influenza-antigen stimulated cell-mediated immunity, both before challenge (Figures 7 and 8) and after influenza challenge (Figures 10–12), the later in old animals, the vaccine regimen containing adjuvants that enhance both humoral, virus-neutralizing, and binding antibodies in serum and respiratory mucosa, together with interferon-gamma secreted cell-mediated immunity seem to result in long-lasting protective immunity in both strains of mice, but perhaps more in out-bred than in inbred animals.

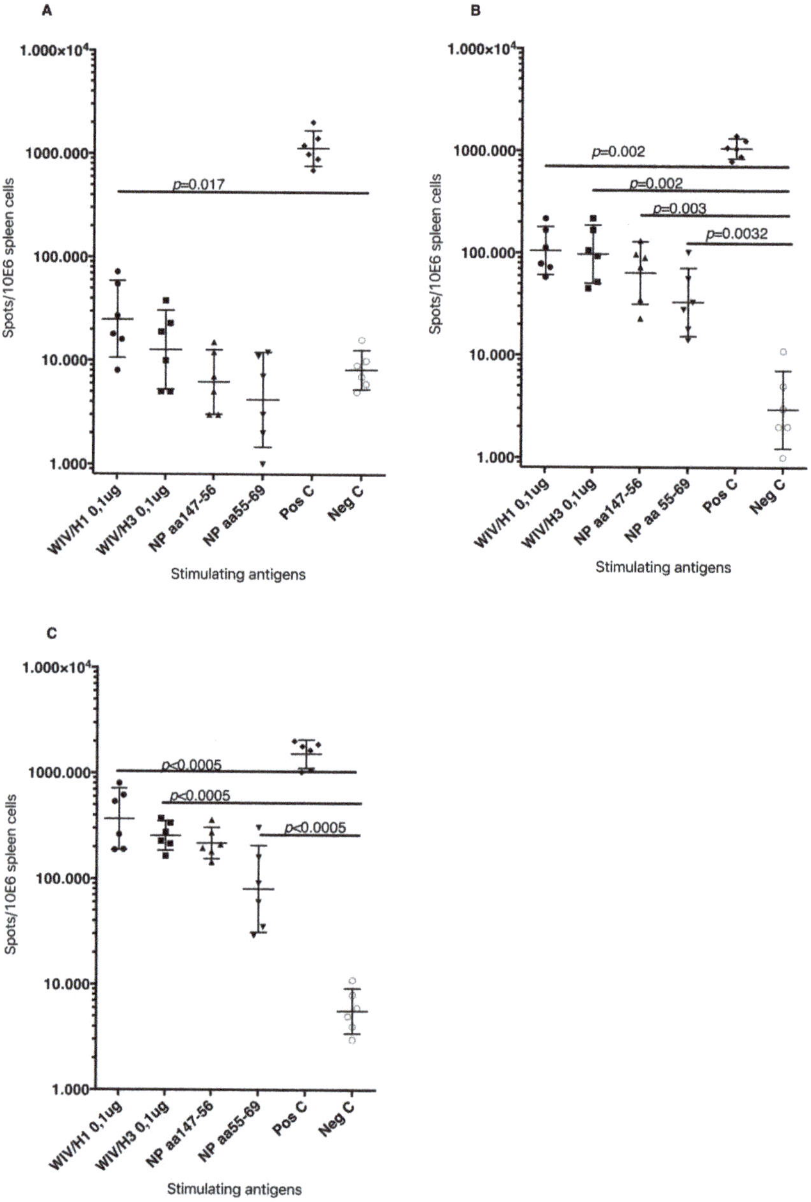

Figure 10. Cell-mediated immunity against influenza antigens after A/H1N1/California.pdm09 challenge was shown as IFN-gamma responses in stimulated spleen cells in vitro in three study groups of vaccinated NMRI mice (Figure 10A–C). (**A**) illustrates the GMT (95% C.I) IFN-gamma ELIspot responses in WIV vaccinated mice (no adjuvant) at day the day of sacrifice day 9–18, (**B**) the WIV with N3 as adjuvant, at the day of sacrifice, at days 12–30, and (**C**) the WIV with N3 and FliC-DNA as adjuvant, at day of sacrifice, at day 29–30. The frequencies of spots/million were evaluated against WIV/Influenza A/H1 and A/H3, as well as against two CTL-peptides from the NP-protein. Significant differences are indicated by nonparametric Mann–Whitney U analysis *p*-values.

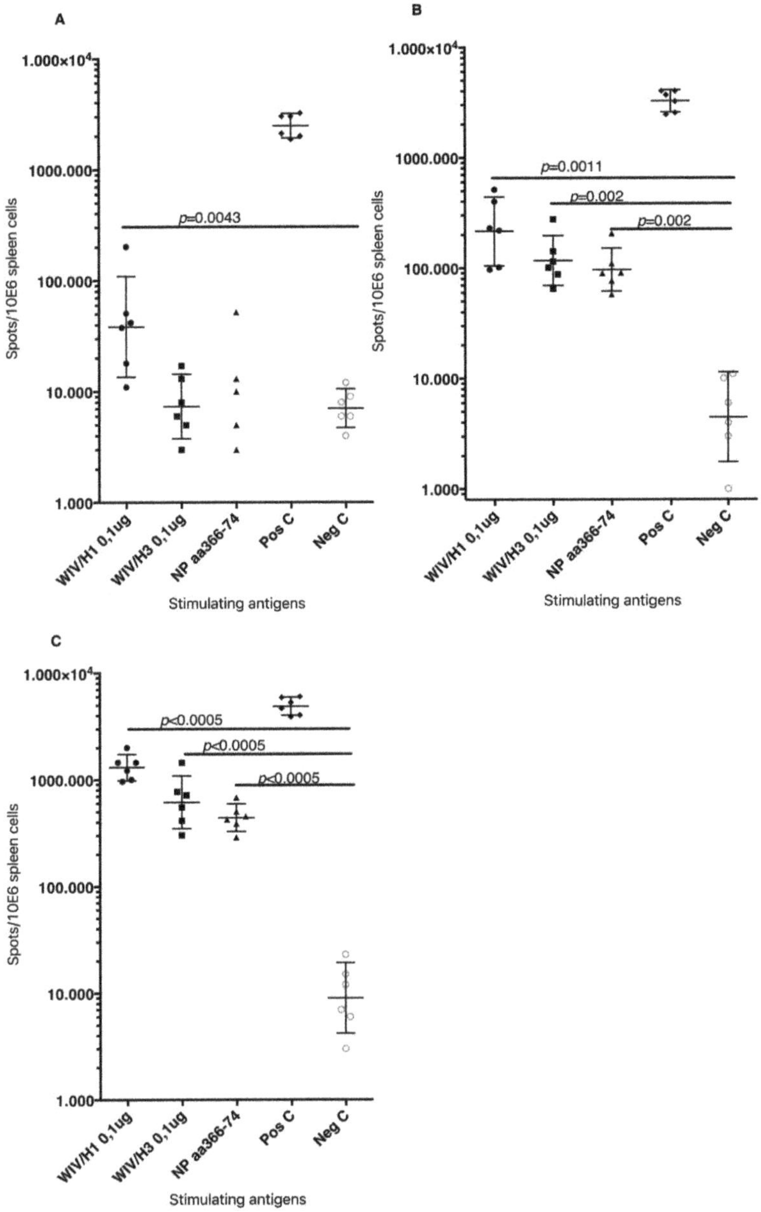

Figure 11. Cell-mediated immunity against influenza antigens after challenge was shown as IFN-gamma responses in stimulated spleen cells in vitro in three study groups of vaccinated C57BL6 mice (**A**–**C**). (**A**) illustrates the GMT (95% C.I) IFN-gamma ELIspot responses in WIV vaccinated mice (no adjuvant) at day of sacrifice at days 6, 9, and 12, (**B**) the WIV with N3 as adjuvant, at day of sacrifice at days 9, 18, and 30 and (**C**) the WIV with N3 and FliC-DNA as adjuvant, at day of sacrifice at days 12, 21, and 30. Frequencies of spots/million were evaluated against WIV/Influenza A/H1 and A/H3, as well as against one CTL-peptide from the NP-protein. Significant differences are indicated by nonparametric Mann–Whitney U analysis *p*-values.

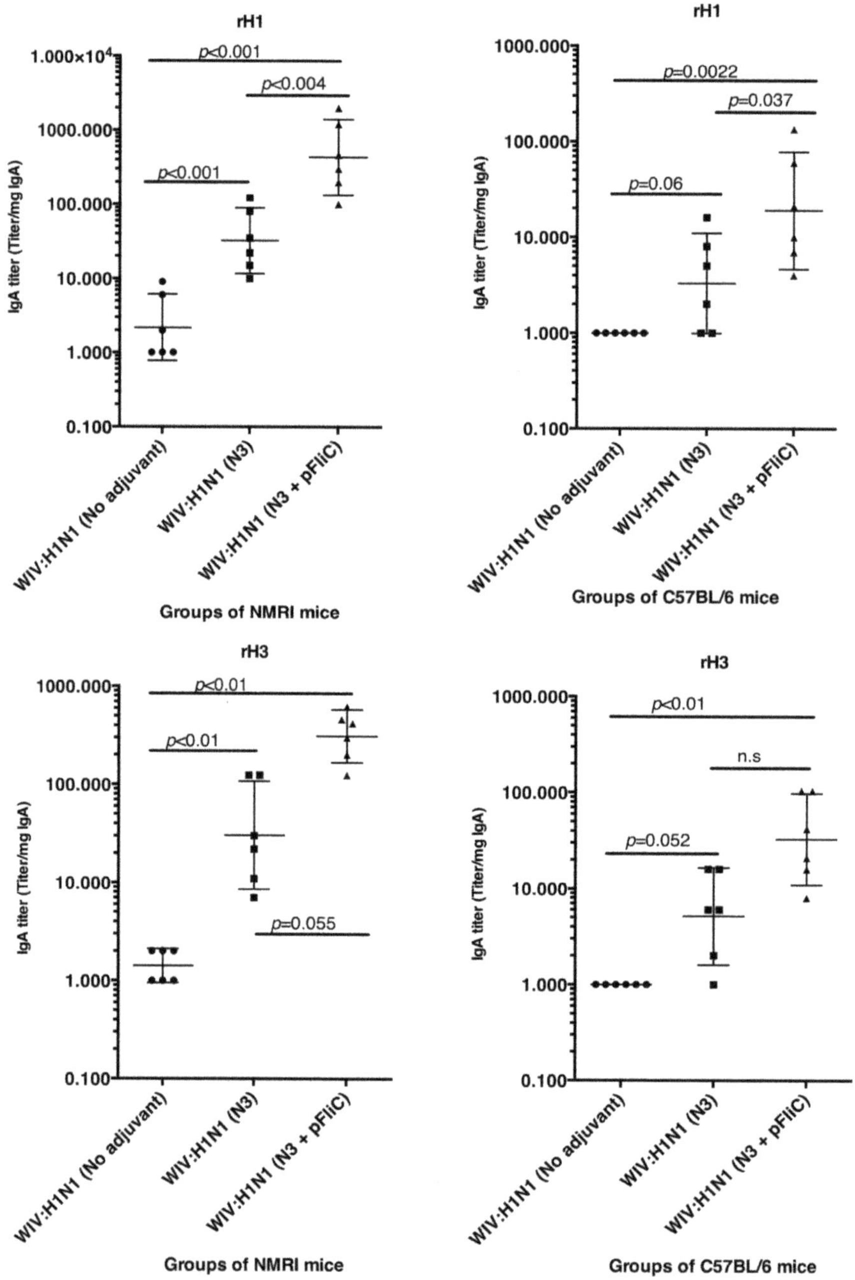

Figure 12. Mucosal lung IgA in lung wash fluids from NMRI and C57BL6 mice, post challenge. IgA anti-recombinant HA/H1/CA09 antigen (**A**,**B**) and anti-recombinant HA/H3/CA (**C**,**D**) ELISA titer analysis. Significant differences are indicated by nonparametric Mann–Whitney U analysis *p*-values.

4. Discussion

A single-dose vaccination would be highly useful, especially in emergency situations with rapid spread of influenza, as most inactivated influenza vaccines require two immunizations to provide full and protective immunity [30,31]. Previous mouse studies with formalin-inactivated WIV have shown that the rapid development of B cell responses in serum and upper airway mucosa is sufficient to protect from mortality. We assessed the use of two potential mucosal adjuvants in combination with WIV intranasal vaccination to improve upon these results and observed the induction of mucosal B cell responses as well as heterosubtypic systemic cellular responses that were detectable after only one dose. Immune reactivity is further enhanced after a nasal booster immunization. Thus, to investigate the development of long-term immunity, vaccinated animals were studied over nine months post-booster immunization before a heterologous influenza A/H1N1 challenge experiment was performed, in mice reaching 21–23 months of age.

Nasal administration of inactivated influenza A antigen with N3 and DNA-encoded flagellin from *Salmonella typhimurium* or from flagellin isolated from human flora *Escherichia coli* significantly increased the influenza A specific immune responses. The observed immunogenicity of this low HA dose, influenza vaccine (25 μg total protein/mouse containing 1.5 μg HA) in each mouse strain induced similar levels of serum antibody, which suggested that the basic antibody responses were comparable. With addition of either N3 or N3 and pFliC(-gly) adjuvants responses were significantly enhanced in both NMRI and C57BL/6 mice after a single immunization. However, the ability of N3 and pFliC(-gly) to promote enhanced serum responses over that of N3 alone was not observed.

After the booster immunization, significantly higher serum IgG or IgA titer toward influenza antigens was only seen in the mice receiving N3 adjuvant alone or N3 and pFliC(-gly). An analysis of serum IgG isotypes revealed that the inclusion of pFliC(-gly) in the adjuvant composition enhanced IgG2a responses when compared to the use of N3 alone, demonstrating its ability to promote a Th1-type or a mixed Th1/Th2-type immune response. Apart from being an indicator of the degree of cell-mediated cytotoxic immune responses, the IgG2 antibodies have also been described to be more beneficial antiviral isotype antibodies. They may enhance antigen uptake and cross-presentation due to their higher capacity to bind to Fc-receptors on antigen-presenting cells, as well as demonstrating better C′-activating properties via the C1q-pathway [32]. The capacity of non-coding plasmid DNA formulated with vaccine antigens to improve or strengthen Th1- or mixed Th1/Th2-type antibody and cell mediated immune responses has been documented [33,34]. However, when compared to our previous study that demonstrated a specific adjuvant effect by the FliC open-reading frame [25], our results suggest that FliC is exerting similar immune enhancing responses observed here.

It is not a straightforward task to understand how such a vaccine formulation functions due to the complex nature of our antigen adjuvant formulation(s). However, we favor a model where the nasal delivery of a cationic adjuvant N3 affects the mucus at mucosal surface layers to better penetrate and deliver the influenza vaccine, together with pFliC(-gly). This would allow for larger amounts of WIV antigen to be taken up by antigen-presenting cells, leading to antigen processing as well as the potential for viral ssRNA to stimulate TLR7 [35]. This enhancement may account for the adjuvant effect of N3 alone. When combined with pFliC(-gly), the N3 may allow for pFliC(-gly) "transfection" of cells in the mucosa triggering multiple innate immune receptors by way of activating dsDNA sensors, as well as sequence-specific CpG DNA sensors [35]. Additionally, as a consequence of FliC polypeptide production, NLRC4-triggered inflammasome activation and inflammatory cell death could occur in the permissive cells [36]. The secretion of flagellin from living or release from dying cells may also activate TLR5 [36,37]. Irregardless of the mechanism, we clearly observe that adjuvant the inclusion of pFliC(-gly) stimulates a mixed Th1/Th2-immune response pattern in both inbred and outbred mice, indicating its benefit in broadening immune responses to WIV.

The use of adjuvants in influenza vaccinations may be especially valuable in elderly individuals that otherwise fail to respond or lack strong influenza virus-specific cell-mediated immunity after traditional adjuvant free vaccination. However, one need to bear in mind is that influenza vaccines with adjuvants have also previously resulted in significant side effects, such as the Berna vaccine incidents where bacterial toxoid subunits, with the ganglioside GM1-binding properties were used as adjuvants for nasal immunization with the risk of resulting in Bells palsy [38,39]. The most recent serious side-effects with the intramuscularly administered influenza A/H1N1/pdm09 vaccine being given with the ASO3-adjuvant, resulting in hundreds of children responding with narcolepsy as a side-effect [40]. Obviously, every new adjuvant combined with influenza-vaccine will need to be analyzed for these undesirable side effects. One should bear in mind that this study has the main goal of providing long-lasting immunity that persists in protective immune responses at higher ages, instead of in children. The influenza strain that was used in the primary immunization belongs to the seasonal influenza strains, but the data obtained show that these influenza strains can provide protection against pandemic influenza A strains, such as A/H1N1/pdm09. Thus, the suggestion in this work is to immunize adults, to develop a robust enough immunity with the capacity to remain protective at higher ages, as exemplified in this report.

The humoral mucosal immunity that was observed in the respiratory tract of immunized mice was clearly enhanced by the presence of cationic N3 adjuvant in the inactivated influenza vaccine mixture. However, the highest lung wash IgA and IgG titers against influenza was seen in the mice of both mouse strains after immunization with N3 and pFliC(-gly). This combination of adjuvant N3 with pFliC(-gly) significantly enhanced the systemic and the mucosal immune responses (41). However, slightly different immune reaction patterns were observed between the two strains of mice when the samples were analyzed by HAI. The putatively protective and neutralizing serum HAI titer among the outbred NMRI mice initially (Day 21) shows equivalent titers for the group vaccinated with WIV alone and groups vaccinated with WIV and adjuvant (Figure 4A). After the booster immunization, the HAI-titers increased to significantly higher titers in N3, and N3 and pFliC(-gly) combination immunized groups (day 90). C57BL/6 mice more robustly responded to WIV with adjuvant after one immunization, which was likely because of strain-specific differences. Although these results indicate that immunization in outbred populations may require two doses, importantly they indicate that these adjuvants have the potential to function effectively in outbred veterinary animal populations as well as humans to promote WIV mucosal immune responses. The inclusion of these adjuvants in an intra-nasal non-living vaccine could provide enhanced protection of the upper mucosa. The most common route of influenza A transmission [41].

In vitro analysis of IL-5 secretion by splenocytes that were stimulated with WIV H1N1 from WIV and N3 immunized mice showed that cells from NMRI mice secreted significantly higher amounts of IL-5 than C57BL/6 mice. This interleukin is normally considered to be a Th2-type, which suggests that the NMRI mouse strain may be more Th2-skewed than C57BL/6. Direct comparison of our trends of IL-5 secretion to the serum IgG and IgA titers and IgG isotypes also established that higher IL-5 levels correlate with Th2-type immunity. Importantly, our observed IL-5 levels peaked at different time points in the two mouse strains. The NMRI spleen cell secretion of IL-5 peaked at 44–48 h while cells from C57BL/6 mice peaked at 70–72 h after stimulation. These differences could be due to natural differences in the immune kinetics in each strain, differences in the total responding cell populations, or fewer spleen cells being capable of IL-5 secretion in the C57BL/6 mice. The IL-5 response following mucosal vaccination illustrates its correlation to immunological aging that could not be seen in younger mice in previous reports looking at the effects of aging and cytokine responses [42] (McDonald JU et al. 2017). Despite these strain-specific differences in their ability to produce IL-5 in response to immunization with WIV and N3, this trend could be altered by the addition of pFliC(-gly) adjuvant, demonstrating its ability to skew the immune responses towards a broader and possibly more robust anti-influenza A immunity.

Preclinical influenza vaccine studies use the influenza virus HAI as a gold standard test to identify the immunization regimes that reveal most favourable vaccine candidates. Although this is not a true influenza A neutralization assay, it correlates well with clinical antibody mediated protection from infection and mortality in man and animals. Ideally, the best measure would be to perform a challenge study with the live influenza virus on influenza vaccinated ferret or man to investigate if protection can be obtained. In our study, we did not have access to a mouse-attenuated pathogenic influenza A/H1N1/SI strain, which is why homologous challenge studies were not performed. Instead, a mouse pathogenic heterologous influenza A/H1N1/pdm09 was performed at days 180 and 270 post final immunization. In lieu of this, HAI analyses with the Salomon Island strain was performed with serum from the various influenza vaccinated groups of mice. Sera with the highest HAI titers against the homologous H1N1 influenza strain were also subjected to an HAI assay against A/H3N2/Wuhan, but they were negative. Putatively protective (≥40) average serum HAI titers to the influenza vaccine strain was already seen after one immunization in the groups that received WIV with N3 or N3 and pFliC(-gly), suggesting a more rapid B cell response toward the HA antigen. These HAI titers were further elevated after the booster immunization and after boost also present in the WIV vaccinated mice given N3 together with pFliC(-gly). Interestingly, the serum and lung wash antibody ELISA titers are shown to increase, even when the HAI titers do not change or increase in a similar manner. Thus, it is important to remember that the binding antibody titers, as measured with ELISA, do not provide any information regarding how their functional activities against influenza A virus or influenza-infected cells. Instead, they may function as surrogate biomarkers of immunogenicity or (at least in mice) suggest Th1/Th2-type immune patterns against the studied antigens.

The choice of vaccination route is important to induce an effective immune response at a specific site. The inactivated vaccines that are currently used are usually intramuscularly injected, but it would be beneficial to administer the vaccines without needles. It would entail easier and faster administration, less expense, and discomfort with needles would be avoided. However, the alternative administration methods have limitations and they do not always lead to an adequate antibody response [31]. The injectable influenza vaccines are protective, because of their ability to induce influenza neutralizing serum antibodies as well as ADCC active antibodies, mainly IgG [33]. They can prevent the pathogen from spreading and be protective at the mucosal surfaces of the lower respiratory airways. However, resistance to influenza infection is connected to systemic and mucosal immunity. Serum IgA antibodies are produced to HA and NA in the upper respiratory tract, and IgG antibodies are also protective in the lower respiratory tract. In comparison to an injectable vaccine, the amount of local IgA antibodies in nasal washings is higher after nasal vaccination, but the amount of serum antibody titers is lower [36,37,41].

Our observations indicate that intra-nasal immunization with a formulation of WIV and N3 lipid alone is able to greatly enhance HAI-specific IgG and IgA in the upper respiratory tract, demonstrating that this approach can elicit effective antibodies at the location where influenza A infects. This effect can be enhanced with the addition of pFliC(-gly). Importantly, pFliC(-gly) strongly promotes a skewing of IgG isotypes towards IgG2a/c, as well as an enhancement in homotypic and heterotypic cellular immune responses. A subclass IgG1/IgG2 pattern mirroring what was seen in serum was seen also in the lung wash IgG content. However, it is unclear how well this indicates the local cell-mediated immunity in the lung tissues. Cellular immunity to influenza A has been long speculated to provide a role in limiting the pathology of influenza A infection, and recent evidence indicates that this is indeed the case [16]. Although it remains to be seen whether the promising anti-viral immune responses that we observe in mice can also be induced in humans, the approach that is delineated here indicates that it is possible to develop a non-living influenza A intranasal vaccine that is capable of eliciting both mucosal humoral antibody, as well as strong systemic cellular responses.

We kept groups of mice during a six and nine months follow up time to address the issue of long-term immunity as well as the protective capacity from disease and illness, and then nasally challenged them with a heterologous influenza A/H1N1 virus. At nine months, especially among the out bred NMRI mice, a complete protection (100%) was obtained, while the inbred C57Bl6 mice obtained 75% protective immunity, long-term, if both cationic N3 and FliC-DNA was used as adjuvant. The immune parameters that were seen in the best protected animals were cell-mediated IFN-gamma responses against a broader repertoire of influenza antigens, than in the other groups. Furthermore, mucosal IgA and serum IgG with a broad influenza A hemagglutinin antigen binding capacity was only seen in these groups and significantly more among the NMRI mice than in C57Bl6 mice, post-challenge. The fact that we used inactivated full virion antigen may explain this phenomena, as, in other studies where the FluMist vaccine was tested together with ritatolimoid (a TLR3-agonist), a broadened secretory IgA response was obtained [43]. Otherwise, no inactivated whole virion influenza vaccines are available on the vaccine markets. Thus, it is possible that the combined Th2/Th1 balanced immunity that was developed in the WIV N3+FliC groups provided a lasting protective immune mixture containing not only a cell-mediated IFN-gamma immunity against conserved NP-epitopes and mucosal broadly HA-binding IgA, but also serum IgG with influenza-specific ADCC-activity, often requiring antibodies with high binding affinity. ADCC have been described as an important immune parameter in protecting mice from severe influenza infection under experimental conditions [44]. In conclusion, the results suggest that a seasonal influenza A/H1N1/Salomon Island/2006, whole inactivated virion combined with cationic oil-in-water adjuvant with DNA-expressed Flagellin C *S. Typhimurium* given twice nasally provide protective immunity in 22 months old in- and out-bred mice against heterologous influenza A/H1N1/California/2009 challenge over nine months. However, with the recent experiences with side-effects when new adjuvants were combined with parenteral influenza vaccination, a thorough safety monitoring will be essential before aiming towards large-scale vaccination campaigns.

Author Contributions: For research articles with several authors, a short paragraph specifying their individual contributions must be provided. The following statements should be used conceptualization, J.H. and S.E.A.; methodology, J.H., S.E.A., S.N., A.B., C.D.; software, J.H., S.E.A., S.N., A.B.; validation, J.H., S.E.A. and A.B.; formal analysis, J.H., S.E.A., S.N., C.D.; investigation, S.E.A., J.H.; resources, S.E.A., J.H., C.D.; writing—original draft preparation, S.E.A., J.H.; writing—review and editing, S.E.A., J.H.; visualization, J.H., C.D.; supervision, J.H., S.E.A. CD; project administration, J.H., S.E.A.; funding acquisition, J.H.

Funding: This research was funded by Vinnova, grant number D09-01 and Hälsofonden 09-4.

Acknowledgments: Ulf Schröder and Jorma Hinkula share the IP rights for the N3 adjuvant. We acknowledge Eurocine Vaccines for the supply of N3 adjuvant. We thank Mona Hedenskog at Swedish Institute for Infectious Disease Control, Solna Sweden, and Erik Hedman, Kristina Kinnunen and Sofie Berger at Linköping University for assistance with HAI, ELISA and ELIspot analyses. This work was financially supported by Hälsofonden and VINNOVA.

Conflicts of Interest: Eurocine Vaccines AB have IP-rights and economical interests in the N3 adjuvant. J.H. declares financial support and IP share. S.E.A. declares interests of patents pending for DNA-encoded flagellin adjuvant technology. The remaining authors declare no conflict of interest.

References

1. Tong, S.; Xueyong, Z.; Li, Y.; Shi, M.; Buergois, M.; Yang, H.; Chen, X.; Recuenco, S.; Gomez, J.; Chen, L.M.; et al. New world bats harbor diverse influenza A viruses. *PLoS Pathog.* **2013**, *9*, e1003657. [CrossRef] [PubMed]
2. Nichol, K.L.; Treanor, J.J. Vaccines for seasonal and pandemic influenza. *J. Infect. Dis.* **2006**, *194*, S111–S118. [CrossRef] [PubMed]
3. Minutello, M.; Senatore, F.; Cecchinelli, G.; Bianchi, M.; Andreani, T.; Podda, A.; Crovari, P. Safety and immunogenicity of an inactivated subunit influenza virus vaccine combined with MF59 adjuvant emulsion in elderly subjects, immunized for three consecutive influenza seasons. *Vaccine* **1999**, *17*, 99–104. [CrossRef]
4. Samdal, H.H.; Bakke, H.; Oftung, F.; Holst, J.; Haugenb, I.L.; Korsvld, G.E.; Kristoffersen, A.C.; Krogh, G.; Nord, K.; Pappuoli, R.; et al. A non-living nasal influenza vaccine can induce major humoral and cellular immune responses in humans without the need for adjuvants. *Hum. Vaccin* **2005**, *1*, 85–90. [CrossRef] [PubMed]
5. Lovgren, K.; Kaberg, H.; Morein, B. An experimental influenza subunit vaccine (iscom): Induction of protective immunity to challenge infection in mice after intranasal or subcutaneous administration. *Clin. Exp. Immunol.* **1990**, *82*, 435–439. [CrossRef] [PubMed]

6. De Haan, A.; Geerligs, H.J.; Huchshorn, J.P.; van Scharrenburg, G.J.M.; Palache, A.M.; Wilschut, J. Mucosal immunoadjuvant activity of liposomes: Induction of systemic IgG and secretory IgA responses in mice by intranasal immunization with an influenza subunit vaccine and coadministered liposomes. *Vaccine* **1995**, *13*, 155–162. [CrossRef]
7. Takada, A.; Matsushita, S.; Ninomiya, A.; Kawaoka, Y.; Kida, H. Intranasal immunization with formalin-inactivated virus vaccine induces a broad spectrum of heterosubtypic immunity against influenza A virus infection in mice. *Vaccine* **2003**, *21*, 3212–3218. [CrossRef]
8. Tamura, S.; Tanimoto, T.; Kurata, T. Mechanisms of broad cross-protection provided by influenza virus infection and their application to vaccines. *Jpn. J. Infect. Dis.* **2005**, *58*, 195–207.
9. Tumpey, T.M.; Renshaw, M.; Clements, J.D.; Katz, J.M. Mucosal delivery of inactivated influenza vaccine induces B-cell-dependent heterosubtypic cross-protection against lethal influenza A H5N1 virus infection. *J. Virol.* **2001**, *75*, 5141–5150. [CrossRef]
10. Quan, F.S.; Compans, R.W.; Nguyen, H.H.; Kang, S.M. Induction of heterosubtypic immunity to influenza virus by intranasal immunization. *J. Virol.* **2008**, *82*, 1350–1359. [CrossRef]
11. Quan, F.S.; Huang, C.; Compans, R.W.; Kang, S.M. Virus-like particle vaccine induces protective immunity against homologous and heterologous strains of influenza virus. *J. Virol.* **2007**, *81*, 3514–3524. [CrossRef] [PubMed]
12. Mozdzanowska, K.; Zharikova, D.; Cudic, M.; Otvos, L.; Gerhard, W. Roles of adjuvant and route of vaccination in antibody response and protection engendered by a synthetic matrix protein 2-based influenza A virus vaccine in the mouse. *Virol. J.* **2007**, *4*, 118. [CrossRef] [PubMed]
13. Lee, L.Y.H.; Ha, D.L.A.; Simmons, C.; De Jong, M.D.; Chau, N.V.V.; Schumacher, R.; Peng, Y.C.; McMichael, A.J.; Farrar, J.J.; Smith, G.L.; et al. Memory T cells established by seasonal human influenza A infection cross-react with avian influenza A (H5N1) in healthy individuals. *J. Clin. Investig.* **2008**, *118*, 3478–3490. [CrossRef] [PubMed]
14. Swain, S.L.; Agrewala, J.N.; Brown, D.M.; Jelley-Gibbs, D.M.; Golech, S.; Huston, G.; Jones, S.C.; Kamperschroer, C.; Lee, W.H.; McKinstry, K.K.; et al. CD4+ T-cell memory: Generation and multi-faceted roles for CD4+ T cells in protective immunity to influenza. *Immunol. Rev.* **2006**, *211*, 8–22. [CrossRef] [PubMed]
15. Jelley-Gibbs, D.M.; Strutt, T.M.; McKinstry, K.K.; Swain, S.L. Influencing the fates of CD4 T cells on the path to memory: Lessons from influenza. *Immunol. Cell Biol.* **2008**, *86*, 343–352. [CrossRef] [PubMed]
16. Wilkinson, T.M.; Li, C.K.; Chui, C.S.; Huang, A.K.; Perkins, M.; Liebner, J.C.; Williams, R.L.; Gilbert, A.; Oxford, J.; Nicholas, B.; et al. Preexisting influenza-specific CD4+ T cells correlate with disease protection against influenza challenge in humans. *Nat. Med.* **2012**, *18*, 274–280. [CrossRef]
17. Doherty, P.C.; Kelso, A. Toward a broadly protective influenza vaccine. *J. Clin. Investig.* **2008**, *118*, 3273–3275. [CrossRef]
18. Garten, R.J.; Davis, C.T.; Russell, C.A.; Shu, B.; Lindstrom, S.; Balish, A.; Sessions, W.M.; Xu, X.; Spepner, E.; Deyde, V.; et al. Antigenic and genetic characteristics of swine-origin 2009 A(H1N1) influenza viruses circulating in humans. *Science* **2009**, *325*, 197–201. [CrossRef]
19. Corrigan, E.M.; Clancy, R.L. Is there a role for a mucosal influenza vaccine in the elderly? *Drugs Aging* **1999**, *15*, 169–181. [CrossRef]
20. Mizel, S.B.; Bates, J.T. Flagellin as an adjuvant: Cellular mechanisms and potential. *J. Immunol.* **2010**, *185*, 5677–5682. [CrossRef]
21. Flores-Langarica, A.; Marshall, J.L.; Hitchcock, J.; Cook, C.; Jobanputra, J.; Bobat, S.; Ross, E.A.; Coughlan, R.E.; Henderson, R.; Uematsu, S.; et al. Systemic flagellin immunization stimulates mucosal CD103+ dendritic cells and drives foxp3+ regulatory T cell and IgA responses in the mesenteric lymph node. *J. Immunol.* **2012**, *189*, 5745–5754. [CrossRef] [PubMed]
22. Geeraedts, F.; Goutagny, N.; Hornung, V.; Severa, M.; de Haan, A.; Pool, J.; Wilschut, J.; Fizgald, K.A.; Huckriede, A. Superior immunogenicity of inactivated whole virus H5N1 influenza vaccine is primarily controlled by Toll-like receptor signalling. *PLoS Pathog.* **2008**, *4*, e1000138. [CrossRef] [PubMed]
23. Schroder, U.; Svenson, S.B. Nasal and parenteral immunizations with diphtheria toxoid using monoglyceride/fatty acid lipid suspensions as adjuvants. *Vaccine* **1999**, *17*, 2096–2103. [CrossRef]

24. Ljungberg, K.; Kolmskog, C.; Wahren, B.; van Amerongen, G.; Baars, M.; Osterhaus, A.; Linde, A.; Rimmelzwaan, G. DNA vaccination of ferrets with chimeric influenza A virus hemagglutinin (H3) genes. *Vaccine* **2002**, *20*, 2045–2052. [CrossRef]
25. Applequist, S.E.; Rollman, E.; Wareing, M.D.; Lidén, M.; Rozell, B.; Hinkula, J.; Ljunggren, H.G. Activation of innate immunity, inflammation, and potentiation of DNA vaccination through mammalian expression of the TLR5 agonist flagellin. *J. Immunol.* **2005**, *175*, 3882–3891. [CrossRef] [PubMed]
26. Falkeborn, T.; Hinkula, J.; Oliver, M.; Lindberg, A.; Maltais, A.K. The intranasal adjuvant Endocine enhanced both systemic and mucosal immune responses in aged mice immunized with influenza antigen. *Virol. J.* **2017**, *14*, 44. [CrossRef] [PubMed]
27. Lundholm, P.; Asakura, Y.; Hinkula, J.; Lucht, E.; Wahren, B. Induction of mucosal IgA by a novel jet delivery technique for HIV-1 DNA. *Vaccine* **1999**, *17*, 2036–2042. [CrossRef]
28. Noah, D.L.; Hill, H.; Hines, D.; White, E.L.; Wolff, M.C. Qualification of the hemagglutination inhibition assay in support of pandemic influenza vaccine licensure. *Clin. Vaccine Immunol.* **2009**, *16*, 558–566. [CrossRef]
29. Cox, R.J.; Brokstad, K.A.; Ogra, P. Influenza virus: Immunity and vaccination strategies. Comparison of the immune response to inactivated and live, attenuated influenza vaccines. *Scand. J. Immunol.* **2004**, *59*, 1–15. [CrossRef]
30. Van Reeth, K.; Labarque, G.; Pensaert, M. Serological profiles after consecutive experimental infections of pigs with European H1N1, H3N2, and H1N2 swine influenza viruses. *Viral. Immunol.* **2006**, *19*, 373–382. [CrossRef]
31. Subbarao, E.K.; Kawaoka, Y.; Ryan-Poirier, K.; Clements, M.L.; Murphy, B.R. Comparison of different approaches to measuring influenza A virus-specific hemagglutination inhibition antibodies in the presence of serum inhibitors. *J. Clin. Microbiol.* **1992**, *30*, 996–999. [PubMed]
32. Amorij, J.P.; Huckriede, A.; Wilschut, J.; Frijlink, H.W.; Hinrichs, W.L.J. Development of stable influenza vaccine powder formulations: Challenges and possibilities. *Pharm. Res.* **2008**, *25*, 1256–1273. [CrossRef] [PubMed]
33. Feng, J.Q.; Mozdzanowska, K.; Gerhard, W. Complement component C1q enhances the biological activity of influenza virus hemagglutinin-specific antibodies depending on their fine antigen specificity and heavy-chain isotype. *J. Virol.* **2002**, *76*, 1369–1378. [CrossRef] [PubMed]
34. Lay, M.; Callejo, B.; Chang, S.; Hong, D.K.; Lewis, D.B.; Carroll, T.D.; Matzinger, S.; Fritts, L.; Miller, C.J.; Warner, J.F.; et al. Cationic lipid/DNA complexes (JVRS-100) combined with influenza vaccine (Fluzone) increases antibody response, cellular immunity, and antigenically drifted protection. *Vaccine* **2009**, *27*, 3811–3820. [CrossRef] [PubMed]
35. Epstein, S.L.; Kong, W.P.; Misplon, J.A.; Lo, C.Y.; Tumpey, T.M.; Xu, L.; Nabel, G.J. Protection against multiple influenza A subtypes by vaccination with highly conserved nucleoprotein. *Vaccine* **2005**, *23*, 5404–5410. [CrossRef] [PubMed]
36. Desmet, C.J.; Ishii, K.J. Nucleic acid sensing at the interface between innate and adaptive immunity in vaccination. *Nat. Rev. Immunol.* **2012**, *12*, 479–491. [CrossRef] [PubMed]
37. Miao, E.A.; Leaf, I.A.; Treuting, P.M.; Mao, D.P.; Dors, M.; Sarkar, A.; Warren, S.E.; Wewers, M.; Aderem, A. Caspase-1-induced pyroptosis is an innate immune effector mechanism against intracellular bacteria. *Nat. Immunol.* **2010**, *11*, 1136–1142. [CrossRef] [PubMed]
38. Holmgren, J.; Lonnroth, I.; Svennerholm, L. Tissue receptor for cholera exotoxin: Postulated structure from studies with GM1 gangliosids and related glycolipids. *Infect. Immun.* **1973**, *8*, 208–214. [PubMed]
39. Mutsch, M.; Zhou, W.; Rhodes, P.; Bopp, M.; Chen, R.T.; Linder, T.; Spyr, C.; Steffen, R. Use of the inactivated intranasal influenza vaccine and the risk of Bells palsy. *N. Engl. J. Med.* **2004**, *350*, 896–903. [CrossRef]
40. Lind, A.; Ramelius, A.; Olsson, T.; Arnheim-Dahlström, L.; Lamb, F.; Khademi, M.; Ambati, A.; Maurer, M.; Nilsson, A.L.; Bomfim, I.L.; et al. A/H1N1 antibodies and TRIB2 autoantibodies in narcolepsy patients diagnosed in conjunction with the Pandemrix vaccination campaign in Sweden 2009–2010. *J. Autoimmun.* **2014**, *50*, 99–106. [CrossRef]
41. Liew, F.Y.; Russell, S.M.; Appleyard, G.; Brand, C.M.; Beale, J. Cross-protection in mice infected with influenza A virus by the respiratory route is correlated with local IgA antibody rather than serum antibody or cytotoxic T cell reactivity. *Eur. J. Immunol.* **1984**, *14*, 350–356. [CrossRef] [PubMed]
42. McDonald, J.U.; Zhong, Z.; Groves, H.T.; Tregoning, J.S. Inflammatory responses to influenza vaccination at thje extremes of age. *Immunology* **2017**, *151*, 451–463. [CrossRef] [PubMed]

43. Overton, E.T.; Goenfert, P.A.; Cunningham, P.; Carter, W.A.; Horvath, J.; Young, D.; Strayer, D.R. Intranasal seasonal influenza vaccine and a TLR-3 agonist, rintatolimod, induced cross-reactive IgA antibody formation against avian H5N1 and H7N9 influenza HA in humans. *Vaccine* **2014**, *32*, 5490–5495. [CrossRef] [PubMed]
44. Tan, G.S.; Leon, P.E.; Albrecht, R.A.; Margine, I.; Hirsh, A.; Bahl, J.; Krammer, F. Broadly-reactive neutralizing and non-neutralizing antibodies directed against the H7 influenza virus hemagglutinine reveal divergent mechanisms of protection. *PLoS Pathog.* **2016**, *12*, e1005578. [CrossRef]

vaccines

MDPI

Article

Designed DNA-Encoded IL-36 Gamma Acts as a Potent Molecular Adjuvant Enhancing Zika Synthetic DNA Vaccine-Induced Immunity and Protection in a Lethal Challenge Model

Lumena Louis [1], Megan C. Wise [2], Hyeree Choi [1], Daniel O. Villarreal [3], Kar Muthumani [1] and David B. Weiner [1,*]

1 Vaccine and Immunotherapy Center, The Wistar Institute, Philadelphia, PA 19104, USA; llouis@wistar.org (L.L.); hychoi@wistar.org (H.C.); kmuthumani@wistar.org (K.M.)
2 Inovio Pharmaceuticals, Plymouth Meeting, PA 19462, USA; megan.wise@inovio.com
3 Incyte Corporation, Wilmington, DE 19803, USA; dovill33@gmail.com
* Correspondence: dweiner@wistar.org

Received: 4 April 2019; Accepted: 18 May 2019; Published: 22 May 2019

Abstract: Identification of novel molecular adjuvants which can boost and enhance vaccine-mediated immunity and provide dose-sparing potential against complex infectious diseases and for immunotherapy in cancer is likely to play a critical role in the next generation of vaccines. Given the number of challenging targets for which no or only partial vaccine options exist, adjuvants that can address some of these concerns are in high demand. Here, we report that a designed truncated Interleukin-36 gamma (IL-36 gamma) encoded plasmid can act as a potent adjuvant for several DNA-encoded vaccine targets including human immunodeficiency virus (HIV), influenza, and Zika in immunization models. We further show that the truncated IL-36 gamma (opt-36γt) plasmid provides improved dose sparing as it boosts immunity to a suboptimal dose of a Zika DNA vaccine, resulting in potent protection against a lethal Zika challenge.

Keywords: IL-36; adjuvant; DNA; Zika

1. Introduction

The most successful approach to controlling infectious diseases on a global scale has been through vaccination. Vaccines have led to control, eradication, or near eradication of several infectious diseases, positively impacting both human longevity and the quality of life. However, much work remains in this area. For many targets, current studies have suggested the need for adjuvants which can provide a number of benefits, including improved vaccine effectiveness, as discussed in several papers and reviews [1–9]. Adjuvants can boost overall immune responses to a specific vaccine, thereby requiring either a lower dose or fewer immunizations, improving protection and compliance as well as increasing the global vaccine supply for a particular product [3]. Adjuvants can also help skew and tailor the immune response, which may be useful in scenarios where specific correlates of protection are understood [10–12]. Furthermore, adjuvants can boost immunity and shorten the time to induce a protective vaccine response in populations that traditionally have a difficult time mounting protective responses, including the elderly and immunocompromised patients [3]. Alum, the most widely used adjuvant among current licensed vaccines, is well documented to enhance humoral immunity [9,13]. Newer vaccine adjuvants including MF59 and the Adjuvant Systems group 03 and 04 (AS03, AS04, respectively) have also been licensed and shown to improve antibody responses to antigens as well as provide dose-sparing effects (among other benefits) for humoral responses [14–18]. Shingrix, the latest vaccine approved to protect against reactivation of herpes zoster and postherpetic neuralgia (shingles), is a recombinant vaccine made of glycoprotein E and AS01$_B$ adjuvant [5,19,20]. This vaccine demonstrated an efficacy of over 95% against herpes zoster, with greater efficacy compared to a live attenuated vaccine, ZostaVax, highlighting the impact that adjuvants can have on vaccine outcomes. However, in spite of this success, there is still a major need in the clinic for adjuvants that can improve cytotoxic T lymphocyte (CTL) responses [7], and there is a lot of exciting work being done in this field. Some of this work includes nontraditional adjuvants such as pathogen-recognition receptor agonists, liposomes, nanoparticles, and gene-encoded adjuvants that can potentially jumpstart the innate immune system and work in concert with the adaptive immune arm to drive lasting memory against antigen [6]. One cytokine, Interleukin-12 (IL-12), has garnered much attention in the field for its adjuvant properties in a number of preclinical models [21–27]. In addition, data from a clinical study showed that inclusion of plasmid IL-12 as part of a human immunodeficiency virus (HIV) synthetic DNA vaccine increased T cell magnitude and response rates in people [28]. These data encourage further investigation of additional less well-studied cytokines as DNA or other potential adjuvants to further broaden immunity and improve cellular as well as humoral immunity for DNA-encoded antigens.

The IL-36 family is made up of the pro-inflammatory mediators alpha, beta, and gamma, as well as antagonist IL-36Ra [29,30]. This relatively novel cytokine family remains poorly understood, although recent important studies have begun to shed light on their mechanism of action. The IL-36 family is a part of the IL-1 superfamily, of which alpha, beta, and gamma are agonists. Upon binding to the IL-36 receptor (IL-36R) and recruitment of the interleukin-1 receptor accessory protein (IL-1RAcP), these cytokines activate the nuclear factor-kappa-light-chain-enhancer of activated B cells (NF-κB) and mitogen-activated protein kinases (MAPK) pathway, resulting in the stimulation of pro-inflammatory intracellular responses, whereas binding of the antagonist, IL-36Ra, prevents recruitment of IL-1RAcP and does not lead to intracellular response [31–33]. IL-36R is primarily expressed on naïve $CD4^+$ T cells, but is also found on dendritic cells, while the cytokines are expressed mainly in skin keratinocytes and epithelium, although they are also expressed at low levels in the lung, kidneys, and intestine [29,34–36]. Given reports of IL-36 beta's ability to amplify Th1 responses [37,38], we sought to understand whether these cytokines could act as adjuvants for DNA vaccination models. Here, we describe that a novel designed truncated IL-36 gamma (opt-36γt), as a co-formulated adjuvant plasmid, boosts humoral as well as $CD4^+$ and $CD8^+$ T cell immunity against three model synthetic DNA antigens including HIV envelope (Env), Influenza hemagglutinin 1 (HA1), and Zika premembrane and envelope (prME). Furthermore, opt-36γt enhanced protection by improving both clinical symptoms and mortality against a Zika virus (ZIKV) challenge and provided significant dose sparing for the Zika vaccine as studied using a suboptimal vaccine dose model. This not only supports the potential of opt-36γt as a gene adjuvant, but also highlights an underappreciated area of importance for protective cellular immune responses in Zika virus pathogenesis. Further investigation into opt-36γt as a potential new adjuvant for enhancing immunity against vaccine antigens is warranted.

2. Materials and Methods

2.1. DNA Constructs

The HIV consensus clade C envelope, Influenza HA1, and Zika prME DNA vaccines used in these studies are as previously described [39–41]. Figures 1A, 4A, and 5A have been adapted from figures from these studies.

The sequences for murine IL-36 alpha, beta, and gamma were obtained from Uniprot (Q9JLA2-1, Q9D6Z6-1, Q8R460-1). These sequences have been modified to be RNA and codon-optimized in order to exploit the host's natural codon preference and enhance protein expression. Furthermore, a highly efficient IgE leader sequence was inserted at the 5′ end of the IL-36 gene to promote efficient secretion of the protein. These full-length optimized IL-36 cytokine plasmids are known henceforth as opt-36α, opt-36β, and opt-36γ.

Recent work by Towne et al. has demonstrated the need for truncation of IL-36 cytokines nine amino acids N-terminal to a conserved *A-X-Asp* motif, for full activity [42]. The second set of IL-36 plasmids have been truncated according to the data presented in the paper and are henceforth known as opt-36αt, opt-36βt, and opt-36γt. All inserts were modified as previously explained above for enhanced expression and cloned into the pGX0001 backbone (Genscript, Piscataway, NJ, USA) [43].

2.2. Western Blot

Transfections were performed using the TurboFectin 8.0 reagent, following the manufacturer's protocols (OriGene, Rockville, MD, USA). Briefly, U2OS cells were grown to 80% confluence in 6-well tissue culture plates and transfected with 2 μg of opt-36αt, opt-36βt, or opt-36γt. The cells were collected 2 days after transfection, washed twice with PBS and lysed with cell lysis buffer (Cell Signaling Technology, Danvers, MA, USA). Gradient (4–12%) Bis-Tris NuPAGE gels (Life Technologies, Carlsbad, CA, USA) were loaded with transfected cell lysates and transferred to polyvinylidene difluoride (PDVF) membrane. The membranes were blocked in PBS Odyssey blocking buffer (LI-COR Biosciences, Lincoln, NE, USA) for 1 h at room temperature. To detect plasmid expression, the anti-HA (A01244 Clone 5E11D8, GenScript, Piscataway, NJ, USA) antibody was diluted 1:1000 and anti–β-actin antibody diluted 1:5000 in Odyssey blocking buffer with 0.2% Tween 20 (Bio-Rad, Hercules, CA, USA) and incubated with the membranes overnight at 4 °C. The membranes were washed with PBST and then incubated with the appropriate secondary antibody (goat anti-mouse IRDye680CW; LI-COR Biosciences) at a 1:15,000 dilution in Odyssey Blocking Buffer for 1 h at room temperature. After washing, the membranes were imaged on the Odyssey infrared imager (LI-COR Biosciences).

2.3. Immunofluorescence Assay (IFA)

For the immunofluorescence assay, U2OS cells were grown in 6-well tissue culture plates and transfected with 2 μg of opt-36αt, opt-36βt, or opt-36γt. Two days after transfection, the cells were fixed with 4% paraformaldehyde for 15 min. Nonspecific binding was then blocked with normal goat serum diluted in PBS at room temperature for 1 h. The plates were then washed in PBS for 5 min and subsequently incubated with anti-HA antibody at a 1:1000 (mouse anti-HA, GenScript) dilution overnight at 4 °C. The plates were washed as described above and incubated with appropriate secondary antibody (goat anti-mouse IgG-AF488, Sigma, St. Louis, MO, USA) at 1:200 dilutions at room temperature for 1 h. After washing, DAPI (Millipore Sigma) was added to stain the nuclei of all cells following manufacturer's protocol. Wells were washed and maintained in PBS, and observed under a microscope (EVOS Cell Imaging Systems; Life Technologies, Carlsbad, CA, USA).

2.4. Animals

All mice were housed in compliance with the NIH, the University of Pennsylvania School of Medicine and the Wistar Institutional Animal Care and Use Committee (IACUC). Six-to-eight-week-old female C57BL/6 mice were purchased from Jackson Laboratory (Bar Harbor, ME, USA). Six-to-eight-week-old female BALB/c mice were purchased from Charles River Laboratory (Wilmington, MA, USA). Five-to-six-week-old male and female Interferon-alpha/beta receptor $(IFNAR)^{-/-}$ mice from the Mutant Mouse Resource and Research Center (MMRRC) repository–Jackson Laboratory were also housed and treated in accordance to the above parties.

2.5. Animal Immunizations

For HIV dosing studies, C57BL/6 mice were immunized three times at three-week intervals with either 2.5 μg of HIV Env DNA only or 2.5 μg of HIV Env DNA and 11, 20, or 30 μg of opt-36βt in a total volume of 30 μL of water. Mice were injected using the intramuscular (IM) route in the shaved tibialis anterior muscle followed by electroporation (EP) using the CELLECTRA® 3P (Inovio Pharmaceuticals, Plymouth Meeting, PA, USA) as previously described [44]. For HIV plasmid comparison studies, C57BL/6 mice were immunized three times at three-week intervals with either 2.5 μg of HIV Env DNA only or 2.5 μg of HIV Env DNA and 11 μg of opt-36αt, opt-36βt, or opt-36γt in a total volume of 30 μL of water. For influenza studies, BALB/c mice were immunized two times at two-week intervals with 1 μg of HA1 DNA plasmid alone or 1 μg of HA1 DNA plasmid and 11 μg of opt-36αt, opt-36βt, or opt-36γt in a total volume of 30 μL of water delivered intramuscularly as described above. For Zika studies, IFNAR$^{-/-}$ mice were immunized once with 0.5 μg of Zika prME alone or 0.5 μg of Zika prME and 11 μg of opt-36γt in 30 μL of water delivered intramuscularly as described above.

2.6. *Animal Challenge Studies*

For the Zika challenge studies, IFNAR$^{-/-}$ mice (n = 12–14/group) were immunized once with 0.5 μg of Zika prME vaccine or 0.5 μg of Zika prME and 11 μg of opt-36γt. The mice were challenged with 1×10^5 PFU ZIKV-PR209 virus via intraperitoneal (IP) injection on day 15. Post challenge, the animals were weighed daily. In addition, they were observed for clinical signs of disease twice daily (decreased mobility; hunched posture; hind-limb knuckle walking (partial paralysis); and/or paralysis of one hind limb or both hind limbs). The criteria for euthanasia on welfare grounds consisted of 20% weight loss or prolonged paralysis in one or both hind limbs.

2.7. *ELISpot Assay*

Precoated anti-IFN-γ 96-well plates (MabTech, Cincinnati, OH, USA) were used to quantify IFN-γ responses to vaccine.

2.7.1. For HIV Studies

Spleens were isolated from C57BL/6 mice either 10 days post final vaccination for acute time points or 50 days post final vaccination for memory timepoint. Single-cell suspensions of splenocytes were made by homogenizing and processing the spleens through a 40-μm cell strainer. Cells were then re-suspended in ACK Lysing buffer (Gibco^{TM}) for 5 min to lyse red blood cells before two washes with PBS and final re-suspension in RPMI complete media (RPMI 1640 + 10% FBS + 1% penicillin–streptomycin). Two hundred thousand splenocytes were added to each well and stimulated overnight at 37 °C in 5% CO_2 with R10 (negative control), concanavalin A (3 μg/mL; positive control), or 15-mer HIV envelope clade C peptides overlapping by 11 amino acids (NIH AIDS Research & Reference Reagent Program). Peptide pools consisted of 15-mer residues overlapping by 11 amino acids, representing the entire protein consensus sequence of HIV-1 clade C, were obtained from the NIH AIDS Research and Reference Reagent Program. The Env peptides were pooled at a concentration of 2 μg/mL/peptide into four pools, and three of the four pools were used as antigens for specific stimulation of IFN-γ release.

2.7.2. For Influenza Study

Spleens were isolated from BALB/c mice 14 days post vaccination. Single-cell suspensions of splenocytes were made by homogenizing and processing the spleens through a 40-μm cell strainer. Cells were then re-suspended in ACK Lysing buffer (Gibco^{TM}, Gaithersburg, MD, USA) for 5 min to lyse red blood cells before two washes with PBS and final re-suspension in RPMI complete media (RPMI 1640 + 10% FBS + 1% penicillin–streptomycin). Two hundred thousand splenocytes were added to each well and stimulated overnight at 37 °C in 5% CO_2 with R10 (negative control), concanavalin A (3 μg/mL; positive control), or 15 mer influenza hemagglutinin peptides overlapping by 11 amino acids spanning the length of the consensus HA1 hemagglutinin protein (GenScript). The HA1 peptides were pooled at a concentration of 1 mg/mL/peptide into four pools as antigens for specific stimulation of IFN-γ release.

2.7.3. For Zika Studies

Spleens were isolated from IFNAR$^{-/-}$ mice 14 days post-final vaccination. Single-cell suspensions of splenocytes were made by homogenizing and processing the spleens through a 40-μm cell strainer.

Cells were then re-suspended in ACK Lysing buffer (Gibco™) for 5 min to lyse red blood cells before two washes with PBS and final re-suspension in RPMI complete media (RPMI 1640 + 10% FBS + 1% penicillin–streptomycin). Two hundred thousand splenocytes were added to each well and stimulated overnight at 37 °C in 5% CO_2 with R10 (negative control), concanavalin A (3 μg/mL; positive control), or 15-mer Zika peptides overlapping by 9 amino acids spanning the length of the Zika prME protein. The Zika prME peptides were pooled at a concentration of 1 mg/mL/peptide into six pools as antigens for specific stimulation of IFN-γ release.

After 18 h of stimulation, the plates were washed and developed following manufacturer's protocol. The plates were then rinsed with distilled water and dried at room temperature overnight. Spots were counted by an automated ELISpot reader (Cellular Technology Ltd., Shaker Heights, OH, USA).

2.8. *Flow Cytometry:*

For intracellular cytokine staining, two million cells were stimulated in 96-well plates with overlapping peptide pools of either HIV Env, Influenza HA1, or Zika prME protein, media alone (negative control), or phorbol 12-myristate 13-acetate (PMA) and ionomycin (BD Biosciences, San Jose, CA, USA) (positive control) for 6 h at 37 °C + 5% CO_2 in the presence of GolgiPlug and GolgiStop™ (BD Biosciences, Franklin Lakes, NJ, USA). These are the same peptides pools described in the ELISpot sections. After 6 h, cells were collected and stained in FACS buffer with a panel of surface antibodies containing live dead eFluor V450, FITC anti-CD4, Alexa Fluor 700 anti-CD44, and APC-Cy7 anti-CD8 for 30 min at 4 °C. Cells were washed and then fixed with Foxp3/Transcription Factor Fixation/Permeabilization (ThermoFischer Scientific, Waltham, MA, USA) for 20 min at 4 °C. Cells were washed with Perm/Wash buffer before intracellular staining with PE-Cy7 anti-IL-2, PerCP-Cy5.5 anti-CD3ε, PE anti-TNFα, and APC anti-IFNγ for 1 h at 4 °C. Cells were then washed with Perm/Wash buffer before suspension in Perm/Wash buffer and acquisition on a BD LSRII. All results were analyzed using FlowJo™ v.10.0.

2.9. *ELISA*

The HIV ELISA was performed using 1 μg/mL HIV consensus C gp120 (Immune Technology Corp., New York, NY, USA) in PBS with 0.5% Tween 20 (PBS-T). After a blocking step, serum was diluted to 1:50 and then 4-fold from there in 1% FBS in PBS-T. Each sample was run in duplicate. After a 1 h incubation, plates washed and incubated with goat anti-mouse IgG-HRP (Santa Cruz Biotechnology, Dallas, TX, USA) at a 1:5000 dilution in 1% FBS in PBS-T. Plates were then developed as described above, and the OD450 values were obtained.

Avidity Index ELISA: The avidity of the humoral response was assessed against universal hemagglutinin at 10 days post final vaccination for influenza studies. Plates were coated with 1 μg/mL of hemagglutinin ((H1N1) (A/New Caledonia/20/99) Immune Technology Corp., New York, NY, USA) in PBS. After a blocking step, serum was diluted to 1:50 or, for the dilution curves, 1:50 and then 4-fold from there in 1% FBS in PBS-T. Each sample was run in duplicate with half of the wells treated and half left untreated. After a 1-h incubation, plates were washed five times with PBS-T. Half of the wells for each sample were incubated with denaturing reagent (8 M urea) for 5 min while the others were incubated with PBS. Plates were washed and incubated with goat anti-mouse IgG-HRP (Santa Cruz Biotechnology) at a 1:5000 dilution in 1% FBS in PBS-T. Plates were then developed as described above, and the OD450 values were obtained. The avidity index was determined by dividing the OD450 values of the treated samples by those of the untreated samples and multiplying by 100.

2.10. *Statistical Analysis*

Statistical analysis was performed using a one-way modified ANOVA with a Turkey post-hoc test for immunogenicity studies and Mantel–Cox test for challenge studies. All analysis was performed using GraphPad Prism Software (La Jolla, CA, USA). Horizontal bars represent mean with error bars expressing the standard error. p-Values < 0.05 were considered as statistically significant.

3. Results

3.1. Opt-36βt Co-Formulation Leads to Enhanced Immune Responses against HIV Env DNA Vaccine Compared to Opt-36β

While the IL-36 family was discovered in 1999 [29,30,34,35,45], members of this family remain poorly understood and continue to be investigated. In the initial studies of their biology, large quantities of IL-36 ligands were needed, in greater excess than those traditionally used for cytokines, to observe their activity [32,46]. With recent reports of IL-36 cytokines gaining activity after N-terminal residue truncation [42,47,48], we studied whether truncation was important for an IL-36 in vivo produced gene adjuvant to impact immune profile of DNA vaccine antigens in an HIV Env (Figure 1A) in vivo DNA vaccine model system. We chose to initially start our studies with IL-36 beta, as IL-36 beta has been reported to amplify Th1 responses [37], making it a potential cellular adjuvant candidate. We designed two DNA constructs encoding either full-length (opt-36β) or truncated (opt-36βt) IL-36 beta (Figure 1B) for these comparative studies. We added a highly efficient IgE leader sequence to both of the sequences as well as RNA and codon optimized them in order to enhance protein expression. We then immunized C57BL/6 (B6) (n = 5) mice with 2.5 μg of HIV Env DNA alone or with 2.5 μg of HIV Env and 11 μg opt-36β or opt-36βt, three times at three-week intervals using the 3P electrode driven by an adaptive electroporation CELLECTRA (EP) device (Figure 1C). Spleens were harvested 10 days post-final vaccination for analysis of antigen-specific responses. We observed a significant increase in the number of antigen-specific $CD4^+$ T cells that secreted IFN-γ and TNF-α in the animals whose vaccine included opt-36βt compared to opt-36β (Figure 1D). There was a trend towards a similar pattern of enhancement for the antigen-induced $CD8^+$ T cell responses, but in contrast to the $CD4^+$ T cell responses, this did not reach significance. A dosing study was next performed, focusing primarily on T cell induction to determine the optimal dose of opt-36βt. We found no significant difference in T cell response with higher doses and, in fact, there appeared to be a trend towards decreased immune response at the 30-μg dose of opt-36βt (Figure 1E). Going forward, we maintained our established dose of 11 μg for adjuvant plasmids for the remainder of the studies.

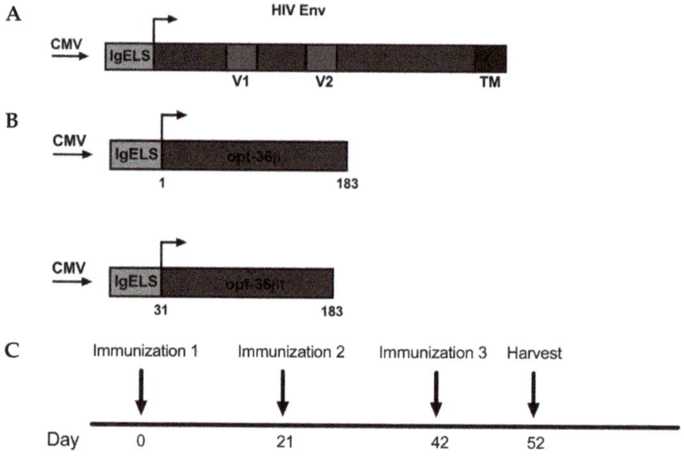

Figure 1. *Cont.*

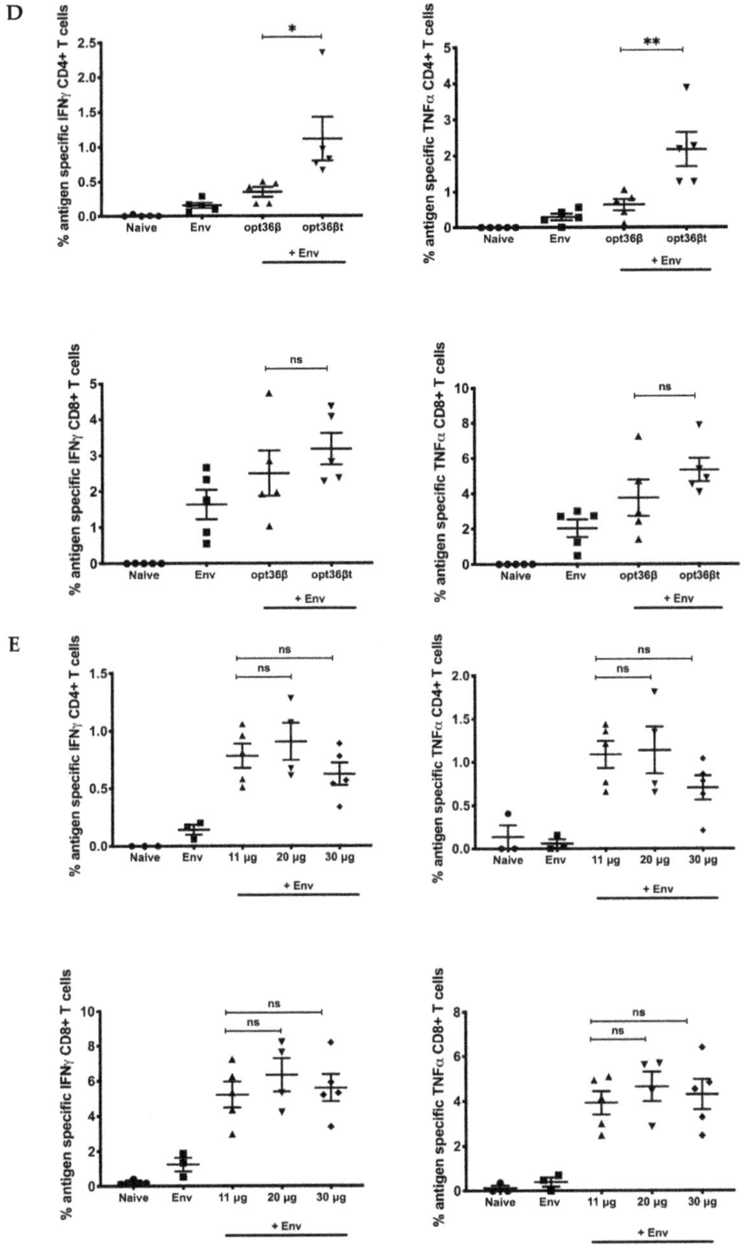

Figure 1. Truncation of IL-36 beta enhances immune responses to HIV Env DNA vaccine. (**A** and **B**) Map of plasmid construct design. HIV Consensus Clade C vaccine plasmid, full length IL-36 beta plasmid and IL-36 beta truncated 9 amino acids N-terminal to anchoring residue. Each construct contains a cytomegalovirus (CMV) promoter followed by an IgE leader sequence. (**C**) Immunization delivery schedule. C57BL/6 mice were immunized three times at three week intervals. (**D**) Env specific $CD4^+$ and $CD8^+$ T cell responses by intracellular cytokine staining after peptide stimulation. E Opt-36βt dosing study of Env specific $CD4^+$ and $CD8^+$ T cell responses by intracellular cytokine staining after peptide stimulation. * $p < 0.05$, ** $p < 0.005$, *** $p < 0.0005$, **** $p < 0.0001$.

Given these results, we next examined the rest of the IL-36 family as truncated cytokines. In this regard, even less is known about IL-36 alpha or gamma compared to beta, so we wanted to evaluate the immune responses in mice adjuvanted with each of the three cytokines in comparative studies. We also assessed the durability of the immune responses elicited by each of the IL-36 ligands post vaccination at a memory time point. Truncated IL-36 alpha (opt-36αt) and IL-36 gamma (opt-36γt) were designed and modified as illustrated (Figure 2A) [49,50]. An HA tag was added to the C-terminus of the sequences to facilitate in vitro detection. Construct expression in vitro was confirmed using Western blot and IFA (Figure 2B,C).

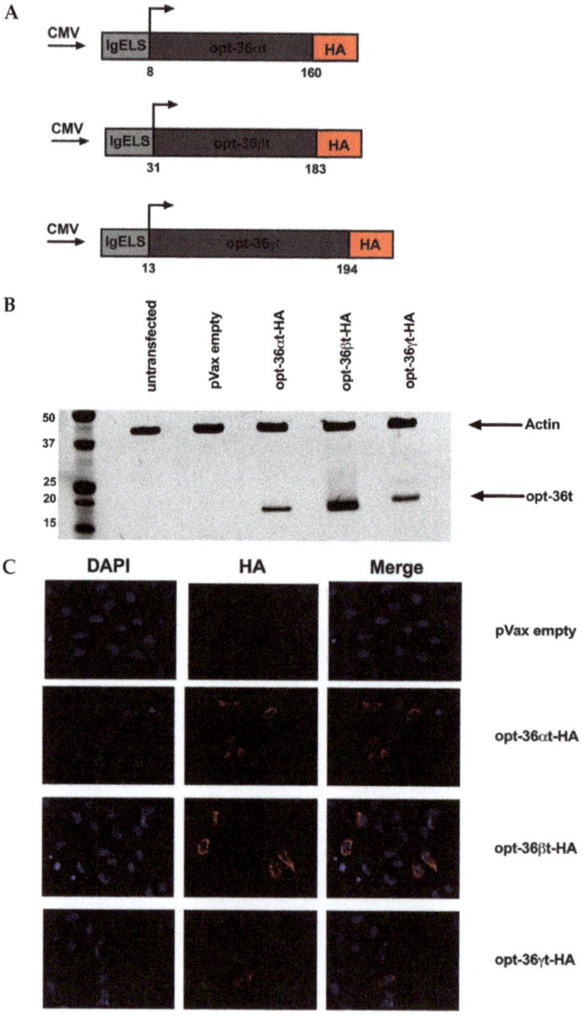

Figure 2. Expression of truncated IL-36 constructs. (**A**) Map of plasmid construct design for IL-36 sequences. Each sequence was truncated 9 amino acids N-terminal to conserved A-X-Asp residue. Each construct contains a cytomegalovirus (CMV) promoter followed by an IgE leader sequence besides the IL-36 sequence, and a HA tag at the C-terminus. (**B**) U2OS cells were transfected with each truncated IL-36 plasmids that contain a HA tag for detection. Lysates from these cells were used in Western blot for detection of plasmid expression. (**C**) Immunofluorescence (IFA) was performed on U2OS cells transfected with truncated IL-36 plasmids to verify plasmid expression.

3.2. *Opt-36βt and opt-36γt Enhance Immune Responses against HIV Env DNA Vaccine at a Memory Time Point*

A major concern in the vaccine field is the generation of vaccine candidates that can provide durable, long-term immune responses, and so we examined whether immune responses following DNA vaccination would be maintained into memory. B6 mice (n = 5/group) were immunized using 2.5 µg of HIV Env DNA alone or a formulation with 11 µg of opt-36αt, opt-36βt, or opt-36γt three times at three-week intervals with CELLECTRA 3P electroporation (EP) (Figure 3A). Spleens were harvested 50 days post-final vaccination to analyze antigen specific responses at a memory time point. A quantitative ELISpot was performed to determine the number of Env-specific IFN-γ secreting T cells that responded to vaccination (Figure 3B). We observed that mice immunized with the HIV vaccine alone produced an average of 775 spot-forming units (SFU)/million splenocytes, while mice adjuvanted with opt-36αt, opt-36βt, and opt-36γt had an average of 1242, 1460, and 1610 SFU/million splenocytes, respectively, supporting an enhanced response to the vaccine was driven by the adjuvants. Similar to the results observed at an acute time point, we found that mice adjuvanted with opt-36βt showed a significant increase in the percent of $CD4^+$ T cells that expressed IFN-γ and TNF-α compared to vaccine only. Interestingly, mice adjuvanted with opt-36γt showed a 3-fold enhancement in the percent of antigen-specific $CD8^+$ T cells which expressed IFN-γ and TNF-α (Figure 3C). We further observed that mice vaccinated with vaccine and opt-36γt had a significant increase in the percent of $CD107a^+$ IFN-γ^+ $CD8^+$ T cells, suggesting the cytolytic potential of these cells (Figure 3C). We also examined the humoral response induced post vaccination, and observed that mice adjuvanted with opt-36αt and opt-36γt exhibited higher average antibody titers compared to mice immunized with Env alone, although this did not reach significance (Supplementary Materials Figure S1). Of note, mice adjuvanted with opt-36βt exhibited suppressed antibody binding compared to vaccine alone.

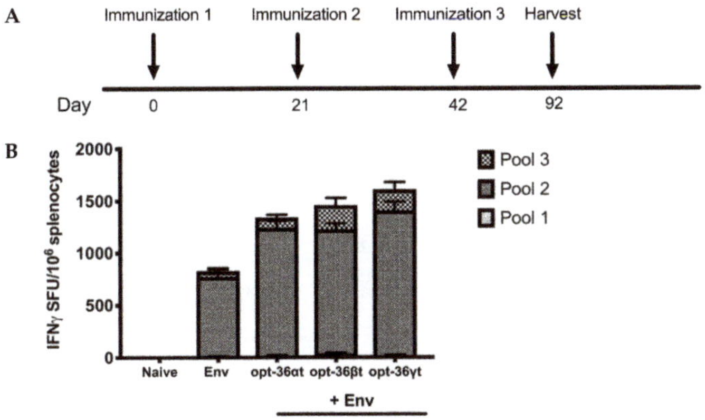

Figure 3. *Cont.*

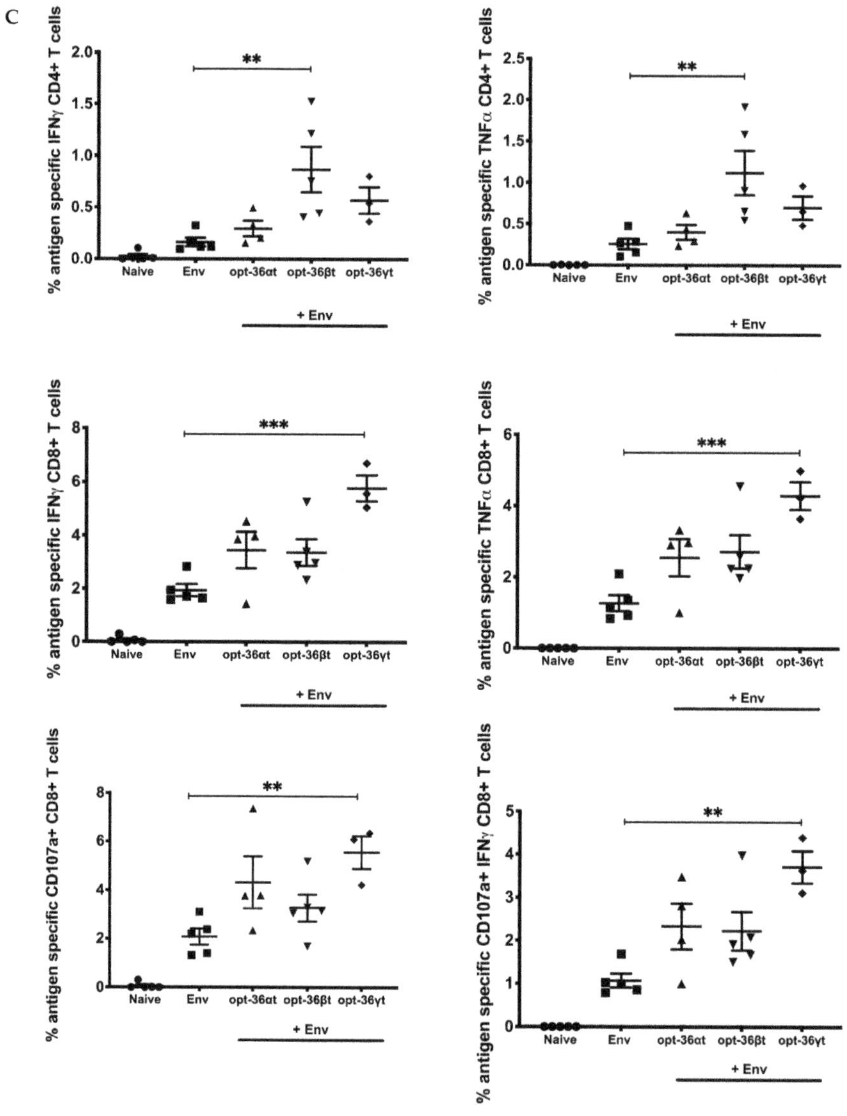

Figure 3. Codelivery of truncated IL-36 beta and gamma enhance immune responses against HIV Env DNA vaccine. (**A**) Immunization delivery schedule. B6 mice were immunized three times 3 weeks apart with Env alone or Env adjuvanted with the opt-36αt, opt-36βt, or opt-36γt. Sera and spleens were harvested 50 days post final vaccination to analyze antigen specific immune responses. (**B**) The frequency of Env specific IFN-γ responses (spot forming units per million splenocytes) induced after vaccination was determined by IFN-γ ELISpot assay in response to pooled Env peptides. (**C**) Env specific CD4 and CD8 T cell responses by intracellular cytokine staining after peptide stimulation. *, $p < 0.05$, ** $p < 0.005$, *** $p < 0.0005$, **** $p < 0.0001$.

3.3. *Opt-36γt Enhances Humoral Immunity in Influenza DNA Vaccine Model*

We next sought to extend this finding to additional antigens with a different DNA vaccine antigen. We studied opt-36αt, opt-36βt, and opt-36γt's ability to impact immune responses driven by an HA1

Syncon influenza DNA vaccine [40]. Given the potency of the adjuvant response in the previous studies, we focused on a two-dose regimen to evaluate the vaccine-induced immune response in a dose-sparing model. BALB/c mice (n = 5/group) were immunized two times at two-week intervals with either 1 μg of HA1 DNA alone (Figure 4A) or 1 μg of HA1 and 11 μg of opt-36αt, opt-36βt, or opt-36γt followed by in vivo EP (Figure 4B). Ten days post final immunization, we observed both opt-36βt and opt-36γt significantly enhanced cellular responses compared to the low-dose vaccine alone (Figure 4C). We observed increased cellular responses in mice adjuvanted with opt-36αt; however, this was not as pronounced as the responses with the other two cytokines. As antibodies are known to be critical for prevention from influenza infection, we studied the binding antibodies generated post vaccination. Opt-36γt elicited significant higher endpoint binding titers compared naïve mice (Figure 4D). We further examined the quality of these antibodies by performing an ELISA based avidity test [51] to examine strength of binding to a HA1 influenza protein. Interestingly, we observed that antibodies from mice that received opt-36γt had greater antigen binding and maintained avidity compared to the antibodies from mice that received opt-36αt and opt-36βt, supporting the induction of improved magnitude of humoral responses (Figure 4E). We also examined the isotypes of the antibodies generated post vaccination, and while all immunized groups exhibited class switching, we did not observe a significant shift in IgG_1 vs. IgG_{2a} ratios among the different groups (Supplementary Materials Figure S2).

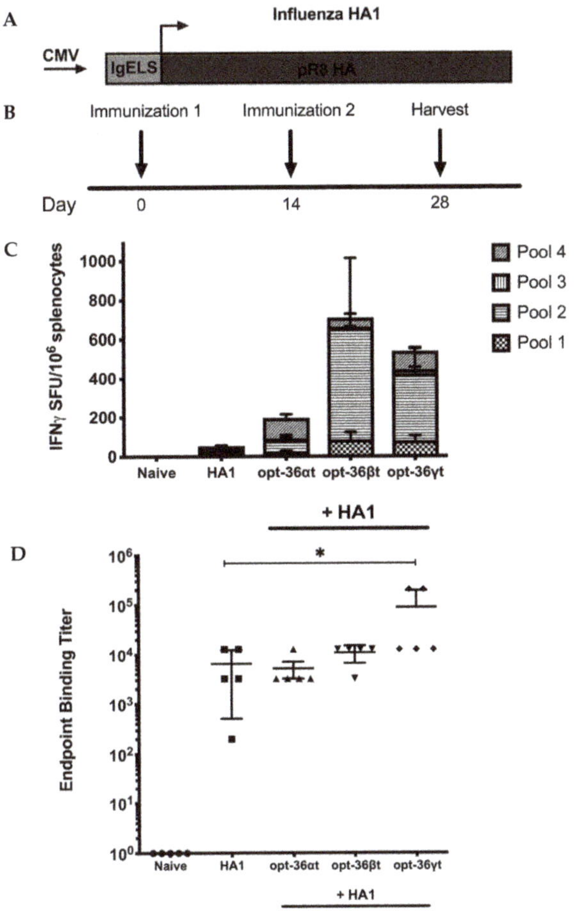

Figure 4. *Cont.*

E

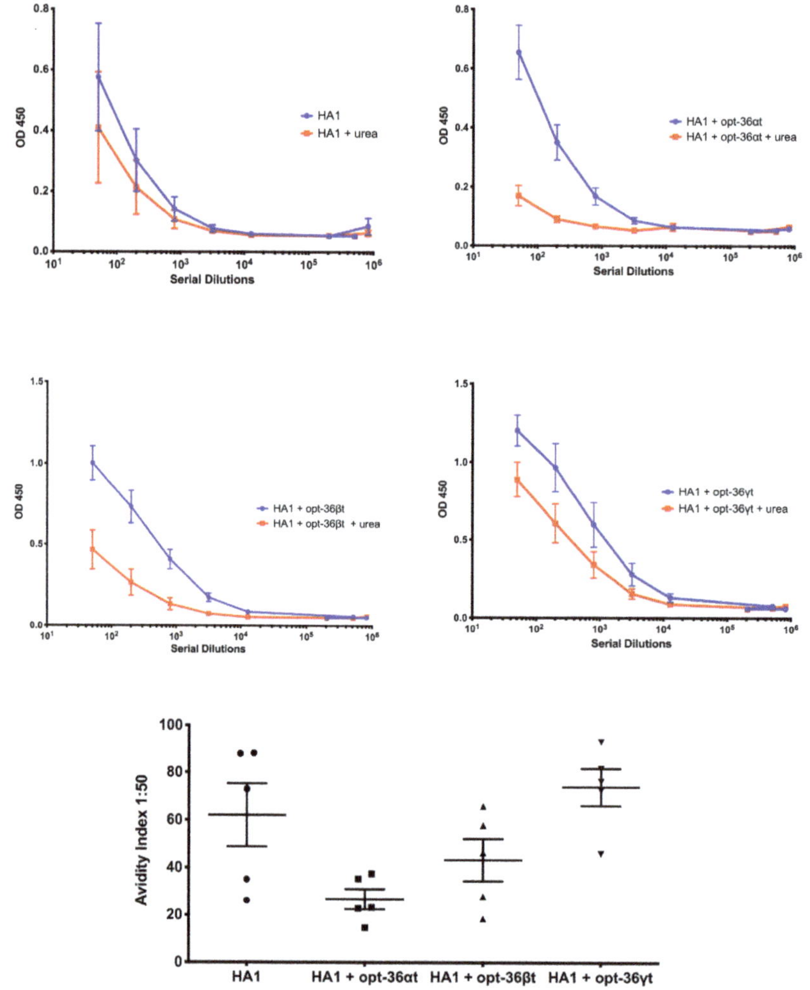

Figure 4. Codelivery of truncated IL-36 gamma enhances binding antibody while maintaining antibody integrity. (**A**) Map of plasmid construct design. Influenza hemagglutinin (HA) (from strain H1N1 A/PR/8/34) vaccine plasmid. Vaccine construct contains a cytomegalovirus (CMV) promoter followed by an IgE leader sequence. (**B**) Immunization delivery schedule. BALB/c mice were immunized two times two weeks apart with influenza HA1 alone or HA1 adjuvanted with opt-36αt, opt-36βt, or opt36γt. Sera and spleens were harvested two weeks post final vaccination to analyze antigen specific responses. (**C**) The frequency of HA specific IFN-γ responses (spot forming units per million splenocytes) induced after vaccination was determined by IFN-γ ELISpot assay in response to pooled HA peptides. (**D**) Endpoint binding titers post vaccination HA1 alone or HA1 + truncated IL-36 adjuvant. (**E**) The avidity of antibodies generated after vaccination at 1:50 dilution. *, $p < 0.05$, **, $p < 0.005$, ***, $p < 0.0005$, ****, $p < 0.0001$.

3.4. Opt-36γt Enhances Cellular Immune Responses Induced by a Zika DNA Vaccine Resulting in Enhanced Protection against Zika Challenge

Based on the data generated in the two DNA vaccine models above, we now focused on studying opt-36γt in combination with a DNA vaccine against Zika and how vaccine-induced immune response impacted challenge outcome. This model allows us to confirm the relevance of the improved immunity and dose-sparing potential driven by the opt-36γt adjuvant. We immunized immunocompromised IFNAR$^{-/-}$ mice (n = 5–6 mice/group) once with an exceptionally low dose (0.5 μg) of Zika prME DNA vaccine alone (Figure 5A) or a combination of both. Two weeks following vaccination, we harvested spleens and blood (Figure 5B). We observed that mice immunized with vaccine only did not generate significant IFN-γ ELISpot responses, but the combination of the vaccine and opt-36γt resulted in a synergy resulting in 700 SFU/million splenocytes (Figure 5C). Immunization with opt-36γt alone did not generate significant cellular responses (Figure S3). Using intracellular cytokine staining, mice adjuvanted with opt-36γt exhibited increased IFN-γ and TNF-α expressing $CD4^+$ T cells as well as IFN-γ expressing $CD8^+$ T cells compared to the vaccine-only treated mice (Figure 5D). Overall antibody responses were very low in all groups (Supplementary Materials Figure S4). This suggests a need for an additional vaccine boost or using higher vaccine doses to further characterize the humoral immunity induced in this model.

We next repeated the study and this time performed a challenge using an immunocompromised mouse challenge model, IFNAR$^{-/-}$ mice (n = 12–14/ group), with a lethal dose of a validated Zika virus stock, strain PR 209. Challenge was performed two weeks after an immunization with either 0.5 μg of Zika prME alone or in combination with 11 μg of opt-36γt (Figure 6A). The animals were followed for two weeks post challenge. One of the side effects of ZIKV challenge typically observed in this mouse strain is weight loss [41]. Significant weight loss was observed in both the naïve and mice immunized with the suboptimal dose of the Zika prME vaccine alone, demonstrating substantial morbidity from the challenge (Figure 6B). Naïve mice appeared to be the most impacted, with many mice losing up to 20% of their starting body weight. The low-dose vaccine only group fared a bit better compared to the naive but still lost a considerable amount of weight. Strikingly, mice immunized with Zika prME in combination with opt-36γt were protected against weight loss, gaining weight during the course of the study. Additionally, mice were monitored for clinical symptoms during the challenge. Mice in both the naïve and vaccine-only groups became progressively sicker (i.e., hunched posture and paralysis of hind limbs) between days 5 and 7. However, the adjuvanted mice remain healthy and show no sign of disease following challenge (Figure 6C). As animals succumbed to disease they were sacrificed at predefined humane endpoints as described in the methods [41]. Mice immunized with Zika prME and opt-36γt exhibited a robust 92% survival rate, compared to 28% for mice immunized with the Zika prME only and 13% for naïve mice (Figure 6D). This data illustrates a significant benefit of the opt-36γt adjuvant in the context of this ZIKV IFNAR$^{-/-}$ challenge model. Study in additional models is important.

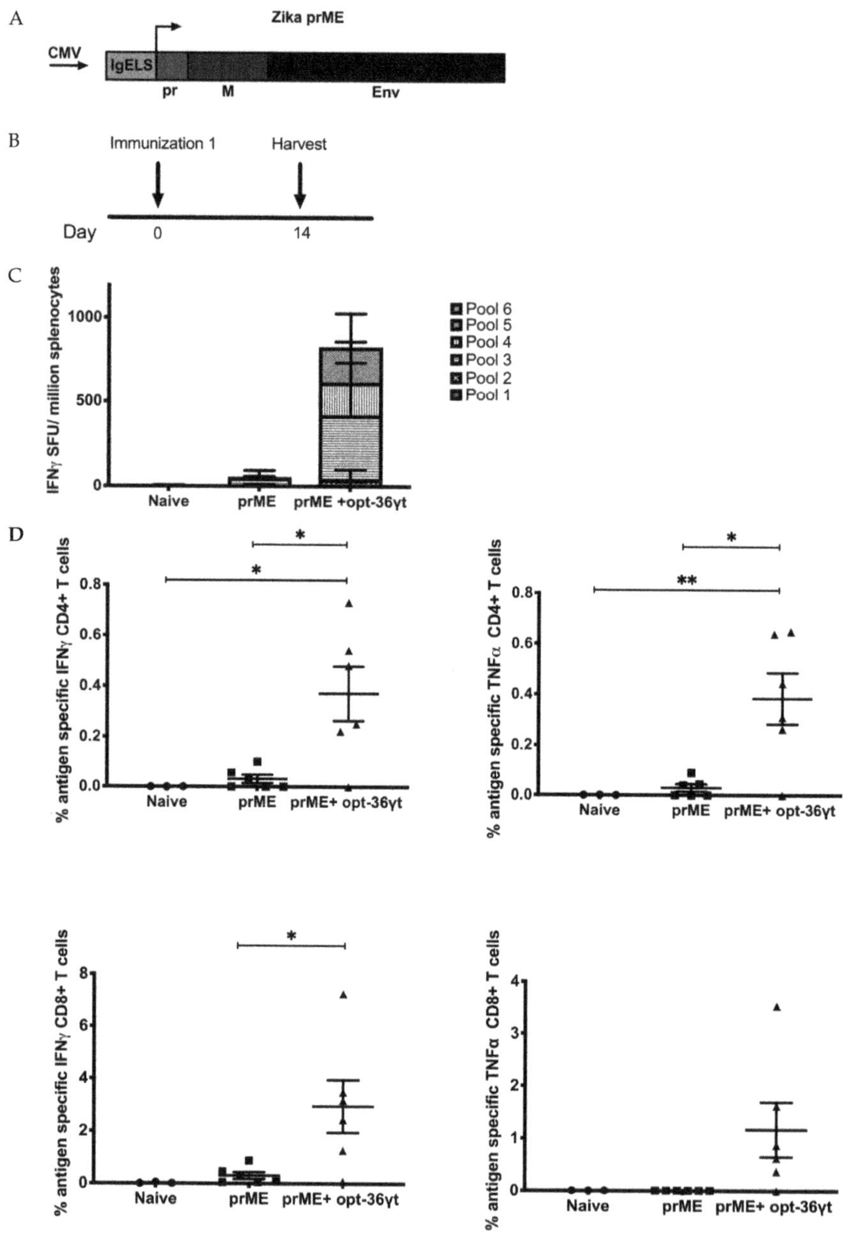

Figure 5. Codelivery of truncated IL-36 gamma enhances immune response to DNA prME vaccine. (**A**) Map of plasmid construct design. Consensus sequence of Zika precursor membrane and Envelope. (**B**) Immunization schedule for Zika vaccine immunization. IFNAR$^{-/-}$ mice were immunized once either vaccine alone or vaccine + opt-36γt (n = 5–6 per group). Spleens were harvested two weeks post vaccination to analyze antigen specific T cell responses. (**C**) The frequency of spot forming units per million splenocytes determined by IFN-γ ELISpot assay in response to pooled Zika prME peptides. (**D**) Zika prME specific CD4 and CD8 T cell responses by intracellular cytokine staining. * $p < 0.05$, ** $p < 0.005$, *** $p < 0.0005$, **** $p < 0.0001$.

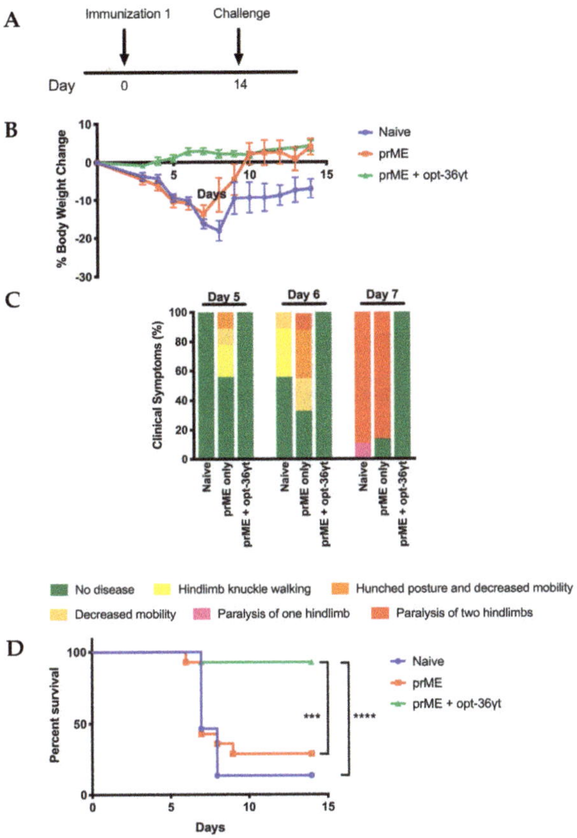

Figure 6. Truncated IL-36 gamma is able to protect against Zika challenge induced weight loss and mortality. (**A**) Immunization delivery schedule. IFNAR$^{-/-}$ mice were immunized with Zika prME plasmid or prME + opt-36γt once and challenged with Zika PR209 virus two weeks later. (**B**) Mouse body weight was tracked over two-week challenge period. (**C**) Clinical symptoms of immunized mice days 5–7 post challenge. (**D**) Survival curves of mice post Zika challenge over 14 days. * $p < 0.05$, ** $p < 0.005$, *** $p < 0.0005$, **** $p < 0.0001$.

4. Discussion

While the IL-36 cytokine family was first discovered nearly two decades ago, it is only recently that roles for these cytokines have begun to be elucidated. The IL-36 family, members of a larger proinflammatory IL-1 family, has been primarily implicated for their potential role in pustular psoriasis and inflammation of the skin and joints [29,30,52,53]. Dysregulation of the natural IL-36 receptor antagonist or overexpression of IL-36 in the skin has been implicated in a number of skin diseases and conditions [53–67]. However, some of these proinflammatory properties have also piqued the scientific community's interest regarding some of the other roles that these cytokines might play. Following reports that IL-36 beta could amplify Th1 responses in CD4$^+$ T cells [37], a number of studies have shown the induction of IL-36 cytokine expression, especially IL-36 gamma, in response to infections including pneumonia, herpes simplex virus (HSV), and candidiasis [68–73], suggesting that IL-36 cytokines may play a significant role in host immunity.

To our knowledge, this is the first study to compare the effects of all three truncated IL-36 cytokines in a vaccination model. In these studies we provide additional insight into the ability of truncated

IL-36 gamma's (opt-36γt) ability to boost immune responses using three DNA vaccine antigens. As previously demonstrated by Towne et al. [42], we found that truncation of the IL-36 cytokines' nine amino acids at the N-terminal region was critical for their activity to enhance vaccine-induced immune responses. For future investigations of IL-36 cytokines in protective immunity studies, the truncated forms of these cytokines will almost certainly be necessary to exploit their full potential.

In the DNA vaccine models we tested, we found that mice immunized with opt-36βt and opt-36γt were both able to enhance vaccine-induced cellular immune responses. However, where opt-36βt was able to significantly increase the number of antigen-specific IFN-γ^+ and TNF-α^+ CD4$^+$ T cells, opt-36γt significantly increased the number of antigen-specific IFN-γ^+, TNF-α^+, and CD107a$^+$ CD8$^+$ T cells, suggesting an impact of opt-36γt to improve cytolytic activity of these cells. Further work must be done to understand the differences between the two cytokines' seemingly preferential action on various cell compartments. Regarding humoral immunity in the influenza DNA vaccination model, we found that opt-36γt was able to increase antibody-binding titers, while opt-36βt appeared to induce antibodies that have weaker avidity. Thus, in our models, opt-36γt can improve both arms of immune response, which is likely important for many of the challenging disease targets that remain. We also found that the synergy of a non-protective dose of Zika DNA vaccine with opt-36γt was able to protect mice against a lethal ZIKV challenge, highlighting the potential of opt-36γt to affect challenge outcome and drive protection. Furthermore, opt-36γt enhanced antibody binding in both the HIV and influenza DNA models, while overall humoral responses in the Zika DNA model were lower than the other models, possibly due to the low amount of plasmid used for immunization. Other differences among the models such as mouse genotype may also be relevant and could be examined in further studies.

There is still much work to be done to fully understand the roles that the IL-36 cytokines play under both homeostatic and pathologic conditions in the host immune system. Multiple studies in mice have shown that the IL-36 cytokines may have distinct functions in response to different inflammatory stimuli. Understanding how opt-36βt and opt-36γt may exert their activities on different cell populations and against additional vaccine targets will be important for further harnessing their potential. Given their ability to enhance CD4$^+$ and CD8$^+$ T cell responses, opt-36γt and opt-36βt look especially promising for disease models in which cellular responses are important, such as cancer where driving CD8$^+$ immunity is important to clear tumors. Studies examining the effects of opt-36γt on driving tumor-infiltrating lymphocytes (TILS) would be relevant. Work by Wang et al. has demonstrated that tumor growth was significantly inhibited in B16 melanoma IL-36 expressing cells compared to control B16 cells that did not express IL-36 gamma in mice [74]. Wang et al. also found that IL-36 gamma could promote early activation and expansion of naïve CD8$^+$ T cells, in line with what we have observed in our DNA vaccine models.

Furthermore, the induction of higher binding antibodies while maintaining avidity by opt-36γt as we observed in the influenza studies may have important implications in diseases in which high avidity and affinity antibody titers are important. As more emphasis is being focused to identify immunogens that can elicit broadly neutralizing antibodies (bNabs) for HIV and influenza, adjuvants that can further refine the antibody response may prove important.

Although there appears to be a deleterious effect on skin health when IL-36 signaling is left unchecked [55], localized controlled delivery of opt-36γt as an adjuvant during intradermal vaccination could enhance vaccine responses and recruitment of cells to the site of infection. This could be especially important for infectious diseases that breach the skin's natural barrier including herpes, malaria, and Leishmania, among others. As the largest organ in the human body, with a rich source of antigen-presenting cells (APCs) and Langerhans cells, as well as nearly 20 billion T cells, the skin is a particularly attractive site to administer an opt-36γt adjuvanted vaccine. Enhanced CTL responses in the skin can help control the spread of an infection before it is able to disseminate to other locations in the body, while greater antibody responses may help with prevention of infection. Studies that examine the delivery of opt-36γt in the skin compared to intramuscular delivery may shed light on another route to impact vaccine immune outcome as well as protection against infection.

As the global population and the demand for vaccines increase worldwide, the need to maximize immune responses while minimizing the effective dose necessary to induce protective responses will continue to grow. Here we describe the first study of an optimized plasmid encoding for a truncated form of IL-36 as a plasmid adjuvant, opt-36γt. We observed that opt-36γt exhibited a dose-sparing effect as well as enhancement of humoral and cellular immune responses to several antigens and improved challenge outcome in a well-studied mouse model system of viral challenge. Additional study of opt-36γt as a genetically encoded adjuvant is likely important.

5. Conclusions

As the next generation of vaccines are developed, they will likely benefit from the identification of novel adjuvants with unique immune modulating properties. Here we evaluated the adjuvant activity of 3 optimized versions IL-36 (opt-36αt, opt-36βt, and opt-36γt), novel members of the IL-1 gene family, previously reported to be involved in proinflammatory activity. We report that truncation of the IL-36 beta form (opt-36βt) enhanced immunization induced immune responses against a HIV Env DNA vaccine, compared to unadjuvanted HIV Env or the same vaccine adjuvanted by full length IL-36 beta (opt-36β). When memory responses were examined, the opt-36βt enhanced antigen specific $CD4^+$ T cell responses while opt-36γt more robustly enhanced antigen specific $CD8^+$ T cell responses. When these adjuvants were studied in an influenza vaccine model, opt-36γt codelivery increased antibody titers against the hemagglutinin protein. These antibody responses exhibited higher binding avidity compared to the control vaccine alone arm. We also evaluated opt-36γt's DNA vaccine dose sparing potency in a lethal Zika vaccine challenge model. Codelivery of opt-36γt with a very low dose Zika DNA vaccine was able to potently enhance IFN-γ T cell responses resulting in potent protection against the ZIKV challenge compared to vaccine only immunized or naïve mice. This study provides proof-of-concept that an optimized plasmid encoding truncated IL-36 gamma is an important new gene adjuvant which can simultaneously enhance both humoral and cellular immunity and positively impact challenge. Further study of this promising genetic adjuvant is warranted.

Supplementary Materials: The following are available online at http://www.mdpi.com/2076-393X/7/2/42/s1, Figure S1: (A) ELISA analysis measuring binding antibody production (measured by OD450 values) in immunized mice. The C57BL/6 mice (n = 5) were immunized intramuscularly three times three weeks apart with 2.5 μg of HIV Env plasmid or 2.5 μg of Env plasmid and 11 μg of opt-36αt, opt-36βt, or opt-36γt. Binding to consensus C gp120 was analyzed with sera from animals post final vaccination. (B) Average endpoint titers, Figure S2: (**A**) ELISA analysis measuring isotype binding antibody production (measured by OD 450 values) in immunized mice. BALB/c mice (n = 4–5) were immunized twice two weeks apart with 1 μg of HA1 DNA plasmid or HA1 DNA plasmid and 11 μg of opt-36αt, opt-36βt, or opt-36γt. Isotypes of antibodies generated were analyzed with sera from animals post final vaccination. (**B**) IgG_{2a}/IgG_1 antibody ratio was analyzed by dividing the OD450 values of IgG_{2a} by the OD450 values of IgG_1, Figure S3: Induction of Zika specific cellular immune responses following vaccination with either Zika prME DNA vaccine alone or opt-36γt alone. ELISpot analysis measuring IFN-γ secretion in splenocytes after one immunization, Figure S4: Induction of antigen specific antibody responses following immunization with either Zika prME DNA vaccine alone or Zika prME DNA vaccine and opt-36γt after one immunization.

Author Contributions: Conceptualization, L.L. and D.O.V.; methodology, L.L. and M.C.W.; validation, L.L.; formal analysis, L.L.; investigation, L.L., H.C.; resources, K.M. and D.B.W.; writing—original draft preparation, L.L.; writing—review and editing, L.L., M.C.W, H.C., D.O.V., and D.B.W.; visualization, L.L.; supervision, L.L., D.B.W.

Funding: This research was funded by an NIH Pharmacology training grant, grant number T32 GM008076, an NIH Training in HIV Pathogenesis grant, grant number T32 AI007632, and an NIAID grant, grant number U19 AI 109646.

Acknowledgments: We thank Sagar Kudchodkar, Piyush Borole, and Kanika Asija for their technical assistance in early Zika studies. We thank Imaging Facility Core at the Wistar Institute for assistance with confocal microscopy experiments. We thank Jeffery Faust and the Flow cytometry Core at the Wistar Institute for their advice on flow cytometry experiments.

Conflicts of Interest: M.C.W. is an employee of Inovio Pharmaceuticals and as such receives salary and benefits including ownership of stock and stock options from the company. K.M. receives grants and consulting fees from Inovio related to DNA vaccine development. D.B.W. has grant funding, participates in industry collaborations, has received speaking honoraria and fees for consulting. This service includes serving on scientific review committees and advisory boards. Remuneration includes direct payments and/or stock or stock options and in the interest of disclosure; therefore, he notes potential conflicts associated with this work with Inovio where he serves on the BOD, Merck, VGXI, OncoSec, Roche, Aldevron and possibly others. The remaining authors declare no conflict of interest.

References

1. Lahiri, A.; Das, P. Chakravortty D. Engagement of TLR signaling as adjuvant: Towards smarter vaccine and beyond. *Vaccine* **2008**, *26*, 6777–6783. [CrossRef] [PubMed]
2. McKee, A.S.; Munks, M.W.; Marrack, P. How Do Adjuvants Work? Important Considerations for New Generation Adjuvants. *Immunity* **2007**, *27*, 687–690. [CrossRef]
3. Reed, S.G.; Orr, M.T.; Fox, C.B. Key roles of adjuvants in modern vaccines. *Nat. Med.* **2013**, *19*, 1597–1608. [CrossRef] [PubMed]
4. Mosca, F.; Tritto, E.; Muzzi, A.; Monaci, E.; Bagnoli, F.; Iavarone, C.; O'Hagan, D.; Rappuoli, R.; De Gregorio, E. Molecular and cellular signatures of human vaccine adjuvants. *Proc. Natl. Acad. Sci. USA* **2008**, *105*, 10501–10506. [CrossRef]
5. Ragupathi, G.; Gardner, J.R.; Livingston, P.O.; Gin, D.Y. Natural and synthetic saponin adjuvant QS-21 for vaccines against cancer. *Expert Rev. Vaccines* **2011**, *10*, 463–470. [CrossRef]
6. Shah, R.R.; Hassett, K.J.; Brito, L.A. Overview of Vaccine Adjuvants: Introduction, History, and Current Status. *Vaccine Adjuv.* **2017**, *1494*, 1–13.
7. Harandi, A.M. Systems analysis of human vaccine adjuvants. *Semin. Immunol.* **2018**, *39*, 30–34. [CrossRef]
8. Boyle, J.; Eastman, D.; Millar, C.; Camuglia, S.; Cox, J.; Pearse, M.; Good, J.; Drane, D. The utility of ISCOMATRIX^{TM} adjuvant for dose reduction of antigen for vaccines requiring antibody responses. *Vaccine* **2007**, *25*, 2541–2544. [CrossRef]
9. Brito, L.A.; Malyala, P.; O'Hagan, D.T. Vaccine adjuvant formulations: A pharmaceutical perspective. *Semin. Immunol.* **2013**, *25*, 130–145. [CrossRef] [PubMed]
10. Vesikari, T.; Knuf, M.; Wutzler, P.; Karvonen, A.; Kieninger-Baum, D.; Schmitt, H.-J.; Baehner, F.; Borkowski, A.; Tsai, T.F.; Clemens, R. Oil-in-Water Emulsion Adjuvant with Influenza Vaccine in Young Children. *N. Engl. J. Med.* **2011**, *365*, 1406–1416. [CrossRef]
11. Podda, A. The adjuvanted influenza vaccines with novel adjuvants: experience with the MF59-adjuvanted vaccine. *Vaccine* **2001**, *19*, 2673–2680. [CrossRef]
12. Khurana, S.; Chearwae, W.; Castellino, F.; Manischewitz, J.; King, L.R.; Honorkiewicz, A.; Rock, M.T.; Edwards, K.M.; Giudice, G.D.; Rappuoli, R.; et al. Vaccines with MF59 Adjuvant Expand the Antibody Repertoire to Target Protective Sites of Pandemic Avian H5N1 Influenza Virus. *Sci. Transl. Med.* **2010**, *2*. [CrossRef] [PubMed]
13. Wen, Y.; Shi, Y. Alum: An old dog with new tricks. *Emerg. Microbes Infect.* **2016**, *5*, e25. [CrossRef] [PubMed]
14. Morel, S.; Didierlaurent, A.; Bourguignon, P.; Delhaye, S.; Baras, B.; Jacob, V.; Planty, C.; Elouahabi, A.; Harvengt, P.; Carlsen, H.; et al. Adjuvant System AS03 containing α-tocopherol modulates innate immune response and leads to improved adaptive immunity. *Vaccine* **2011**, *29*, 2461–2473. [CrossRef]
15. Yam, K.K.; Gupta, J.; Winter, K.; Allen, E.; Brewer, A.; Beaulieu, É.; Mallett, C.P.; Burt, D.S.; Ward, B.J. AS03-Adjuvanted, Very-Low-Dose Influenza Vaccines Induce Distinctive Immune Responses Compared to Unadjuvanted High-Dose Vaccines in BALB/c Mice. *Front. Immunol.* **2015**. [CrossRef]
16. Galli, G.; Medini, D.; Borgogni, E.; Zedda, L.; Bardelli, M.; Malzone, C.; Nuti, S.; Tavarini, S.; Sammicheli, C.; Hilbert, A.K.; et al. Adjuvanted H5N1 vaccine induces early CD4+ T cell response that predicts long-term persistence of protective antibody levels. *Proc. Natl. Acad. Sci. USA* **2009**, *106*, 3877–3882. [CrossRef]
17. Garçon, N.; Di Pasquale, A. From discovery to licensure, the Adjuvant System story. *Hum. Vaccines Immunother.* **2016**, *13*, 19–33. [CrossRef] [PubMed]
18. Garçon, N.; Vaughn, D.W.; Didierlaurent, A.M. Development and evaluation of AS03, an Adjuvant System containing α-tocopherol and squalene in an oil-in-water emulsion. *Expert Rev. Vaccines* **2012**, *11*, 349–366. [CrossRef]
19. Bharucha, T.; Ming, D.; Breuer, J. A critical appraisal of 'Shingrix', a novel herpes zoster subunit vaccine (HZ/Su or GSK1437173A) for varicella zoster virus. *Hum. Vaccines Immunother.* **2017**, *13*, 1789–1797. [CrossRef]
20. Sly, J.R.; Harris, A.L. Recombinant Zoster Vaccine (Shingrix) to Prevent Herpes Zoster. *Nurs. Womens Health* **2018**, *22*, 417–422. [CrossRef]

21. Jalah, R.; Patel, V.; Kulkarni, V.; Rosati, M.; Alicea, C.; Ganneru, B.; von Gegerfelt, A.; Huang, W.; Guan, Y.; Broderick, K.E.; et al. IL-12 DNA as molecular vaccine adjuvant increases the cytotoxic T cell responses and breadth of humoral immune responses in SIV DNA vaccinated macaques. *Hum. Vaccines Immunother.* **2012**, *8*, 1620–1629. [CrossRef]
22. Chong, S.-Y.; Egan, M.A.; Kutzler, M.A.; Megati, S.; Masood, A.; Roopchard, V.; Garcia-Hand, D.; Montefiori, D.C.; Quiroz, J.; Rosati, M.; et al. Comparative ability of plasmid IL-12 and IL-15 to enhance cellular and humoral immune responses elicited by a SIVgag plasmid DNA vaccine and alter disease progression following SHIV89.6P challenge in rhesus macaques. *Vaccine* **2007**, *25*, 4967–4982. [CrossRef]
23. Khosroshahi, K.H.; Ghaffarifar, F.; Sharifi, Z.; D'Souza, S.; Dalimi, A.; Hassan, Z.M.; Khoshzaban, F. Comparing the effect of IL-12 genetic adjuvant and alum non-genetic adjuvant on the efficiency of the cocktail DNA vaccine containing plasmids encoding SAG-1 and ROP-2 of *Toxoplasma gondii*. *Parasitol. Res.* **2012**, *111*, 403–411. [CrossRef]
24. Boyer, J.D.; Robinson, T.M.; Kutzler, M.A.; Parkinson, R.; Calarota, S.A.; Sidhu, M.K.; Muthumani, K.; Lewis, M.; Pavlakis, G.; Felber, B.; et al. SIV DNA vaccine co-administered with IL-12 expression plasmid enhances CD8 SIV cellular immune responses in cynomolgus macaques. *J. Med. Primatol.* **2005**, *34*, 262–270. [CrossRef]
25. Sin, J.-I.; Kim, J.J.; Arnold, R.L.; Shroff, K.E.; McCallus, D.; Pachuk, C.; McElhiney, S.P.; Wolf, M.W.; Bruin, S.J.P.; Higgins, T.J.; et al. IL-12 Gene as a DNA Vaccine Adjuvant in a Herpes Mouse Model: IL-12 Enhances Th1-Type $CD4^+$ T Cell-Mediated Protective Immunity Against Herpes Simplex Virus-2 Challenge. *J. Immunol.* **1999**, *162*, 2912–2921. [PubMed]
26. Kim, J.J.; Ayyavoo, V.; Bagarazzi, M.L.; Chattergoon, M.A.; Dang, K.; Wang, B.; Boyer, J.D.; Weiner, D.B. In vivo engineering of a cellular immune response by coadministration of IL-12 expression vector with a DNA immunogen. *J. Immunol.* **1997**, *158*, 816–826. [PubMed]
27. Kalams, S.A.; Parker, S.; Jin, X.; Elizaga, M.; Metch, B.; Wang, M.; Hural, J.; Lubeck, M.; Eldridge, J.; Cardinali, M.; et al. Safety and Immunogenicity of an HIV-1 Gag DNA Vaccine with or without IL-12 and/or IL-15 Plasmid Cytokine Adjuvant in Healthy, HIV-1 Uninfected Adults. *PLoS ONE* **2012**, *7*, e29231. [CrossRef]
28. Kalams, S.A.; Parker, S.D.; Elizaga, M.; Metch, B.; Edupuganti, S.; Hural, J.; De Rosa, S.; Carter, D.K.; Rybczyk, K.; Frank, I.; et al. Safety and Comparative Immunogenicity of an HIV-1 DNA Vaccine in Combination with Plasmid Interleukin 12 and Impact of Intramuscular Electroporation for Delivery. *J. Infect. Dis.* **2013**, *208*, 818–829. [CrossRef]
29. Gresnigt, M.S.; van de Veerdonk, F.L. Biology of IL-36 cytokines and their role in disease. *Semin. Immunol.* **2013**, *25*, 458–465. [CrossRef] [PubMed]
30. Clavel, G.; Thiolat, A.; Boissier, M.-C. Interleukin newcomers creating new numbers in rheumatology: IL-34 to IL-38. *Joint Bone Spine* **2013**, *80*, 449–453. [CrossRef]
31. Smith, D.E.; Renshaw, B.R.; Ketchem, R.R.; Kubin, M.; Garka, K.E.; Sims, J.E. Four New Members Expand the Interleukin-1 Superfamily. *J. Biol. Chem.* **2000**, *275*, 1169–1175. [CrossRef]
32. Towne, J.E.; Garka, K.E.; Renshaw, B.R.; Virca, G.D.; Sims, J.E. Interleukin (IL)-1F6, IL-1F8, and IL-1F9 Signal through IL-1Rrp2 and IL-1RAcP to Activate the Pathway Leading to NF-κB and MAPKs. *J. Biol. Chem.* **2004**, *279*, 13677–13688. [CrossRef]
33. Kumar, S.; McDonnell, P.C.; Lehr, R.; Tierney, L.; Tzimas, M.N.; Griswold, D.E.; Capper, E.A.; Tal-Singer, R.; Wells, G.I.; Doyle, M.L.; et al. Identification and Initial Characterization of Four Novel Members of the Interleukin-1 Family. *J. Biol. Chem.* **2000**, *275*, 10308–10314. [CrossRef]
34. Dinarello, C.A. Overview of the interleukin-1 family of ligands and receptors. *Semin. Immunol.* **2013**, *25*, 389–393. [CrossRef]
35. Dietrich, D.; Martin, P.; Flacher, V.; Sun, Y.; Jarrossay, D.; Brembilla, N.; Mueller, C.; Arnett, H.A.; Palmer, G.; Towne, J.; et al. Interleukin-36 potently stimulates human M2 macrophages, Langerhans cells and keratinocytes to produce pro-inflammatory cytokines. *Cytokine* **2016**, *84*, 88–98. [CrossRef]
36. Yazdi, A.S.; Ghoreschi, K. The Interleukin-1 Family. *Regul. Cytokine Gene Expr. Immun. Dis.* **2016**, *941*, 21–29.
37. Vigne, S.; Palmer, G.; Martin, P.; Lamacchia, C.; Strebel, D.; Rodriguez, E.; Olleros, M.L.; Vesin, D.; Garcia, I.; Ronchi, F.; et al. IL-36 signaling amplifies Th1 responses by enhancing proliferation and Th1 polarization of naive $CD4^+$ T cells. *Blood* **2012**, *120*, 3478–3487. [CrossRef]

38. Vigne, S.; Palmer, G.; Lamacchia, C.; Martin, P.; Talabot-Ayer, D.; Rodriguez, E.; Ronchi, F.; Sallusto, F.; Dinh, H.; Sims, J.E.; et al. IL-36R ligands are potent regulators of dendritic and T cells. *Blood* **2011**, *118*, 5813–5823. [CrossRef] [PubMed]
39. Yan, J.; Corbitt, N.; Pankhong, P.; Shin, T.; Khan, A.; Sardesai, N.Y.; Weiner, D.B. Immunogenicity of a novel engineered HIV-1 clade C synthetic consensus-based envelope DNA vaccine. *Vaccine* **2011**, *29*, 7173–7181. [CrossRef] [PubMed]
40. Scott, V.L.; Patel, A.; Villarreal, D.O.; Hensley, S.E.; Ragwan, E.; Yan, J.; Sardesai, N.Y.; Rothwell, P.J.; Extance, J.P.; Caproni, L.J.; et al. Novel synthetic plasmid and Doggybone^{TM} DNA vaccines induce neutralizing antibodies and provide protection from lethal influenza challenge in mice. *Hum. Vaccines Immunother.* **2015**, *11*, 1972–1982. [CrossRef] [PubMed]
41. Muthumani, K.; Griffin, B.D.; Agarwal, S.; Kudchodkar, S.B.; Reuschel, E.L.; Choi, H.; Kraynyak, K.A.; Duperret, E.K.; Keaton, A.A.; Chung, C.; et al. In vivo protection against ZIKV infection and pathogenesis through passive antibody transfer and active immunisation with a prMEnv DNA vaccine. *NPJ Vaccines* **2016**, *1*, 16021. [CrossRef]
42. Towne, J.E.; Renshaw, B.R.; Douangpanya, J.; Lipsky, B.P.; Shen, M.; Gabel, C.A.; Sims, J.E. Interleukin-36 (IL-36) Ligands Require Processing for Full Agonist (IL-36α, IL-36β, and IL-36γ) or Antagonist (IL-36Ra) Activity. *J. Biol. Chem.* **2011**, *286*, 42594–42602. [CrossRef]
43. Kumar, S.; Yan, J.; Muthumani, K.; Ramanathan, M.P.; Yoon, H.; Pavlakis, G.N.; Felber, B.K.; Sidhu, M.; Boyer, J.D.; Weiner, D.B. Immunogenicity Testing of a Novel Engineered HIV-1 Envelope Gp140 DNA Vaccine Construct. *DNA Cell Biol.* **2006**, *25*, 383–392. [CrossRef]
44. Choi, H.; Kudchodkar, S.B.; Reuschel, E.L.; Asija, K.; Borole, P.; Ho, M.; Wojtak, K.; Reed, C.; Ramos, S.; Bopp, N.E.; et al. Protective immunity by an engineered DNA vaccine for Mayaro virus. *PLoS Negl. Trop. Dis.* **2019**, *13*, e0007042. [CrossRef]
45. Catalan-Dibene, J.; McIntyre, L.L.; Zlotnik, A. Interleukin 30 to Interleukin 40. *J. Interferon Cytokine Res.* **2018**, *38*, 423–439. [CrossRef]
46. Debets, R.; Timans, J.C.; Homey, B.; Zurawski, S.; Sana, T.R.; Lo, S.; Wagner, J.; Edwards, G.; Clifford, T.; Menon, S.; et al. Two Novel IL-1 Family Members, IL-1δ and IL-1ε, Function as an Antagonist and Agonist of NF-κB Activation Through the Orphan IL-1 Receptor-Related Protein 2. *J. Immunol.* **2001**, *167*, 1440–1446. [CrossRef]
47. Henry, C.M.; Sullivan, G.P.; Clancy, D.M.; Afonina, I.S.; Kulms, D.; Martin, S.J. Neutrophil-Derived Proteases Escalate Inflammation through Activation of IL-36 Family Cytokines. *Cell Rep.* **2016**, *14*, 708–722. [CrossRef]
48. Clancy, D.M.; Henry, C.M.; Davidovich, P.B.; Sullivan, G.P.; Belotcerkovskaya, E.; Martin, S.J. Production of biologically active IL-36 family cytokines through insertion of N-terminal caspase cleavage motifs. *FEBS Open Bio* **2016**, *6*, 338–348. [CrossRef]
49. André, S.; Seed, B.; Eberle, J.; Schraut, W.; Bültmann, A.; Haas, J. Increased Immune Response Elicited by DNA Vaccination with a Synthetic gp120 Sequence with Optimized Codon Usage. *J. Virol.* **1998**, *72*, 1497–1503.
50. Deml, L.; Bojak, A.; Steck, S.; Graf, M.; Wild, J.; Schirmbeck, R.; Wolf, H.; Wagner, R. Multiple Effects of Codon Usage Optimization on Expression and Immunogenicity of DNA Candidate Vaccines Encoding the Human Immunodeficiency Virus Type 1 Gag Protein. *J. Virol.* **2001**, *75*, 10991–11001. [CrossRef]

51. Wise, M.C.; Hutnick, N.A.; Pollara, J.; Myles, D.J.F.; Williams, C.; Yan, J.; LaBranche, C.C.; Khan, A.S.; Sardesai, N.Y.; Montefiori, D.; et al. An Enhanced Synthetic Multiclade DNA Prime Induces Improved Cross-Clade-Reactive Functional Antibodies when Combined with an Adjuvanted Protein Boost in Nonhuman Primates. *J. Virol.* **2015**, *89*, 9154. [CrossRef]
52. Ding, L.; Wang, X.; Hong, X.; Lu, L.; Liu, D. IL-36 cytokines in autoimmunity and inflammatory disease. *Oncotarget* **2017**, *9*, 2895–2901. [CrossRef] [PubMed]
53. Foster, A.M.; Baliwag, J.; Chen, C.S.; Guzman, A.M.; Stoll, S.W.; Gudjonsson, J.E.; Ward, N.L.; Johnston, A. IL-36 promotes myeloid cell infiltration, activation and inflammatory activity in skin. *J. Immunol.* **2014**, *192*, 6053–6061. [CrossRef]
54. Traks, T.; Keermann, M.; Prans, E.; Karelson, M.; Loite, U.; Kõks, G.; Silm, H.; Kõks, S.; Kingo, K. Polymorphisms in IL36G gene are associated with plaque psoriasis. *BMC Med. Genet.* **2019**, *20*. [CrossRef] [PubMed]
55. Ellingford, J.M.; Black, G.C.M.; Clayton, T.H.; Judge, M.; Griffiths, C.E.M.; Warren, R.B. A novel mutation in IL36RN underpins childhood pustular dermatosis. *J. Eur. Acad. Dermatol. Venereol.* **2016**, *30*, 302–305. [CrossRef]
56. Mahil, S.K.; Catapano, M.; Meglio, P.D.; Dand, N.; Ahlfors, H.; Carr, I.M.; Smith, C.H.; Trembath, R.C.; Peakman, M.; Wright, J.; et al. An analysis of IL-36 signature genes and individuals with IL1RL2 knockout mutations validates IL-36 as a psoriasis therapeutic target. *Sci. Transl. Med.* **2017**, *9*, eaan2514. [CrossRef] [PubMed]
57. Ainscough, J.S.; Macleod, T.; McGonagle, D.; Brakefield, R.; Baron, J.M.; Alase, A.; Wittmann, M.; Stacey, M. Cathepsin S is the major activator of the psoriasis-associated proinflammatory cytokine IL-36γ. *Proc. Natl. Acad. Sci. USA* **2017**, *114*, E2748–E2757. [CrossRef]
58. Meier-Schiesser, B.; Feldmeyer, L.; Jankovic, D.; Mellett, M.; Satoh, T.K.; Yerly, D.; Navarini, A.; Abe, R.; Yawalkar, N.; Chung, W.-H.; et al. Culprit Drugs Induce Specific IL-36 Overexpression in Acute Generalized Exanthematous Pustulosis. *J. Investig. Dermatol.* **2019**, *139*, 848–858. [CrossRef] [PubMed]
59. Boutet, M.-A.; Bart, G.; Penhoat, M.; Amiaud, J.; Brulin, B.; Charrier, C.; Morel, F.; Lecron, J.-C.; Rolli-Derkinderen, M.; Bourreille, A.; et al. Distinct expression of interleukin (IL)-36α, β and γ, their antagonist IL-36Ra and IL-38 in psoriasis, rheumatoid arthritis and Crohn's disease. *Clin. Exp. Immunol.* **2016**, *184*, 159–173. [CrossRef] [PubMed]
60. Johnston, A.; Xing, X.; Wolterink, L.; Barnes, D.H.; Yin, Z.; Reingold, L.; Kahlenberg, J.M.; Harms, P.W.; Gudjonsson, J.E. IL-1 and IL-36 are dominant cytokines in generalized pustular psoriasis. *J. Allergy Clin. Immunol.* **2017**, *140*, 109–120. [CrossRef] [PubMed]
61. Di Caprio, R.; Balato, A.; Caiazzo, G.; Lembo, S.; Raimondo, A.; Fabbrocini, G.; Monfrecola, G. IL-36 cytokines are increased in acne and hidradenitis suppurativa. *Arch. Dermatol. Res.* **2017**, *309*, 673–678. [CrossRef]
62. Towne, J.; Sims, J. IL-36 in psoriasis. *Curr. Opin. Pharmacol.* **2012**, *12*, 486–490. [CrossRef]
63. Hashiguchi, Y.; Yabe, R.; Chung, S.-H.; Murayama, M.A.; Yoshida, K.; Matsuo, K.; Kubo, S.; Saijo, S.; Nakamura, Y.; Matsue, H.; et al. IL-36α from Skin-Resident Cells Plays an Important Role in the Pathogenesis of Imiquimod-Induced Psoriasiform Dermatitis by Forming a Local Autoamplification Loop. *J. Immunol.* **2018**, *201*, 167–182. [CrossRef]
64. Wang, W.; Yu, X.; Wu, C.; Jin, H. IL-36γ inhibits differentiation and induces inflammation of keratinocyte via Wnt signaling pathway in psoriasis. *Int. J. Med. Sci.* **2017**, *14*, 1002–1007. [CrossRef]
65. Kanazawa, N.; Nakamura, T.; Mikita, N.; Furukawa, F. Novel IL36RN mutation in a Japanese case of early onset generalized pustular psoriasis. *J. Dermatol.* **2013**, *40*, 749–751. [CrossRef]
66. Tortola, L.; Rosenwald, E.; Abel, B.; Blumberg, H.; Schäfer, M.; Coyle, A.J.; Renauld, J.-C.; Werner, S.; Kisielow, J.; Kopf, M. Psoriasiform dermatitis is driven by IL-36–mediated DC-keratinocyte crosstalk. *J. Clin. Investig.* **2012**, *122*, 3965–3976. [CrossRef]
67. Arakawa, A.; Vollmer, S.; Besgen, P.; Galinski, A.; Summer, B.; Kawakami, Y.; Wollenberg, A.; Dornmair, K.; Spannagl, M.; Ruzicka, T.; et al. Unopposed IL-36 Activity Promotes Clonal $CD4^+$ T-Cell Responses with IL-17A Production in Generalized Pustular Psoriasis. *J. Investig. Dermatol.* **2018**, *138*, 1338–1347. [CrossRef]
68. Verma, A.H.; Zafar, H.; Ponde, N.O.; Hepworth, O.W.; Sihra, D.; Aggor, F.E.Y.; Ainscough, J.S.; Ho, J.; Richardson, J.P.; Coleman, B.M.; et al. IL-36 and IL-1/IL-17 Drive Immunity to Oral Candidiasis via Parallel Mechanisms. *J. Immunol.* **2018**, *201*, 627–634. [CrossRef]
69. Winkle, S.M.; Throop, A.L.; Herbst-Kralovetz, M.M. IL-36γ Augments Host Defense and Immune Responses in Human Female Reproductive Tract Epithelial Cells. *Front. Microbiol.* **2016**, *7*. [CrossRef]

70. Gardner, J.K.; Herbst-Kralovetz, M.M. IL-36γ induces a transient HSV-2 resistant environment that protects against genital disease and pathogenesis. *Cytokine* **2018**, *111*, 63–71. [CrossRef]
71. Kovach, M.A.; Singer, B.; Martinez-Colon, G.; Newstead, M.W.; Zeng, X.; Mancuso, P.; Moore, T.A.; Kunkel, S.L.; Peters-Golden, M.; Moore, B.B.; et al. IL-36γ is a crucial proximal component of protective type-1-mediated lung mucosal immunity in Gram-positive and -negative bacterial pneumonia. *Mucosal. Immunol.* **2017**, *10*, 1320–1334. [CrossRef] [PubMed]
72. Milora, K.A.; Uppalapati, S.R.; Sanmiguel, J.C.; Zou, W.; Jensen, L.E. Interleukin-36β provides protection against HSV-1 infection, but does not modulate initiation of adaptive immune responses. *Sci. Rep.* **2017**, *7*. [CrossRef]
73. Aoyagi, T.; Newstead, M.W.; Zeng, X.; Nanjo, Y.; Peters-Golden, M.; Kaku, M.; Standiford, T.J. Interleukin-36γ and IL-36 receptor signaling mediate impaired host immunity and lung injury in cytotoxic *Pseudomonas aeruginosa* pulmonary infection: Role of prostaglandin E2. *PLoS Pathog.* **2017**, *13*. [CrossRef]
74. Wang, X.; Zhao, X.; Feng, C.; Weinstein, A.; Xia, R.; Wen, W.; Lv, Q.; Zuo, S.; Tang, P.; Yang, X.; et al. IL-36γ transforms the tumor microenvironment and promotes type 1 lymphocyte-mediated antitumor immune responses. *Cancer Cell* **2015**, *28*, 296. [CrossRef] [PubMed]

vaccines MDPI

Article

Genetically Modified Mouse Mesenchymal Stem Cells Expressing Non-Structural Proteins of Hepatitis C Virus Induce Effective Immune Response

Olga V. Masalova [1,*], Ekaterina I. Lesnova [1], Regina R. Klimova [1], Ekaterina D. Momotyuk [1], Vyacheslav V. Kozlov [1], Alla M. Ivanova [1], Olga V. Payushina [2], Nina N. Butorina [3], Natalia F. Zakirova [4], Alexander N. Narovlyansky [1], Alexander V. Pronin [1], Alexander V. Ivanov [4,*] and Alla A. Kushch [1]

1 Gamaleya National Research Center of Epidemiology and Microbiology, Ministry of Health of the Russian Federation, Moscow 123098, Russia; wolf252006@yandex.ru (E.I.L.); regi.k@mail.ru (R.R.K.); edm95r@rambler.ru (E.D.M.); hyperslava@yandex.ru (V.V.K.); 5893211@bk.ru (A.M.I.); narovl@yandex.ru (A.N.N.); proninalexander@yandex.ru (A.V.P.); vitallku@mail.ru (A.A.K.)

2 Federal State Autonomous Educational Institution of Higher Education I.M. Sechenov First Moscow State Medical University of the Ministry of Health of the Russian Federation (Sechenov University), Moscow 119991, Russia; payushina@mail.ru

3 Koltzov Institute of Developmental Biology of Russian Academy of Sciences, Moscow 119334, Russia; nnbut@mail.ru

4 Center for Precision Genome Editing and Genetic Technologies for Biomedicine, Engelhardt Institute of Molecular Biology, Russian Academy of Sciences, Moscow 119991, Russia; nat_zakirova@mail.ru

* Correspondence: ol.mas@mail.ru (O.V.M.); aivanov@yandex.ru (A.V.I.); Tel.: +7-499-190-30-49 (O.V.M.); +7-199-135-60-65 (A.V.I.)

Received: 5 December 2019; Accepted: 31 January 2020; Published: 2 February 2020

Abstract: Hepatitis C virus (HCV) is one of the major causes of chronic liver disease and leads to cirrhosis and hepatocarcinoma. Despite extensive research, there is still no vaccine against HCV. In order to induce an immune response in DBA/2J mice against HCV, we obtained modified mouse mesenchymal stem cells (mMSCs) simultaneously expressing five nonstructural HCV proteins (NS3-NS5B). The innate immune response to mMSCs was higher than to DNA immunization, with plasmid encoding the same proteins, and to naïve unmodified MSCs. mMSCs triggered strong phagocytic activity, enhanced lymphocyte proliferation, and production of type I and II interferons. The adaptive immune response to mMSCs was also more pronounced than in the case of DNA immunization, as exemplified by a fourfold stronger stimulation of lymphocyte proliferation in response to HCV, a 2.6-fold higher rate of biosynthesis, and a 30-fold higher rate of secretion of IFN-γ, as well as by a 40-fold stronger production of IgG2a antibodies to viral proteins. The immunostimulatory effect of mMSCs was associated with pronounced IL-6 secretion and reduction in the population of myeloid derived suppressor cells (MDSCs). Thus, this is the first example that suggests the feasibility of using mMSCs for the development of an effective anti-HCV vaccine.

Keywords: hepatitis C virus (HCV); mesenchymal stem cells (MSC); modified MSC; DNA immunization; nonstructural HCV proteins; immune response; HCV vaccine; myeloid derived suppressor cells (MDSCs)

1. Introduction

Mesenchymal stem cells (MSCs) are successfully used in various fields of regenerative medicine [1]. Cell therapy is based on the ability of MSCs to migrate to the sites of pathology. They are able to exert anti-inflammatory and immunomodulatory effects upon allogeneic transplantation, as well as in autoimmune diseases [2–5]. Obtaining genetically modified MSCs expressing introduced genes significantly expands the possibilities of both cellular and genetic therapy, ensuring the delivery of therapeutic molecules to the sites of damage and inflammation [6,7]. MSCs transduced by the interferon β (IFN-β) gene have been shown to reduce the signs of inflammation and the severity of the disease and to improve the condition of the CNS in experimental multiple sclerosis [8]. Positive results with modified MSCs have been obtained in myocardial infarction [9] and in cancer therapy [10].

These results suggest that obtaining and using modified MSCs (mMSCs) that harbor viral genes could be effective for the development of antiviral vaccines. This approach has a number of advantages over traditional vaccine technologies. mMSCs can express many proteins simultaneously, thus ensuring a wide range of epitopes with the correct post-translational modifications as during natural infection. They are also capable of delivering, expressing, and presenting an antigen for a long time. Indeed, Tomchuck et al. demonstrated in an experimental model of HIV infection that cellular vaccines based on transfected MSCs could be developed [11].

One of the urgent but unresolved problems of biology and medicine is the development of an effective vaccine towards hepatitis C virus (HCV). HCV is considered as one of the main etiological agents of chronic liver disease, including terminal stages – cirrhosis and hepatocarcinoma. In up to 80% of cases, acute hepatitis C transfers into chronic disease, which may be caused by a very high heterogeneity of viral genome and the existence of quasispecies, interference of the virus with innate and adaptive immune response pathways, and the formation of "escape" variants of HCV that are not recognized by the immune system [12,13]. Anti-HCV therapy based on a combination of pegylated recombinant IFN-α and ribavirin eliminates the virus in no more than 50% of patients [14]. Modern therapy using direct-acting antivirals (DAA) that target HCV NS3, NS5A, and NS5B proteins makes it possible to cure up to 99% of patients, but the extremely high cost of DAAs makes access to the treatment limited, as exemplified by higher rates of detection of new cases compared to number of patients treated with these drugs [15] Another factor that limits access to treatment is unawareness of a majority (ca. 80%) of patients of their status. In addition, there is a lot of evidence showing that HCV can remain in the liver cells and peripheral blood mononuclear cells (PBMC) of patients after the disappearance of viral RNA in serum, thus establishing occult infection [16,17]. Such ongoing viral replication in hepatocytes can lead to continuous liver injury and may underlie the absence of improvement in clinical outcomes after a sustained virological response achieved in a majority of patients [16].

The development of anti-HCV vaccines can contribute to global efforts to eradicate the virus. Numerous attempts to develop a vaccine whose action is based on broadly neutralizing antibodies against structural proteins failed, most likely due to very high variability of E1 and E2 glycoproteins and escape of virions due to bound lipoproteins and glycans [18]. Efficient vaccines could be based on the recombinant viral proteins/peptides that contain B- and T-cell epitopes or DNA plasmids/viral vectors, ensuring their expression [19]. However, the optimal set of HCV genes or their fragments that should be present in the vaccine has not yet been determined. Literature data suggest that none of the candidate vaccines triggered a full preventive and therapeutic response against HCV [20,21]. Recently, several vaccines against HCV based on dendritic cells (DC) have been reported [22,23]. DCs are highly specialized antigen-presenting cells (APC), so DC-based vaccination based on ex vivo stimulated and matured DCs loaded with HCV specific antigens is an attractive approach to elicit sustained anti-viral response to HCV proteins. However, generation of DCs can require substantial time and expense. It was shown that induction of T cell immune responses by DC vaccination is highly dependent on efficient antigen loading of the DCs [24]. The trials showed that such vaccines did not clear HCV infection in chronic hepatitis C patients despite induction of pronounced T-cell response [25,26]. Thus, the development of MSC vaccines based on genetic and cellular technologies could be one of the most promising strategies to prevent the spread of infectious diseases.

The aim of this work was to obtain MSCs expressing HCV genes and to analyze the humoral and cellular immune responses of animals to the introduction of these modified MSCs. As a model we chose genes of nonstructural HCV proteins that form viral replicase complex, as they are more conservative than structural proteins and in total comprise two-thirds of the entire HCV proteome [27]. Several lines of evidence show that clearance of acute HCV infection in chimpanzees and humans is temporally associated with early, strong, and broadly reactive T cell responses against multiple non-structural viral proteins [12,28]. The non-structural proteins are considered as the dominant targets for CD8+ and CD4+ cells [27]. A robust HCV-specific CD8+ and CD4+ T cell responses to the non-structural proteins has the potential to restrict infection, eliminate virus-infected cells after challenge, and prevent persistent infection at the very least [29].

2. Materials and Methods

2.1. Animals

Mice of the DBA/2J (H-2d) line (females, 6–8 weeks old) were obtained from the laboratory of the animal breeder Stolbovaya, FMBA, Moscow Region. All animal experiments were carried out in accordance with order 708 of the Ministry of Health of the Russian Federation and with the "Regulations on the ethical attitudes to laboratory animals of N.F. Gamaleya NRCEM (Moscow, Russia)".

2.2. Isolation of Primary MSCs

Mouse primary MSCs were obtained from bone aspirates of DBA mice. Both femurs and tibias from each leg were used. The cell suspension was homogenized and centrifuged at 2000 g for 10 min. Cell pellets were resuspended in high glucose Dulbecco's Modified Eagle Medium (DMEM) containing 10% fetal calf serum (FCS) (Invitrogen, Waltham, MA, USA), 10 μg/mL insulin, 5.5 μg/mL transferrin, 6.7 ng/mL sodium selenite, 10 ng/mL basic fibroblast growth factor, 2 mM L-glutamine, and 50 μg/mL gentamicin. The cells were seeded in culture flasks (Costar, New York, NY, USA) at a concentration of 2×10^6 cells/mL. The next day, as well as every subsequent 3-4 days, the culture medium was replaced. The resulting adhesive cell population was reseeded using a 0.25% trypsin solution. MSCs were cultured at 37°C in a 5% CO_2 atmosphere. Unless otherwise specified, culture media and other reagents were purchased from PanEco, Russia (Moscow, Russia).

2.3. Characterization of MSCs

Cell morphology and the state of the cell monolayer were examined visually using an AX10 inverted microscope (Zeiss, Germany). Immunophenotypic analysis of MSCs was performed by flow cytometry as described below.

2.4. Assessment of Adipogenic and Osteogenic Potencies of MSCs

MSCs isolated from red bone marrow were grown on passage 1 in 12-well plates into an osteogenic medium (growth medium supplemented with 10 nM dexamethasone, 50 μg/mL 2-phospho-L-ascorbate, and 10 mM sodium β-glycerophosphate) at a density of 1 × 104 cells/mL or into an adipogenic medium (standard growth medium supplemented with 10 μM dexamethasone, 0.2 mM indomethacin, 1 IU/mL insulin, and 0.5 mM 3-isobutyl-1-methylxanthine) at a density of 3×10^4 cells/mL. As a control, the cells maintained at the same density in a standard growth medium were used. The medium was changed twice a week; cultivation was continued for 20 days (adipogenesis) or 21 days (osteogenesis). For the analysis of adipogenic differentiation, cells were fixed with 4% formalin in 0.1 M phosphate-buffered saline, pH 7.2-7.4 (PBS), and stained with Oil Red O (Sigma, St. Louis, MO, USA) in order to detect neutral fat inclusions. For the analysis of osteogenic differentiation, the culture was fixed with a mixture of sodium citrate, acetone, and formaldehyde; cytochemical detection of alkaline phosphatase activity was carried out by the method of azo coupling of Fast Red Violet (FRV) with naphthol AS-BI (Sigma, USA), according to the manufacturer's protocol. In addition, in the culture of MSCs subjected to osteogenesis induction, deposits of calcium salts were detected by staining cells fixed with 96% ethanol with Alizarin Red S (Sigma, USA) at pH 4.1. After cytochemical reactions, the cells of all studied cultures were additionally stained with hematoxylin and analyzed using a Primovert inverted light microscope (Zeiss, Germany).

2.5. Plasmid and Transfection of MSC Culture

We used the pcNS3-NS5B plasmid construct encoding five nonstructural HCV proteins (NS3, NS4A, NS4B, NS5A, and NS5B) of genotype 1b that was constructed using a commercially available pcDNA-3.1(+) vector (Invitrogen, USA) [30]. The plasmid was purified from *E. coli* strain *JM109* using a commercial QIAGEN Plasmid Purification Maxi Kit (QIAGEN, Hinden, Germany) according to the manufacturer's instructions.

To obtain genetically transformed cells expressing HCV proteins, we used a primary MSC culture at third-fourth passages. MSCs were seeded on a six-well plate at a density of $5x10^4$ cells/mL. Twenty-four hours after reaching the subconfluent monolayer (70–90% cells/well), complexes of a plasmid with Xfect Transfection Reagent (Clontech Laboratories, Takara, USA) were applied to the cells. The transformed cells were selected in a medium containing 0.5 mg/mL G-418 (Invitrogen, Waltham, MA, USA). Cell viability was analyzed using a standard MTT test [31] and the trypan blue dye exclusion assay [32]. We conducted several rounds of selection, changing the medium with G-418 every 72 h. Cytokine secretion was measured by quantifying their levels in the conditioned medium.

2.6. Immunocytochemical and Immunoblot Detection of Viral Proteins

Expression of HCV proteins in the transfected MSCs was determined by the methods of indirect immunofluorescence and immunoperoxidase staining, using monoclonal antibodies (mAbs) against HCV proteins [33] as primary antibodies and secondary antibodies against mouse immunoglobulins (Ig) conjugated with fluorescein isothiocyanate (FITC) or horseradish peroxidase (HRP) (Dako, Denmark), as previously described [34,35]. Cell nuclei were stained with 4′-6-diamidino-2-phenylindole (DAPI) (immunofluorescence analysis) or with hematoxylin (immunoperoxidase method). The signals were visualized using an Axio Scope A1 microscope (Zeiss, Germany). The proportion of cells expressing viral proteins relative to the total number of cells was counted in at least eight fields of view at a magnification of 400× and expressed as a percentage value. This corresponds to counting at least 1600 cells for each HCV protein.

Western blot analysis was performed as described previously using the same monoclonal antibodies or serum of the rabbits immunized with the respective protein [36].

2.7. Immunization of Animals

To study the parameters of the immune response, we used four groups of DBA mice with 10 animals in each group. The mice from group 1 were injected with genetically modified MSCs (mMSC), mice from group 2 with non-transfected, "native" MSCs, mice from group 3 with pcNS3-NS5B plasmid, and mice from group 4 with saline. MSCs and mMSC (5×10^5 cells) were injected into the tail vein, plasmids (100 µg)—intramuscularly into the quadriceps femoris muscle. Two immunizations with an interval of 2–3 weeks were conducted.

In some experiments, the animals were injected with mMSC treated with a recombinant mouse IFN-γ protein (Abcam, Cambridge, UK) at a concentration of 80 ng/mL for 18 h. The immunization scheme was as described above.

2.8. The Recombinant HCV Proteins

The recombinant HCV proteins were used as antigens to stimulate T-cell responses in vitro and as sorbents in an enzyme-linked immunosorbent assay (ELISA) to evaluate antibody production. The proteins were combined into four pools: NS3 (protease domain with a sequence of 1027–1229 aa, helicase domain 1230–1658 aa, immunodominant region 1356–1459 aa, genotype 1b); NS4 (1677–1754 aa and mosaic protein containing regions 1691–1710, 1712–1733, 1921–1940 aa from genotypes 1, 2, 3, and 5); NS5A (the full-length protein 1973–2419 aa and fragments 2061–2302 aa, 2212–2313 aa, genotypes 1b and 1a); the NS5B protein lacking C-terminal hydrophobic 21 amino acid residues

(2420–2990 aa, genotype 1b); as a negative control, we used the nucleocapsid (core) protein (1–90 aa). The recombinant proteins were expressed in *E.coli* and purified by chromatography on Ni-NTA-agarose or on glutathione sepharose, as described previously [30,37–39].

2.9. *Humoral Immune Response*

The immune response to the injected constructs was assessed 10 days after the second immunization. The activity of antibodies against HCV proteins in mouse sera was determined by indirect ELISA, as described previously [30]. As secondary antibodies, we used antibodies against mouse Ig isotypes IgG1 and IgG2a conjugated to HRP (Jackson Immunoresearch Laboratories, Cambridge, UK). As the serum titer in ELISA, we used the reciprocal of the highest serum dilution, at which the optical density was 2 times higher than that for the control group.

2.10. *T-Cell Proliferation and ELISpot Assays*

T-cell proliferation was assessed by the incorporation of [^{3}H]-thymidine into the DNA of dividing cells. The spleens of 10 mice of each group were pooled, a suspension of splenocytes was seeded in U-bottomed 96-well microculture plates at a density of 5×10^5 cells/well, and specific stimulants (pools of the recombinant HCV NS3, NS4, NS5A, and NS5B proteins at a final concentration of 1 μg/mL) were added. As negative controls, we used medium alone (spontaneous proliferation) and recombinant HCV core protein. Mitogen concanavalin A (ConA, 5 μg/mL, Sigma, USA) was used as an unspecific positive control. All samples were set in at least three replicates. The cells were cultured in a RPMI-1640 medium containing 20% FCS (Invitrogen, USA), 4.5 mg/mL glucose, 2 mM glutamine, 0.2 u/mL insulin, and 50 μg/mL gentamicin at 37 °C in a 5% CO_2 atmosphere. Four days later, aliquots of cell culture fluids were withdrawn and frozen at −20 °C. The remaining cells were labeled with 1 μCi/well [^{3}H]-thymidine (TdR, Amersham-Pharmacia-Biotech) and 18 h later harvested onto the glass-fiber filters. The radioactivity was measured using a MicroBeta2 β-counter (PerkinElmer, Waltham, MA, USA). Results were expressed as stimulation indexes (SI), determined by dividing the mean radioactive ^{3}H incorporation as counts per minute (c.p.m.) in the presence of antigens by means of ^{3}H incorporation in the wells containing medium alone and control antigen.

The number of IFN-γ synthesizing cells was determined using the ELISPOT mouse IFN-γ Kit (BD Biosciences, San Jose, CA, USA) according to the manufacturer's instructions. The results were expressed as the number of spot forming cells (SFC) per 10^6 cells.

2.11. *Detection of Cytokines in Cell Culture Fluids by Sandwich ELISA*

Measurement of cytokine levels (IFN-γ, TNF-α, IL-2, IL-6, IL-10, IL-12) was performed by ELISA in conditioned medium from selection of the MSC cells transfected with pcNS3-NS5B. The concentration of IFN-γ was also determined in medium from the splenocytes stimulated for four days. We used the Mouse IL-6 ELISA development kit (HRP), Mouse IFN-γ ELISA development kit (HRP), Mouse TNF-α ELISA development kit (HRP) (Mabtech, Stockholm, Sweden), Mouse IL-10 DuoSet ELISA, and Mouse IL-12 p70 Duoset ELISA (R&D Systems, Minneapolis, MN, USA). The detection sensitivity for IL-6 was 10 pg/mL, for IFN-γ and TNF-α—2 pg/mL, for IL-2—4 pg/mL, for IL-10 and IL-12—30 pg/mL. The concentrations of cytokines were determined from the calibration curves of standard samples.

2.12. *Flow Cytometry*

For immunophenotyping of MSCs, adhesive cells of the 2nd-3rd passages were collected using Accutase (CLS, Eppelheim, Germany), washed twice in ice-cold PBS, and separately stained (10^6 cells/sample) with primary phycoerythrin (PE)-labeled antibodies against CD73, CD90.1, and CD105 (BD Biosciences, USA) for 45 min, or unlabeled rat antibodies against CD45 and CD34 for 45 min and secondary Rabbit Anti-Rat-FITC conjugate (Abcam, Cambridge, UK) for 30 min at room temperature.

Analysis of dendritic (DC) and myeloid derived suppressor cells (MDSCs) was performed by multicolor flow cytometry. The suspensions of splenocytes from 10 immunized mice of each group

(10^6 cells/sample) were incubated with PE-labeled antibodies against CD11c, FITC-labeled antibodies against Gr-1 (Ly-6G and Ly-6C), and allophycocyanin (APC)-labeled antibodies against CD11b (BD Biosciences, USA). Antibodies to the corresponding isotype controls were included in all experiments. The absolute and relative number of cells carrying the markers was assessed by FACS on a flow cytometer BD FACSCanto II (Beckton Dickinson, Franklin Lakes, NJ, USA) using free software BD FACSDiva, v.6.1.3 (BD Biosciences, San Jose, CA, USA).

2.13. *Determination of Type I IFNs (IFN-α/β) Production by Immune Cells*

Quantification of IFN-α/β was carried out by a biological method in accordance with techniques based on the antiviral effect of interferons [40,41]. Briefly, mice splenocytes and peripheral blood leukocytes from 10 immunized mice of each group were stimulated in vitro by Newcastle disease virus (a standard IFN-α/β inducer) [42,43]. After virus inactivation, serial dilutions of the culture fluids were added to mouse fibroblast L-929 cell culture and 24 h later infected with encephalomyocarditis virus (EMCV). IFN-α/β activity was estimated as the highest reciprocal dilution that caused a 50% decrease in the cytopathogenic effect of 100 tissue culture infectious doses (TCID5O) per ml, and was expressed in international units per ml (IU/mL) using WHO International Standard Interferon alpha-2b (NIBSC cat. #95/566: https://nibsc.org/products/brm_product_catalogue/who_standards.aspx).

2.14. *Phagocytic Activity*

Phagocytic activity was determined by quantification of reactive oxygen species (ROS) production by the luminol-dependent chemiluminescence (CL) method. As a CL activator, we used opsonized zymosan, as described previously [44]. For analysis, we used a suspension of mice splenocytes and peripheral blood leukocytes from 10 immunized mice of each group. Spontaneous and induced CL were measured on a Synergy H1 hybrid multifunction photometer (BioTek, USA). As a quantitative indicator of the level of ROS production, we used an activation index (AI) – the ratio of the intensity of induced CL to the intensity of spontaneous CL.

2.15. *Statistical Analysis*

Statistical analysis was performed with Statistica 6 software (StatSoft Inc., Tulsa, OK, USA). Prism 5 software (GraphPad5, SanDiego, USA) was used to create graphs. Data was presented as means ± SD (standard deviation) of three independent experiments and analyzed by two-tailed Student t-test or one-way analysis of variance (ANOVA), followed by Tukey tests for multiple comparisons, when appropriate ($p < 0.05$ was considered as statistically significant).

3. Results

3.1. *Cells Isolated From the Bone Marrow of Mice Display Features of Mesenchymal Stem Cells*

MSCs isolated from the bone marrow of mice were characterized by adhesiveness and morphology. Light microscopy showed that MSCs were attached to the surface of culture flasks and were polymorphic cells with a fibroblast-like morphology. Cells actively proliferated and formed a monolayer (Figure 1a).

Phenotyping of MSCs of two to three passages by flow cytometry showed that most of them (83–96%) expressed CD73, CD90.1, and CD105 receptors that are markers of MSCs (Figure 1b, upper panel). At the same time, no expression was detected for hematopoietic cell markers CD45 and CD34 (Figure 1b, lower panel).

Analysis of the adipogenic potency of the obtained MSCs revealed that, at the end of 20 days of cultivation, single adipocytes were present in the control culture (Figure 1c, upper left panel); adipocytes located either individually or in small, usually loose groups of 5–10 cells were detected in the induced culture (Figure 1c, middle and upper right panel). Adipocytes differed in morphology and were at different stages of fat droplet accumulation: both mature oval or round adipocytes containing many large lipid vacuoles were found, as well as fibroblast-like cells, in which fat inclusions were smaller and occupied only part of the cytoplasm.

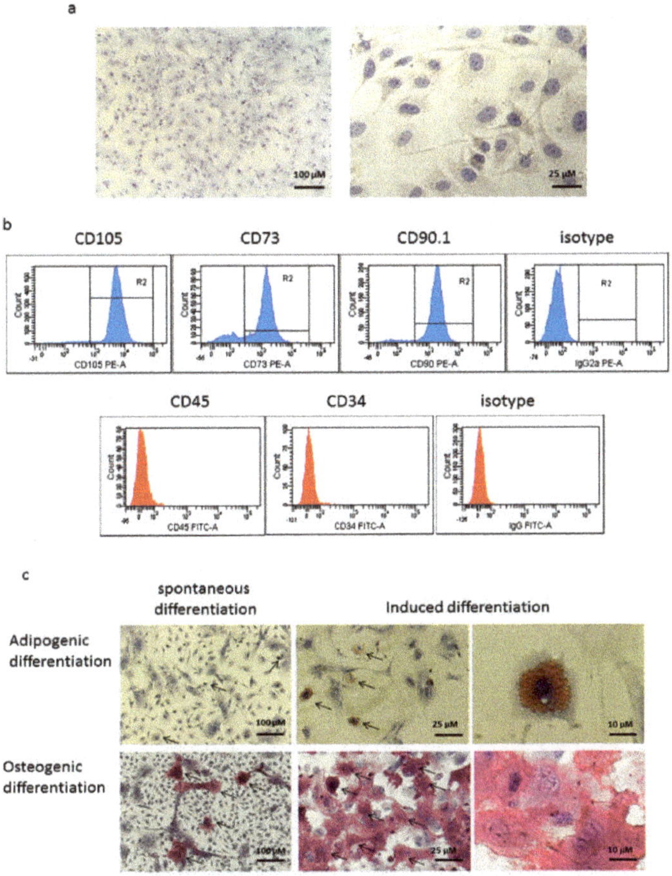

Figure 1. Characterization of mesenchymal stem cells (MSC) isolated from the bone marrow of mice. (**a**) The morphology of MSC isolated from the red bone marrow of mice is polymorphic cells that exhibit a fibroblast-like shape. The cells were seeded on culture flasks, and, after staining the nuclei with hematoxylin, they were visualized by light microscopy, scale bar, 100 µM (left), and 25 µM (right). (**b**) These are typical results of MSCs receptor analysis by flow cytometry. For immunophenotyping of MSCs, adhesive cells of the second and third passages were stained with phycoerythrin (PE)-labeled antibodies against CD73, CD90.1, CD105, or PE-labeled antibodies of the corresponding isotype controls, and unlabeled rat antibodies against CD45 or CD34 followed by rabbit antirat fluoresceine isothiocyanate (FITC) conjugate. The isolated MSCs expressed CD105, CD73, and CD90 (upper panel), but did not express CD45 and CD34 (lower panel). (**c**) The adipogenic (upper panel) and osteogenic (lower panel) differentiation of MSC isolated from the bone marrow of mice. MSCs were grown into an adipogenic or osteogenic medium; the medium was changed twice a week for 20 days (adipogenesis) or 21 days (osteogenesis). Then, MSCs were stained to detect neutral fat inclusions or alkaline phosphatase activity, respectively. Single adipocytes (upper left panel) and osteocytes (lower left panel) were present in the control cultures; arrows indicate spontaneous differentiation, scale bar, 100 µM; induced cultures MSC, arrows indicate fat cells (middle and upper right panel) and osteocytes (middle and lower right panel), (scale bar, 25 µM, and 10 µM, respectively).

A study of the osteogenic differentiation of MSCs showed that, after 21 days of cultivation, the cells in the control culture formed a confluent monolayer of uneven density with cells of fibroblast-like morphology. The cytochemical reaction to alkaline phosphatase, a marker of osteogenic cells, identified just a few cells containing this enzyme in the control culture (Figure 1c, lower left panel). In contrast, in the induced culture, most cells that contained alkaline phosphatase significantly exceeded those in the control culture (85±13 vs. 9±8, respectively, $p<0.001$). Cells with the positive reaction had a fibroblast-like shape and formed clusters of various size and density, in many cases closely contacting each other. The reaction intensity varied in different cells and often was very high (Figure 1c, middle and lower right panel), thus showing that the cells underwent osteogenic differentiation. Therefore, MSCs isolated from mouse bone marrow exhibited moderate capability to differentiate into mature multilocular adipocytes. They also could pass initial stages of osteogenic differentiation. It can be concluded that the isolated and multiplied cells corresponded to the generally accepted minimal characteristics of MSCs [45].

3.2. *Modified MSCs Express Genes of Hepatitis C Virus*

MSCs were transfected with the pcNS3-NS5B plasmid and the expression of viral genes was analyzed by immunocytochemical methods. Transfection efficiency was 55% on average. Figure 2a,d show typical staining of the transfected cells with monoclonal antibody against NS5A protein; expression of the other target HCV proteins was also demonstrated (Figure S1). The cell lines, obtained by selection of the transfected cells in the presence of G-418 for two weeks, also demonstrated expression of the HCV proteins (Figure 2b,e), in contrast to the non-transfected MSC (Figure 2c,f). Finally, expression of the HCV proteins was also confirmed by western blotting (Figure S2).

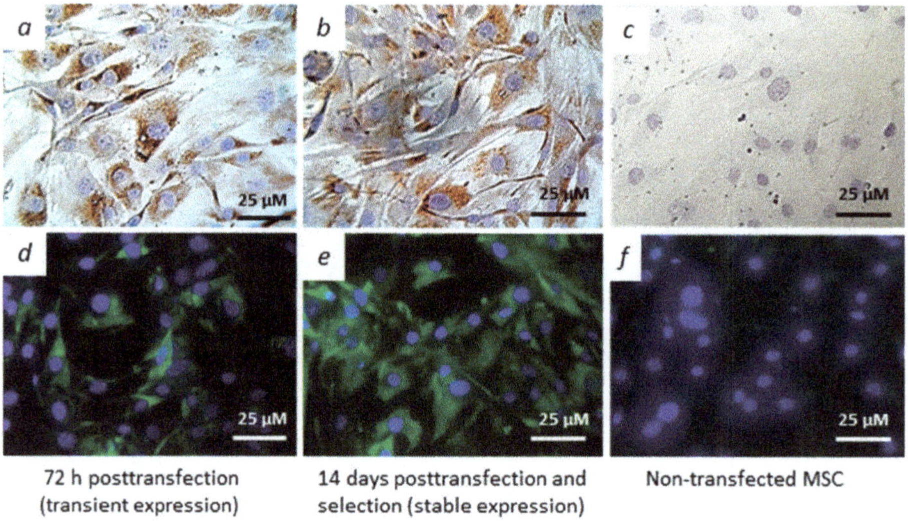

Figure 2. Immunocytochemical staining of hepatitis C virus (HCV) NS5A in MSCs transfected with pcNS3-NS5B. Primary MSC cultures at third-fourth passages were transfected with the pcNS3-NS5B plasmid and later selected with G-418. The cells were stained with monoclonal antibody against HCV NS5A using immunoperoxidase (top panel) and immunofluorescence (bottom panel) methods. NS5A is located in cytoplasm (brown or green, respectively); nuclei were stained with hematoxylin or 4′,6-diamidino-2-phenylindole (DAPI), respectively (blue). (**a**,**d**) 72 h post-transfection; (**b**,**e**) two weeks post-transfection and selection; (**c**,**f**) non-transfected MSC (scale bar, 25 μM).

3.3. Dynamics of Cytokine Production in Transfected MSCs

Next, we measured levels of cytokines IL-2, IL-6, IL-10, IL-12, IFN-γ, and TNF-α secreted by MSCs in vitro after transfection of cells with pcNS3-NS5B and sequential selection using G-418. The nontransfected MSCs secreted three cytokines: IFN-γ, IL-2, and IL-6, whereas the other cytokines were not detected in the conditioned medium. The concentration of IFN-γ increased up to the third day post-transfection, and then gradually decreased until the limit of detection at day 15 (end of cell selection) (Figure 3a). Different kinetics was observed in the case of IL-2: after an initial decrease in its level at day 3, its levels were increased at days 6–9 with a second decrease afterwards (Figure 3b). On the contrary, secretion of IL-6 was significantly increased during the entire observation period and exceeded by eightfold at day 15th the levels in the case of the untransfected MSCs (Figure 3c).

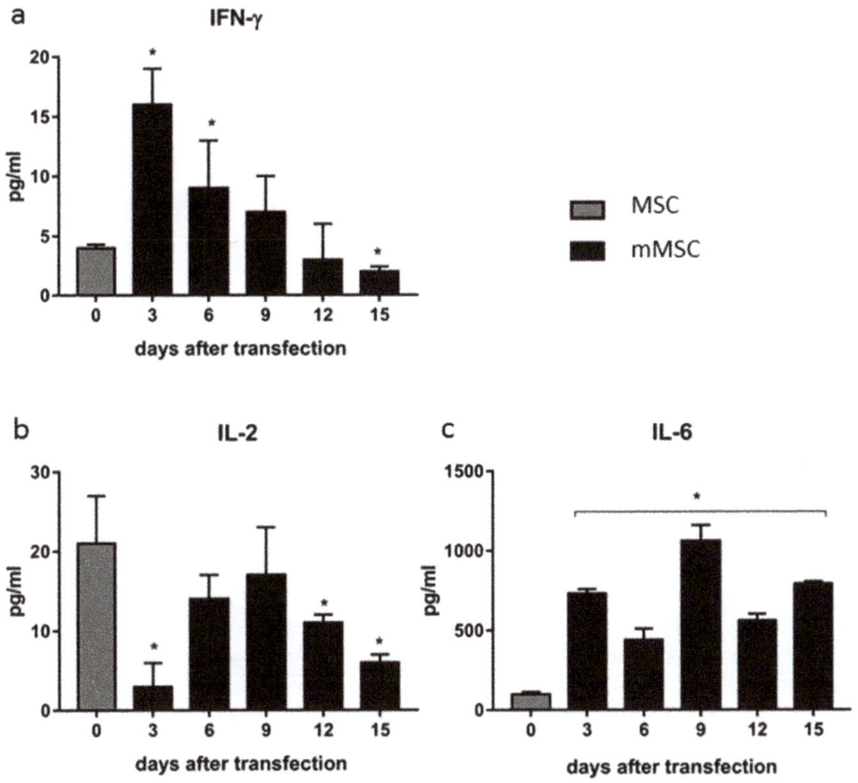

Figure 3. Levels of cytokines secreted by MSC in vitro after transfection with pcNS3-NS5B. The MSCs were transfected with pcNS3-NS5B, selected with G-418 for two weeks with changing medium every three days, and cytokine levels were quantified in a conditioned medium. The concentrations of IFN-γ (**a**), IL-2 (**b**), and IL-6 (**c**) are expressed in pg/ml. Values on each diagram are means ± SD of four measurements done in three independent experiments, * $p < 0.05$ compared to the non-transfected MSC (gray bars).

3.4. Immune Response to Administration of Modified MSCs to Mice Exceeds Immune Response to Plasmid

Our next goal was to evaluate the immune response in mice immunized with the mMSC. Comparative analysis of the humoral immune response in mice showed that mMSC (group 1) induced the formation of antibodies to all viral proteins encoded by the plasmid. Levels of antibodies to NS3, NS4, and NS5A were on average 40-fold higher than in group 3 (immunized with the pNS3-NS5B plasmid) (Table 1). In contrast, levels of antibodies to NS5B were higher in mice immunized with the plasmid than with mMSC (Table 1). The distribution of antibody isotypes for HCV proteins differed between the groups: in groups 1 and 3, the antibodies belonged mainly to the IgG2a isotype; in group 1, IgG1 antibodies to the NS3 protein were also detected. After introduction of naïve MSCs (group 2), IgG2a antibodies were not found, while IgG1 antibodies were detected in only four out of ten mice and were present at a low level. Therefore, differences with the control were not statistically significant.

Table 1. The levels of anti-HCV antibodies in the sera of mice receiving two injections of mMSC, MSC, or plasmid.

HCV Proteins	Group 1 mMSC		Group 2 MSC		Group 3 pcNS3-NS5B		Group 4 Control	
	IgG1	IgG2a	IgG1	IgG2a	IgG1	IgG2a	IgG1	IgG2a
NS3	200 ± 34 # (4/10)	410 ± 27 # (10/10)	20 ± 14 (2/10)	<10 (0/10)	<10 (0/10)	10 (0/10)	<10 (0/10)	<10 (0/10)
NS4	<10 (0/10)	1600 ± 24 # (10/10)	80 ± 63 (4/10)	<10 (0/10)	90 ± 64 (2/10)	40 ± 12 * (9/10)	<10 (0/10)	<10 (0/10)
NS5A	<10 (0/10)	40 ± 7 # (9/10)	10 ± 15 (1/10)	<10 (0/10)	<10 (0/10)	<10 (0/10)	<10 (0/10)	<10 (0/10)
NS5B	<10 (0/10)	80 ± 12 * (10/10)	60 ± 42 (4/10)	<10 (0/10)	<10 (0/10)	249 ± 61 # (10/10)	<10 (0/10)	<10 (0/10)

Four pools of recombinant HCV proteins (described in Materials and Methods) were used as sorbents in ELISA to evaluate antibody production; IgG1 and IgG2a are antibody isotypes. Values show the geometric mean titer ± SD of three measurements done from three independent experiments. * $p < 0.05$ compared to control; # $p < 0.05$ compared to all groups. Numbers of animals in each group that developed antibodies to the HCV proteins to the total numbers of animals are given in brackets.

To assess the cellular response of lymphocytes in vitro, we used recombinant proteins from the HCV non-structural region as specific stimulants. For a negative control, we also assessed the response to the core protein that was not encoded by the pNS3-NS5B plasmid and in mMSCs. For a positive control, ConA was used for stimulation.

All tested non-structural HCV proteins stimulated proliferation of splenocytes in groups 1 and 3, SIs statistically significantly ($p < 0.05$) differed from SIs in groups 2 and 4 (Figure 4a). In group 1, SIs exceeded those in group 3 by 2.5–6.1 times, on average by 4.2 ± 1.6 times. The greatest proliferative response was caused by NS5B, when SI reached 27.

Stimulated lymphocytes secreted IFN-γ (Figure 4b). In group 1, the response was obtained to all specific antigens; the highest cytokine concentration (over 1.7 ng/mL) was stimulated by NS5B. In group 3, the production of IFN-γ was induced by all proteins except NS5A; the NS4 protein showed the highest activity. In groups 1 and 3, the cytokine levels secreted in response to specific antigens varied in a wide range from 3.5 to 60-fold, being on average 30-fold higher than in the case of groups 2 and 4.

In ELISpot assay, the average number of IFN-γ synthesizing cells in response to four specific stimulants in groups 1 and 3 was significantly higher than that in the control groups (Figure 4c). Differences in signal intensity between groups 1 and 3 were 2.6 ± 0.2. The NS5B protein exhibited higher activity than other virus antigens. It should be noted that group 2, which was administered to naïve MSCs, demonstrated immune responses to HCV proteins in contrast to group 4, but their intensity was much lower than in the case of the transfected cells in group 1 (Figure 4b,c).

The ELISpot reaction was also performed with splenocytes from mice that were administered mMSC treated with IFN-γ. A number of IFN-γ producing cells in this group was 11-fold lower than those in group 1. It is noteworthy that the number of spots for NS3 was 13.3 ± 7.1%, for NS4—7.1 ± 2.6%, for NS5A—7.6 ± 1.5%, for NS5B—8.9 ± 4.2% of the corresponding values in group 1.

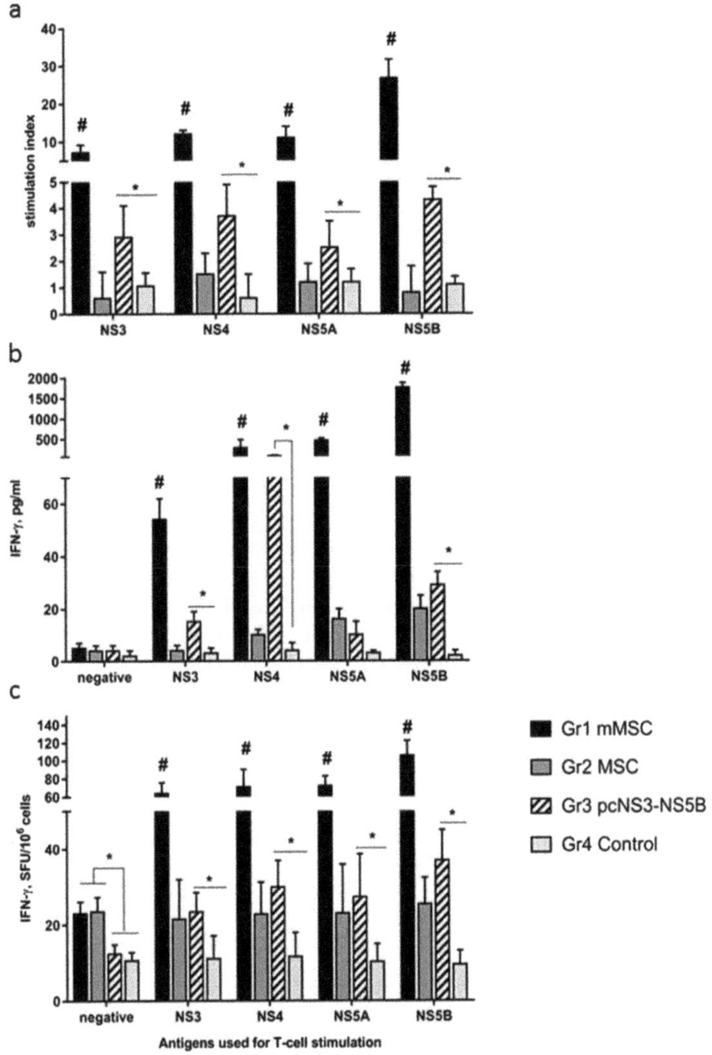

Figure 4. A comparative analysis of the cellular immune response in mice to HCV proteins in vitro after immunization with modified MSC, naïve MSC, and plasmid. Four groups (Gr) of mice were injected twice with mMSC (Gr1), non-transfected MSC (Gr2), plasmid pcNS3-NS5B (Gr3), or saline (Gr4). To assess the cellular response of lymphocytes in vitro, we used purified recombinant proteins from the non-structural region of HCV, which were combined into four pools (NS3, NS4, NS5A, and NS5B). A recombinant HCV core and medium alone were used as negative controls (negative). (**a**) Results of T-cell proliferation are expressed as stimulation indexes (SI); the IFN-γ production by splenocytes in response to HCV antigens was assayed as cytokine concentrations in culture fluids by ELISA, expressed as pg/ml (**b**), or as the number of IFN-γ synthesizing cells by ELISpot in the number of spot forming cells (SFC) per 10^6 cells (**c**). Values on each diagram are means ± SD of three measurements done in three independent experiments. * $p < 0.05$ compared to control; # $p < 0.05$ compared to all groups.

Assessment of the results of T-cell proliferation and ELISpot assays showed that mouse groups 1 and 2, which received MSCs, had a higher level of spontaneous cellular response as well as the response to ConA, compared to groups 3 and 4 ($p < 0.05$, Table 2). Differences in IFN-γ production during ConA stimulation between groups were not statistically significant.

Table 2. Spontaneous and concanavalin A (ConA)-induced cellular response of lymphocytes from immunized mice in vitro.

Assay	Stimulant	Group 1 mMSC	Group 2 MSC	Group 3 pcNS3-NS5B	Group 4 Control
T-cell proliferation (SI)	ConA	320 ± 22	311 ± 26	348 ± 79	240 ± 17
T-cell proliferation (c.p.m.)	medium	164 ± 46 *	273 ± 84 *	73 ± 15	65 ± 9
	ConA	52406 ± 10014 *	84933 ± 15010 *	25432 ± 12031	15602 ± 7025
ELISA, IFN-γ secretion (pg/mL)	medium	5 ± 2	4 ± 2	4 ± 2	2 ± 2
	ConA	1108 ± 242	1336 ± 380	954 ± 314	902 ± 143
ELISpot, IFN-γ synthesis (SFC/10^6 cells)	medium	23.0 ± 3.1*	23.5 ± 3.8*	12.4 ± 2.4	10.6 ± 2.2
	ConA	2400 ± 350*	2250 ± 407*	1200 ± 210	750 ± 156

Values are means ± SD of three measurements done in three independent experiments. * $p < 0.05$ compared to Gr3 and Gr4.

3.5. Decrease in Proportion of Myeloid Derived Suppressor Cells in Spleens of Mice Immunized with MSCs

Using flow cytometry, we compared the number of splenocytes from immunized mice that express CD11b+Gr-1+ markers of MDSCs and do not express CD11c marker of dendritic cells (DC) (Figure 5a). An almost twofold decrease in the relative content of MDSCs in groups 1 and 2 compared with groups 3 and 4 was found ($p = 0.007$ and 0.015, respectively) (Figure 5b). The content of CD11c+ dendritic cells varied from 6.3 to 7.5% and did not differ between groups (results not shown, $p > 0.05$). The lowest MDSCs to dendritic cells ratio was observed in the spleens of mice of group 1 ($p = 0.003$ compare to control) (Figure 5c).

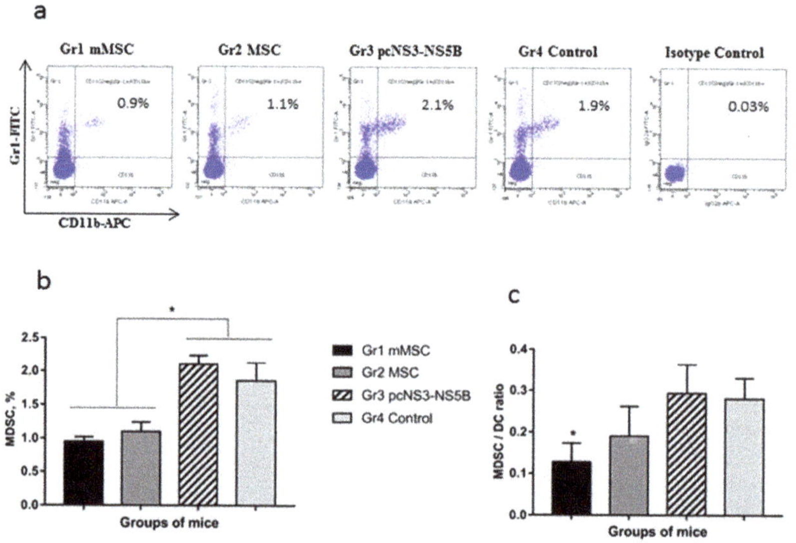

Figure 5. A comparative analysis of the proportion of myeloid derived suppressor cells in spleens of immunized mice. Splenocytes from the immunized mice were stained with anti-CD11c, anti-CD11b, and anti-Gr1 antibodies and analyzed by flow cytometry. Representative dot plots (**a**) and mean values (**b**) of the number of MDSC expressing CD11b and Gr1, and negative for the marker of DC (CD11c) are shown, in the percentages; (**c**) the MDSCs to dendritic cells (DC) ratio. Values on each diagram are means ± SD of three independent analysis, and each of them was performed in triplicate. * $p < 0.05$ compared to Gr3 and Gr4 (**b**) or compared to the control Gr4 (**c**).

3.6. *Changes in Activity of IFN-α/β and in Phagocytic Activity of Immune Cells of Immunized Mice*

Next, the biological activity of type I IFNs and the phagocytic activity of leukocytes in groups of the immunized mice were studied. Activity of type I IFNs was evaluated by measuring relative production of IFN-α/β in response to stimulation of leukocytes by the Newcastle disease virus. There was no statistically significant difference in the production of IFN-α/β by peripheral blood cells between the groups. Mouse splenocytes more actively produced type I IFNs; the highest production was found in group 1, whereas the smallest was in group 3 (Figure 6a).

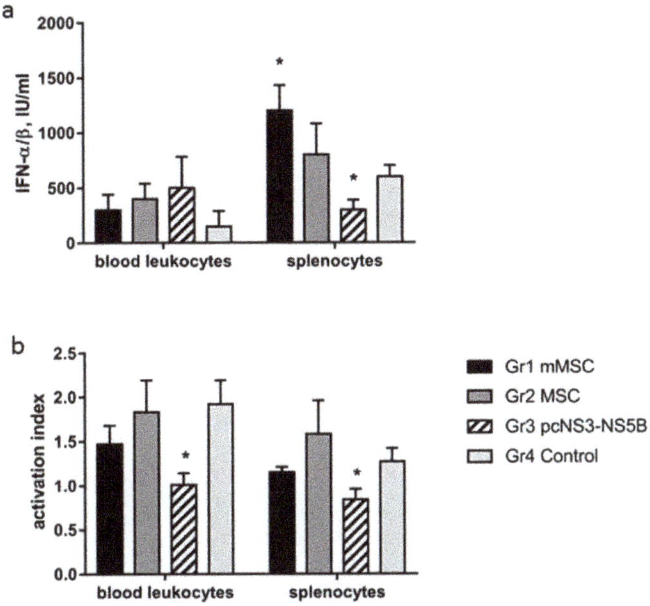

Figure 6. The differences in the biological activity of type I IFNs and phagocytic activity of peripheral blood leukocytes and splenocytes from immunized mice. (**a**) The activity of type I IFNs was evaluated by the production of IFN-α/β in response to stimulation of leukocytes by the Newcastle disease virus in vitro and was expressed in IU/ml; (**b**) phagocytic activity of immune cells was determined by luminol-dependent chemiluminescence (CL) and was expressed as activation index—the ratio of the intensity of induced CL to the intensity of spontaneous CL. The values on each diagram are means ± SD of six measurements done in three independent experiments. * $p < 0.05$ compared to control group 4.

Phagocytic activity between the groups was compared by quantification of the production of reactive oxygen species (ROS), determined by luminol-dependent chemiluminescence (CL). For analysis, we used a suspension of splenocytes and a leukocyte preparation from heparinized whole blood. The activation index (AI) was reduced in the blood and in splenocytes of group 3 mice (Figure 6b) due to an increase in the level of spontaneous CL and a decrease in induced CL. Spontaneous CL shows the level of ROS production by cells, and an excessive increase in CL could be associated with a hazardous effect of ROS towards the cells. Induced CL reflects a potential ability of cells to respond to stimuli. The inability of immune cells to stimulate CL (AI ≤ 1) can point to inhibition of the bactericidal activity of phagocytes upon immunization with a plasmid. In the remaining experimental groups, the AI values were >1 and did not differ from the control group.

4. Discussion

Advances in cell therapy in recent years are associated with the use of the immunosuppressive properties of MSCs in transplantology, oncology, and some other areas of medicine, although many issues remain unresolved [46]. Depending on the microenvironment, MSCs can exhibit both immunosuppressive and immunostimulating properties [47,48]. However, the mechanisms of stimulation of the immune response by MSCs remain vague and have been studied mostly in vitro in mixed leukocyte reactions (MLR) [47,49].

To date there are only two papers investigating immune response to MSCs that express viral proteins. The first one describes the cells that express human immunodeficiency virus (HIV) Gp120 [11]. The second, recently published by Bolhassani et al. (2019) showed immunization of mice by mMSC that express E7 protein of human papillomavirus (HPV E7 antigen) in a complex with small heat shock proteins leads to a strong T-cell immune response and to a partial protection of animals against HPV-induced tumors [50]. Our data present a first evidence that modified MSCs (mMSCs) expressing HCV proteins affect innate and adaptive immune responses in mice. The experimental data show that the administration of naïve or modified MSCs to mice increases both spontaneous and ConA-induced levels of lymphocyte proliferation. Assessment of the proliferative response to mitogens is one of the most universal tests to assess the lymphocyte function; a weak reaction indicates the failure of cellular immunity. The functional activity of activated lymphocytes (production of IFN-γ) increased. The biological activity of IFN-α/β increased, as established in the test with the inhibition of the cytopathogenic effect of the encephalomyocarditis virus. Type I IFNs are known to play an important immunoregulatory role in relation to both the innate and adaptive immune responses to viral infections. For example, IFN-α/β induces the cytotoxicity of NK cells and increases the expression of MHC class I and co-stimulating molecules on antigen-presenting cells (APCs) [51]. A comparison of the effectiveness of these parameters of the innate immune response to mMSC with the response to immunization with a DNA construct shows that in the latter case the immune cells induce IFN-α/β and IFN-γ at a lower level. When mice were immunized with DNA, the phagocytic activities of monocytes/macrophages, neutrophils and dendritic cells decreased as well. In contrast, the functions of phagocytic cells during immunization with MSCs and mMSCs remained at the level of healthy intact mice.

The adaptive immune response to mMSCs was also significantly higher than that to the plasmid. For instance, mMSC induced a humoral response to all viral proteins expressed in MSCs. Almost all antibodies to non-structural HCV proteins were of IgG2a isotype. Switching to the synthesis of IgG2a antibodies is controlled by the Th1 cellular component of the immune response: a correlation between the level of IgG2a, virus-neutralizing properties, and IFN-γ synthesis has been established [52,53]. The DNA construct also caused the formation of IgG2a antibodies, but their activity was less than that in response to modified MSCs. The most significant difference in antibody titers (40-fold) was found in response to HCV NS3 and NS4 proteins. It should be noted that in combination with the gene adjuvant, pcGM-CSF plasmid, the pcNS3-NS5B construct induced a more active formation of IgG2a antibodies [30]. The immunomodulatory orientation of MSCs with respect to the B-cell response has been suggested to depend on the level of stimulation with viral antigens: the weaker the signal, the greater the stimulating potencies of MSCs [54]. A high level of IL-6 produced by mMSC can stimulate an active humoral response to HCV: this cytokine has been shown to be necessary for differentiation of B cells and secretion of immunoglobulins [54,55].

Production of IgG1 antibodies against HCV was detected in groups immunized with the non-transfected MSCs; however, these antibodies were detected sporadically and with low activity. This may be caused by a cross-reaction between the recombinant proteins obtained in the bacterial system and the antibacterial antibodies in the blood sera of mice.

We characterized the cellular response by the proliferation of lymphocytes and their functional activity—secretion and intracellular content of IFN-γ. These methods are considered as the most informative by a majority of authors [17]. The cellular immune response to the modified MSC significantly exceeded the response to the plasmid pcNS3-NS5B in the proliferative response to the

HCV sequence, as well as in the synthesis and secretion of IFN-γ. Differences in the signal intensity between groups 1 and 3 were 2.6–4.2 times in T-cell proliferation and ELISpot and up to 30 times in ELISA when determining the concentrations of produced IFN-γ. All non-structural HCV proteins elicited a cellular response; the maximum response was observed for NS5B. This protein is an RNA-dependent RNA polymerase, the key component of HCV replicase. NS5B is a target for direct-acting antivirals in the treatment of hepatitis C [56]; NS5B has the largest number of conserved T-cell epitopes that are important for vaccine design and induction of an effective immune response [57]. Thus, when immunizing with mMSCs, we achieve a functionally active T-cell response to several HCV proteins simultaneously, including different genotypes. This result is very important as an HCV vaccine should elicit multiantigenic, multigenotypic responses that should protect against challenge with the range of genotypes and subtypes circulating in the community [29]. We also hope that usage of more conserved viral proteins (i.e. nonstructural) will allow induction of a pangenotype response.

One of the mechanisms of the suppressor action of MSCs on the adaptive immune response in inflammation and cancer is believed to be their inhibition of maturation of antigen-presenting dendritic cells under the action of various soluble factors - TGF-β, IL-10, NO, and PD-1 [48]. We showed that when immunizing healthy animals in all experimental groups, the number of dendritic cells did not change compared to the control.

A very interesting fact is the data that immunization with MSCs and mMSC causes a twofold decrease in the number of MDSCs, a heterogeneous population of immature myeloid cells with a powerful suppressor potential. This phenomenon for immunization with MSCs is described for the first time. The role of MDSCs in viral infections has not been adequately studied [58]. In patients infected with HCV, an increase in the MDSC population is observed; these cells inhibit the proliferation of $CD4^+$ and $CD8^+$ lymphocytes, NK cells, and IFN-γ production [59,60]. Similar results have been obtained in the study of cells from patients with HIV and hepatitis B infections [61,62]. Most experimental data show that the administration of MSCs in oncological and autoimmune diseases results in MDSC accumulation and immunosuppression mediated by certain chemokines and growth factors [63–65]. On the other hand, when modeling cancer in mice, a dependence of the immunomodulatory "phenotype" of MSCs on the injection site was found: the simultaneous injection of MSCs with tumor cells led to immunosuppression, distal injection led to immunostimulation; the immune response was shown to correlate with a decrease in the proportion of MDSCs and T-regulatory cells (Treg) [66]. Thus, one of the mechanisms of stimulation of the innate and adaptive immune response to naïve and modified MSCs in our experiments may be the suppression of MDSCs.

During inflammation, the immunosuppressive properties of MSCs are manifested: they suppress both innate and adaptive immunity, weakening the maturation and ability to present antigens by dendritic cells, inducing the polarization of macrophages in the direction of the alternative phenotype, inhibiting the activation and proliferation of T and B lymphocytes and reducing the cytotoxicity of NK cells [48]. We administered MSCs to healthy mice. On the one hand, the biological properties of MSCs depend on the microenvironment; on the other hand, the immunomodulating effect of MSCs themselves is mediated by the secretion of various soluble factors. We compared the production of several cytokines by naïve and modified MSCs in vitro. It turned out that the expression of HCV proteins influenced the production of at least three pro-inflammatory cytokines - IFN-γ, IL-2, and IL-6. For example, after two weeks of cultivation of transfected cultures of MSCs in the presence of G-418, the concentrations of secreted cytokines IFN-γ and IL-2 decreased by 2–3.5 times, and that of IL-6 increased by eight times compared with MSCs. These stably transfected cells were injected into mice. Interestingly, the accumulation of IL-6 leads to the activation of the pro-inflammatory phenotype of the MSC population—MSC-1 [47] and promotes the formation of Th17 cells that activate the immune response [67]. Most likely, fluctuations in cytokine production are associated with the action of viral proteins on cell metabolism but not with changes in MSCs epigenetics because mesenchymal cells have been shown to maintain the genetic stability for at least seven to nine passages [68]. The spectrum of cytokines that are produced by cells transfected with HCV genes has been previously found to change with time, depending on the type of cells and specific viral proteins [69–71].

The data on the effect of exogenous IFN-γ on MSCs are contradictory. Several authors have noted an increase in the antigen-presenting properties of MSCs as a result of IFN-γ pretreatment [72]. Other studies have shown that the "priming" of MSCs in vitro with IFN-γ, TNF-α, or IL-1β leads to the formation of the immunosuppressive phenotype MSC-2 [47,73,74]. Our results showed, for the first time, that after administration in mice, modified MSCs treated with IFN-γ cause a pronounced (tenfold) decrease in the cellular response. This means that an excessive concentration of pro-inflammatory cytokines does not stimulate, but instead inhibits the immune response to antigens presented by MSCs.

The major technique that is recommended for evaluation of T-cell response to novel HCV vaccines is quantification of IFN-γ production by ELISpot assay that shows activity of antiviral response [19,75,76]. Though we have not shown protection against HCV infection using mMSCs, such experiments could be performed in future using the respective models. So, we consider our results as a basis for subsequent preclinical (and clinical) studies of protective effect of mMSCs in future. Human mMSCs that express non-structural HCV proteins could be evaluated as a prophylactic vaccine that triggers a strong T-cell response. A growing trend in human MSC clinical trials is the use of allogenic and culture-expanded cells [1]. Application of mMSC to chronic hepatitis C patients may enhance therapeutic response to direct acting antivirals (DAA) via enhanced T-cell immune response that can clear the infected cells. Studies of a combined usage of various candidate HCV vaccines and antiviral agents including DAA are one of the current trends in the field (as can be exemplified by [77,78]. Despite the fact that the results do not always show enhanced clearance of the infection, this approach is still considered promising [19,79,80].

5. Conclusions

Thus, for the first time, we demonstrated the feasibility of using modified MSCs expressing non-structural HCV proteins as a platform for creating an effective vaccine against hepatitis C. The mMSC induced a higher innate and adaptive immune response than DNA immunization with the same plasmid. The immunostimulating phenotype of these cells is associated with a high level of IL-6 secretion and a reduction in the proportion of myeloid-derived suppressor cells.

Supplementary Materials: The following are available online at http://www.mdpi.com/2076-393X/8/1/62/s1, Figure S1: Immunohistochemical staining of HCV proteins in MSC transfected with pcNS3-NS5B, Figure S2: Immunoblot analysis of HCV protein expression in MSC transfected with pcNS3-NS5B.

Author Contributions: Conceptualization, O.V.M. and A.A.K.; methodology, O.V.M., R.R.K., A.N.N., A.V.P., and A.A.K.; investigation, O.V.M., E.I.L., R.R.K., E.D.M., V.V.K., A.M.I., N.F.Z., O.V.P., N.N.B.; resources, A.N.N., A.V.P., and A.V.I.; data curation, O.V.M. and A.A.K.; writing—original draft preparation, O.V.M., R.R.K., O.V.P., A.N.N., A.V.I., and A.A.K.; writing—review and editing, O.V.M., A.N.N., A.V.I., and A.A.K.; visualization, O.V.M. and A.A.K.; project administration, O.V.M.; funding acquisition, O.V.M. and A.V.I. All authors have read and agreed to the published version of the manuscript.

Funding: This research was funded by the Russian Foundation for Basic Research (grants 17-04-01238 and 17-00-00085). Genetic engineering and production of recombinant proteins were supported by Ministry of Science and Higher Education of the Russian Federation [Agreement No. 075-15-2019-1660].

Conflicts of Interest: The authors declare no conflict of interest.

References

1. Yuan, X.; Logan, T.M.; Ma, T. Metabolism in human mesenchymal stromal cells: A missing link between hmsc biomanufacturing and therapy? *Front. Immunol.* **2019**, *10*, 977. [CrossRef]
2. Dameshghi, S.; Zavaran-Hosseini, A.; Soudi, S.; Shirazi, F.J.; Nojehdehi, S.; Hashemi, S.M. Mesenchymal stem cells alter macrophage immune responses to leishmania major infection in both susceptible and resistance mice. *Immunol. Lett.* **2016**, *170*, 15–26. [CrossRef] [PubMed]

3. Goodarzi, P.; Larijani, B.; Alavi-Moghadam, S.; Tayanloo-Beik, A.; Mohamadi-Jahani, F.; Ranjbaran, N.; Payab, M.; Falahzadeh, K.; Mousavi, M.; Arjmand, B. Mesenchymal stem cells-derived exosomes for wound regeneration. *Adv. Exp. Med. Biol.* **2018**, *1119*, 119–131.
4. Lukashyk, S.P.; Tsyrkunov, V.M.; Isaykina, Y.I.; Romanova, O.N.; Shymanskiy, A.T.; Aleynikova, O.V.; Kravchuk, R.I. Mesenchymal bone marrow-derived stem cells transplantation in patients with HCV related liver cirrhosis. *J. Clin. Transl. Hepatol.* **2014**, *2*, 217–221. [PubMed]
5. Munir, H.; McGettrick, H.M. Mesenchymal stem cell therapy for autoimmune disease: Risks and rewards. *Stem Cells Dev.* **2015**, *24*, 2091–2100. [CrossRef] [PubMed]
6. Cobo, M.; Anderson, P.; Benabdellah, K.; Toscano, M.G.; Munoz, P.; Garcia-Perez, A.; Gutierrez, I.; Delgado, M.; Martin, F. Mesenchymal stem cells expressing vasoactive intestinal peptide ameliorate symptoms in a model of chronic multiple sclerosis. *Cell Transp.* **2013**, *22*, 839–854. [CrossRef] [PubMed]
7. Wyse, R.D.; Dunbar, G.L.; Rossignol, J. Use of genetically modified mesenchymal stem cells to treat neurodegenerative diseases. *Int. J. Mol. Sci.* **2014**, *15*, 1719–1745. [CrossRef]
8. Marin-Banasco, C.; Benabdellah, K.; Melero-Jerez, C.; Oliver, B.; Pinto-Medel, M.J.; Hurtado-Guerrero, I.; de Castro, F.; Clemente, D.; Fernandez, O.; Martin, F.; et al. Gene therapy with mesenchymal stem cells expressing ifn-ss ameliorates neuroinflammation in experimental models of multiple sclerosis. *Br. J. Pharmacol.* **2017**, *174*, 238–253. [CrossRef]
9. Xue, X.; Liu, Y.; Zhang, J.; Liu, T.; Yang, Z.; Wang, H. BCL-XL genetic modification enhanced the therapeutic efficacy of mesenchymal stem cell transplantation in the treatment of heart infarction. *Stem Cells Int.* **2015**, *2015*, 176409. [CrossRef]
10. Haber, T.; Baruch, L.; Machluf, M. Ultrasound-mediated mesenchymal stem cells transfection as a targeted cancer therapy platform. *Sci. Rep.* **2017**, *7*, 42046. [CrossRef]
11. Tomchuck, S.L.; Norton, E.B.; Garry, R.F.; Bunnell, B.A.; Morris, C.A.; Freytag, L.C.; Clements, J.D. Mesenchymal stem cells as a novel vaccine platform. *Front. Cell. Infect. Microbiol.* **2012**, *2*, 140. [CrossRef] [PubMed]
12. Park, S.H.; Rehermann, B. Immune responses to hcv and other hepatitis viruses. *Immunity* **2014**, *40*, 13–24. [CrossRef] [PubMed]
13. Dustin, L.B. Innate and adaptive immune responses in chronic HCV infection. *Curr. Drug Targets* **2017**, *18*, 826–843. [CrossRef] [PubMed]
14. Pawlotsky, J.M. Hepatitis C virus: Standard-of-care treatment. *Adv. Pharmacol.* **2013**, *67*, 169–215.
15. Spearman, C.W.; Dusheiko, G.M.; Hellard, M.; Sonderup, M. Hepatitis C. *Lancet* **2019**, *394*, 1451–1466. [CrossRef]
16. Wang, Y.; Rao, H.; Chi, X.; Li, B.; Liu, H.; Wu, L.; Zhang, H.; Liu, S.; Zhou, G.; Li, N.; et al. Detection of residual HCV-RNA in patients who have achieved sustained virological response is associated with persistent histological abnormality. *EBioMedicine* **2019**, *46*, 227–235. [CrossRef]
17. Elmasry, S.; Wadhwa, S.; Bang, B.R.; Cook, L.; Chopra, S.; Kanel, G.; Kim, B.; Harper, T.; Feng, Z.; Jerome, K.R.; et al. Detection of occult hepatitis C virus infection in patients who achieved a sustained virologic response to direct-acting antiviral agents for recurrent infection after liver transplantation. *Gastroenterology* **2017**, *152*, 550–553. [CrossRef]
18. Di Lorenzo, C.; Angus, A.G.; Patel, A.H. Hepatitis C virus evasion mechanisms from neutralizing antibodies. *Viruses* **2011**, *3*, 2280–2300. [CrossRef]
19. Ahlen, G.; Frelin, L. Methods to evaluate novel hepatitis C virus vaccines. *Methods Mol. Biol.* **2016**, *1403*, 221–244.
20. Verma, R.; Khanna, P.; Chawla, S. Hepatitis C vaccine. Need of the hour. *Hum. Vaccin. Immunother.* **2014**, *10*, 1927–1929. [CrossRef]
21. Garcia, A.; Fernandez, S.; Toro, F.; De Sanctis, J.B. An overview of hepatitis C vaccines. *Recent Pat. Inflamm. Allergy Drug Discov.* **2014**, *8*, 85–91. [CrossRef] [PubMed]
22. Wintermeyer, P.; Gehring, S.; Eken, A.; Wands, J.R. Generation of cellular immune responses to HCV ns5 protein through in vivo activation of dendritic cells. *J. Viral Hepat.* **2010**, *17*, 705–713. [CrossRef]
23. Yu, H.; Babiuk, L.A.; van Drunen Littel-van den Hurk, S. Strategies for loading dendritic cells with hepatitis c ns5a antigen and inducing protective immunity. *J. Viral Hepat.* **2008**, *15*, 459–470. [CrossRef] [PubMed]
24. Zhou, Y.; Zhang, Y.; Yao, Z.; Moorman, J.P.; Jia, Z. Dendritic cell-based immunity and vaccination against hepatitis C virus infection. *Immunology* **2012**, *136*, 385–396. [CrossRef] [PubMed]

25. Chernykh, E.; Leplina, O.; Oleynik, E.; Tikhonova, M.; Tyrinova, T.; Starostina, N.; Ostanin, A. Immunotherapy with interferon-alpha-induced dendritic cells for chronic hcv infection (the results of pilot clinical trial). *Immunol. Res.* **2018**, *66*, 31–43. [CrossRef]
26. Zabaleta, A.; D'Avola, D.; Echeverria, I.; Llopiz, D.; Silva, L.; Villanueva, L.; Riezu-Boj, J.I.; Larrea, E.; Pereboev, A.; Lasarte, J.J.; et al. Clinical testing of a dendritic cell targeted therapeutic vaccine in patients with chronic hepatitis c virus infection. *Mol. Ther. Methods Clin. Dev.* **2015**, *2*, 15006. [CrossRef]
27. Bailey, J.R.; Barnes, E.; Cox, A.L. Approaches, progress, and challenges to hepatitis C vaccine development. *Gastroenterology* **2019**, *156*, 418–430. [CrossRef]
28. Thimme, R.; Oldach, D.; Chang, K.M.; Steiger, C.; Ray, S.C.; Chisari, F.V. Determinants of viral clearance and persistence during acute hepatitis C virus infection. *J. Exp. Med.* **2001**, *194*, 1395–1406. [CrossRef]
29. Wijesundara, D.K.; Gummow, J.; Li, Y.; Yu, W.; Quah, B.J.; Ranasinghe, C.; Torresi, J.; Gowans, E.J.; Grubor-Bauk, B. Induction of genotype cross-reactive, hepatitis C virus-specific, cell-mediated immunity in DNA-vaccinated mice. *J. Virol.* **2018**, *92*. [CrossRef]
30. Masalova, O.V.; Lesnova, E.I.; Ivanov, A.V.; Pichugin, A.V.; Permiakova, K.; Smirnova, O.A.; Tynitskaia, V.L.; Ulanova, T.I.; Burkov, A.N.; Kochetkov, S.N.; et al. Comparative analysis of the immune response to DNA constructions encoding hepatitis c virus nonstructural proteins. *Vopr. Virusol.* **2013**, *58*, 21–28.
31. Tolosa, L.; Donato, M.T.; Gomez-Lechon, M.J. General cytotoxicity assessment by means of the MTT assay. *Methods Mol. Biol.* **2015**, *1250*, 333–348. [PubMed]
32. Schlueter, N.; Lussi, A.; Ganss, C.; Gruber, R. L929 fibroblast bioassay on the in vitro toxicity of SNCL2, h3po4, clearfil se primer and combinations thereof. *Swiss Dent. J.* **2016**, *126*, 566–572. [PubMed]
33. Rechkina, E.A.; Denisova, G.F.; Masalova, O.V.; Lideman, L.F.; Denisov, D.A.; Lesnova, E.I.; Ataullakhanov, R.I.; Gur'ianova, S.V.; Kushch, A.A. Epitope mapping of antigenic determinants of hepatitis C virus proteins by phage display. *Mol. Biol. (Mosk)* **2006**, *40*, 312–323. [CrossRef]
34. Masalova, O.V.; Lesnova, E.I.; Solyev, P.N.; Zakirova, N.F.; Prassolov, V.S.; Kochetkov, S.N.; Ivanov, A.V.; Kushch, A.A. Modulation of cell death pathways by hepatitis C virus proteins in huh7.5 hepatoma cells. *Int. J. Mol. Sci.* **2017**, *18*, 2346. [CrossRef] [PubMed]
35. Masalova, O.V.; Lesnova, E.I.; Pichugin, A.V.; Melnikova, T.M.; Grabovetsky, V.V.; Petrakova, N.V.; Smirnova, O.A.; Ivanov, A.V.; Zaberezhny, A.D.; Ataullakhanov, R.I.; et al. The successful immune response against hepatitis C nonstructural protein 5a (ns5a) requires heterologous DNA/protein immunization. *Vaccine* **2010**, *28*, 1987–1996. [CrossRef]
36. Ivanov, A.V.; Smirnova, O.A.; Ivanova, O.N.; Masalova, O.V.; Kochetkov, S.N.; Isaguliants, M.G. Hepatitis C virus proteins activate nrf2/are pathway by distinct ROS-dependent and independent mechanisms in huh7 cells. *PLoS ONE* **2011**, *6*, e24957. [CrossRef] [PubMed]
37. Mukovnya, A.V.; Tunitskaya, V.L.; Khandazhinskaya, A.L.; Golubeva, N.A.; Zakirova, N.F.; Ivanov, A.V.; Kukhanova, M.K.; Kochetkov, S.N. Hepatitis C virus helicase/ntpase: An efficient expression system and new inhibitors. *Biochemistry (Moscow)* **2008**, *73*, 660–668. [CrossRef]
38. Ivanov, A.V.; Korovina, A.N.; Tunitskaya, V.L.; Kostyuk, D.A.; Rechinsky, V.O.; Kukhanova, M.K.; Kochetkov, S.N. Development of the system ensuring a high-level expression of hepatitis C virus nonstructural ns5b and ns5a proteins. *Protein Expr. Purif.* **2006**, *48*, 14–23. [CrossRef]
39. Ulanova, T.I.; Puzyrev, V.F.; Burkov, A.N.; Obriadina, A.P. Impact of the heterogenicity of amino acid sequence on the immunoreactivity of an antigenic epitopic complex localized within amino acids 1192-1456 of protein ns3 protein of hepatitis c virus. *Vopr. Virusol.* **2006**, *51*, 28–30.
40. Babaiants, A.A.; Manakhova, L.S.; Karganova, G.G.; Porkhovatyi, S.; Kondratenko, I.V. Leukocyte interferon reaction in patients with primary immunodeficiencies. *Vopr. Virusol.* **1985**, *30*, 714–717.
41. Vlaspolder, F.; Donkers, E.; Harmsen, T.; Kraaijeveld, C.A.; Snippe, H. Rapid bioassay of human interferon by direct enzyme immunoassay of encephalomyocarditis virus in hep-2 cell monolayers after a single cycle of infection. *J. Virol. Methods* **1989**, *24*, 153–158. [CrossRef]
42. Fournier, P.; Wilden, H.; Schirrmacher, V. Importance of retinoic acid-inducible gene I and of receptor for type I interferon for cellular resistance to infection by newcastle disease virus. *Int. J. Oncol.* **2012**, *40*, 287–298. [PubMed]
43. Stewart, W.E., II. *The Interferon System*; Springer-Verlag: New York, NY, USA, 1979.

44. Hasegawa, H.; Suzuki, K.; Nakaji, S.; Sugawara, K. Analysis and assessment of the capacity of neutrophils to produce reactive oxygen species in a 96-well microplate format using lucigenin- and luminol-dependent chemiluminescence. *J. Immunol. Methods* **1997**, *210*, 1–10. [CrossRef]
45. Dominici, M.; Le Blanc, K.; Mueller, I.; Slaper-Cortenbach, I.; Marini, F.; Krause, D.; Deans, R.; Keating, A.; Prockop, D.; Horwitz, E. Minimal criteria for defining multipotent mesenchymal stromal cells. The international society for cellular therapy position statement. *Cytotherapy* **2006**, *8*, 315–317. [CrossRef]
46. Zhao, L.; Chen, S.; Yang, P.; Cao, H.; Li, L. The role of mesenchymal stem cells in hematopoietic stem cell transplantation: Prevention and treatment of graft-versus-host disease. *Stem Cell Res. Ther.* **2019**, *10*, 182. [CrossRef]
47. Rivera-Cruz, C.M.; Shearer, J.J.; Figueiredo Neto, M.; Figueiredo, M.L. The immunomodulatory effects of mesenchymal stem cell polarization within the tumor microenvironment niche. *Stem Cells Int.* **2017**, *2017*, 4015039. [CrossRef]
48. Volarevic, V.; Gazdic, M.; Simovic Markovic, B.; Jovicic, N.; Djonov, V.; Arsenijevic, N. Mesenchymal stem cell-derived factors: Immuno-modulatory effects and therapeutic potential. *Biofactors* **2017**, *43*, 633–644. [CrossRef]
49. Crop, M.J.; Baan, C.C.; Korevaar, S.S.; Ijzermans, J.N.; Weimar, W.; Hoogduijn, M.J. Human adipose tissue-derived mesenchymal stem cells induce explosive T-cell proliferation. *Stem Cells Dev.* **2010**, *19*, 1843–1853. [CrossRef]
50. Bolhassani, A.; Shahbazi, S.; Agi, E.; Haghighipour, N.; Hadi, A.; Asgari, F. Modified DCs and MSCs with HPV e7 antigen and small Hsps: Which one is the most potent strategy for eradication of tumors? *Mol. Immunol.* **2019**, *108*, 102–110. [CrossRef]
51. Ank, N.; West, H.; Bartholdy, C.; Eriksson, K.; Thomsen, A.R.; Paludan, S.R. Lambda interferon (ifn-lambda), a type III IFN, is induced by viruses and IFNs and displays potent antiviral activity against select virus infections in vivo. *J. Virol.* **2006**, *80*, 4501–4509. [CrossRef]
52. Jin, J.; Yang, J.Y.; Liu, J.; Kong, Y.Y.; Wang, Y.; Li, G.D. DNA immunization with fusion genes encoding different regions of hepatitis C virus e2 fused to the gene for hepatitis b surface antigen elicits immune responses to both hcv and hbv. *World J. Gastroenterol.* **2002**, *8*, 505–510. [CrossRef] [PubMed]
53. Chmielewska, A.M.; Naddeo, M.; Capone, S.; Ammendola, V.; Hu, K.; Meredith, L.; Verhoye, L.; Rychlowska, M.; Rappuoli, R.; Ulmer, J.B.; et al. Combined adenovirus vector and hepatitis c virus envelope protein prime-boost regimen elicits t cell and neutralizing antibody immune responses. *J. Virol.* **2014**, *88*, 5502–5510. [CrossRef]
54. Rasmusson, I.; Le Blanc, K.; Sundberg, B.; Ringden, O. Mesenchymal stem cells stimulate antibody secretion in human B cells. *Scand. J. Immunol.* **2007**, *65*, 336–343. [CrossRef] [PubMed]
55. Splawski, J.B.; McAnally, L.M.; Lipsky, P.E. Il-2 dependence of the promotion of human B cell differentiation by il-6 (bsf-2). *J. Immunol.* **1990**, *144*, 562–569. [PubMed]
56. Borgia, G.; Maraolo, A.E.; Nappa, S.; Gentile, I.; Buonomo, A.R. Ns5b polymerase inhibitors in phase II clinical trials for HCV infection. *Expert Opin Investig Drugs* **2018**, *27*, 243–250. [CrossRef]
57. Rao, X.; Hoof, I.; van Baarle, D.; Kesmir, C.; Textor, J. HLA preferences for conserved epitopes: A potential mechanism for hepatitis c clearance. *Front. Immunol.* **2015**, *6*, 552. [CrossRef]
58. O'Connor, M.A.; Rastad, J.L.; Green, W.R. The role of myeloid-derived suppressor cells in viral infection. *Viral. Immunol.* **2017**, *30*, 82–97. [CrossRef]
59. Cai, W.; Qin, A.; Guo, P.; Yan, D.; Hu, F.; Yang, Q.; Xu, M.; Fu, Y.; Zhou, J.; Tang, X. Clinical significance and functional studies of myeloid-derived suppressor cells in chronic hepatitis C patients. *J. Clin. Immunol.* **2013**, *33*, 798–808. [CrossRef]
60. Goh, C.C.; Roggerson, K.M.; Lee, H.C.; Golden-Mason, L.; Rosen, H.R.; Hahn, Y.S. Hepatitis c virus-induced myeloid-derived suppressor cells suppress NK cell IFN-gamma production by altering cellular metabolism via arginase-1. *J. Immunol.* **2016**, *196*, 2283–2292. [CrossRef]
61. Qin, A.; Cai, W.; Pan, T.; Wu, K.; Yang, Q.; Wang, N.; Liu, Y.; Yan, D.; Hu, F.; Guo, P.; et al. Expansion of monocytic myeloid-derived suppressor cells dampens T cell function in hiv-1-seropositive individuals. *J. Virol.* **2013**, *87*, 1477–1490. [CrossRef]
62. Pallett, L.J.; Gill, U.S.; Quaglia, A.; Sinclair, L.V.; Jover-Cobos, M.; Schurich, A.; Singh, K.P.; Thomas, N.; Das, A.; Chen, A.; et al. Metabolic regulation of hepatitis b immunopathology by myeloid-derived suppressor cells. *Nat. Med.* **2015**, *21*, 591–600. [CrossRef] [PubMed]

63. Bianchi, G.; Borgonovo, G.; Pistoia, V.; Raffaghello, L. Immunosuppressive cells and tumour microenvironment: Focus on mesenchymal stem cells and myeloid derived suppressor cells. *Histol. Histopathol.* **2011**, *26*, 941–951. [PubMed]
64. Yen, B.L.; Yen, M.L.; Hsu, P.J.; Liu, K.J.; Wang, C.J.; Bai, C.H.; Sytwu, H.K. Multipotent human mesenchymal stromal cells mediate expansion of myeloid-derived suppressor cells via hepatocyte growth factor/C-met and STAT3. *Stem Cell Rep.* **2013**, *1*, 139–151. [CrossRef] [PubMed]
65. Chen, H.W.; Chen, H.Y.; Wang, L.T.; Wang, F.H.; Fang, L.W.; Lai, H.Y.; Chen, H.H.; Lu, J.; Hung, M.S.; Cheng, Y.; et al. Mesenchymal stem cells tune the development of monocyte-derived dendritic cells toward a myeloid-derived suppressive phenotype through growth-regulated oncogene chemokines. *J. Immunol.* **2013**, *190*, 5065–5077. [CrossRef]
66. Zheng, H.; Zou, W.; Shen, J.; Xu, L.; Wang, S.; Fu, Y.X.; Fan, W. Opposite effects of coinjection and distant injection of mesenchymal stem cells on breast tumor cell growth. *Stem Cells Transl. Med.* **2016**, *5*, 1216–1228. [CrossRef]
67. Svobodova, E.; Krulova, M.; Zajicova, A.; Pokorna, K.; Prochazkova, J.; Trosan, P.; Holan, V. The role of mouse mesenchymal stem cells in differentiation of naive t-cells into anti-inflammatory regulatory T-cell or proinflammatory helper T-cell 17 population. *Stem Cells Dev.* **2012**, *21*, 901–910. [CrossRef]
68. Kim, M.; Rhee, J.K.; Choi, H.; Kwon, A.; Kim, J.; Lee, G.D.; Jekarl, D.W.; Lee, S.; Kim, Y.; Kim, T.M. Passage-dependent accumulation of somatic mutations in mesenchymal stromal cells during in vitro culture revealed by whole genome sequencing. *Sci. Rep.* **2017**, *7*, 14508. [CrossRef]
69. Yu, G.Y.; He, G.; Li, C.Y.; Tang, M.; Grivennikov, S.; Tsai, W.T.; Wu, M.S.; Hsu, C.W.; Tsai, Y.; Wang, L.H.; et al. Hepatic expression of hcv RNA-dependent RNA polymerase triggers innate immune signaling and cytokine production. *Mol. Cell.* **2012**, *48*, 313–321. [CrossRef]
70. Nishitsuji, H.; Funami, K.; Shimizu, Y.; Ujino, S.; Sugiyama, K.; Seya, T.; Takaku, H.; Shimotohno, K. Hepatitis C virus infection induces inflammatory cytokines and chemokines mediated by the cross talk between hepatocytes and stellate cells. *J. Virol.* **2013**, *87*, 8169–8178. [CrossRef]
71. Masalova, O.V.; Lesnova, E.I.; Permyakova, K.Y.; Samokhvalov, E.I.; Ivanov, A.V.; Kochetkov, S.N.; Kushch, A.A. Effect of hepatitis C virus proteins on the production of proinflammatory and profibrotic cytokines in huh7.5 human hepatoma cells. *Mol. Biol. (Mosk)* **2016**, *50*, 422–430. [CrossRef]
72. Francois, M.; Romieu-Mourez, R.; Stock-Martineau, S.; Boivin, M.N.; Bramson, J.L.; Galipeau, J. Mesenchymal stromal cells cross-present soluble exogenous antigens as part of their antigen-presenting cell properties. *Blood* **2009**, *114*, 2632–2638. [CrossRef]
73. Lin, T.; Pajarinen, J.; Kohno, Y.; Huang, J.F.; Maruyama, M.; Romero-Lopez, M.; Nathan, K.; Yao, Z.; Goodman, S.B. Trained murine mesenchymal stem cells have anti-inflammatory effect on macrophages, but defective regulation on T-cell proliferation. *FASEB J.* **2019**, *33*, 4203–4211. [CrossRef] [PubMed]
74. Yang, C.; Chen, Y.; Li, F.; You, M.; Zhong, L.; Li, W.; Zhang, B.; Chen, Q. The biological changes of umbilical cord mesenchymal stem cells in inflammatory environment induced by different cytokines. *Mol. Cell Biochem.* **2018**, *446*, 171–184. [CrossRef] [PubMed]
75. Hartnell, F.; Brown, A.; Capone, S.; Kopycinski, J.; Bliss, C.; Makvandi-Nejad, S.; Swadling, L.; Ghaffari, E.; Cicconi, P.; Del Sorbo, M.; et al. A novel vaccine strategy employing serologically different chimpanzee adenoviral vectors for the prevention of HIV-1 and hcv coinfection. *Front. Immunol.* **2018**, *9*, 3175. [CrossRef] [PubMed]
76. Kelly, C.; Swadling, L.; Brown, A.; Capone, S.; Folgori, A.; Salio, M.; Klenerman, P.; Barnes, E. Cross-reactivity of hepatitis C virus specific vaccine-induced T cells at immunodominant epitopes. *Eur. J. Immunol.* **2015**, *45*, 309–316. [CrossRef] [PubMed]
77. Callendret, B.; Eccleston, H.B.; Satterfield, W.; Capone, S.; Folgori, A.; Cortese, R.; Nicosia, A.; Walker, C.M. Persistent hepatitis C viral replication despite priming of functional CD8+ T cells by combined therapy with a vaccine and a direct-acting antiviral. *Hepatology* **2016**, *63*, 1442–1454. [CrossRef]
78. Di Bisceglie, A.M.; Janczweska-Kazek, E.; Habersetzer, F.; Mazur, W.; Stanciu, C.; Carreno, V.; Tanasescu, C.; Flisiak, R.; Romero-Gomez, M.; Fich, A.; et al. Efficacy of immunotherapy with tg4040, peg-interferon, and ribavirin in a phase 2 study of patients with chronic HCV infection. *Gastroenterology* **2014**, *147*, 119–131.e3. [CrossRef]

79. Echevarria, D.; Gutfraind, A.; Boodram, B.; Layden, J.; Ozik, J.; Page, K.; Cotler, S.J.; Major, M.; Dahari, H. Modeling indicates efficient vaccine-based interventions for the elimination of hepatitis C virus among persons who inject drugs in metropolitan chicago. *Vaccine* **2019**, *37*, 2608–2616. [CrossRef]
80. Scott, N.; McBryde, E.; Vickerman, P.; Martin, N.K.; Stone, J.; Drummer, H.; Hellard, M. The role of a hepatitis C virus vaccine: Modelling the benefits alongside direct-acting antiviral treatments. *BMC Med.* **2015**, *13*, 198. [CrossRef]

MDPI
St. Alban-Anlage 66
4052 Basel
Switzerland
Tel. +41 61 683 77 34
Fax +41 61 302 89 18
www.mdpi.com

Vaccines Editorial Office
E-mail: vaccines@mdpi.com
www.mdpi.com/journal/vaccines

www.ingramcontent.com/pod-product-compliance
Lightning Source LLC
LaVergne TN
LVHW070736100526
838202LV00013B/1246
* 9 7 8 3 0 3 6 5 0 3 0 0 4 *